About the author

Hedley Thomas is a senior writer for *The Australian*. His journalism career began in 1985 with a cadetship at the *Gold Coast Bulletin*. He has worked in Brisbane, London and Hong Kong and has reported on the collapse of the Berlin Wall, the bloody revolution in Romania, the first Gulf War, the 1997 handover of Hong Kong to China and the devastating earthquake in the Japanese city of Kobe.

For his investigations, feature-writing and news reporting, Thomas has received numerous awards including three Walkley Awards. His first Walkley was in 1999 (with colleague Paul Whittaker) when he exposed the Net Bet affair; his second was in 2003 for his feature article on fallen chief magistrate, Di Fingleton. His third Walkley was in 2005 for breaking the story about rogue surgeon, Dr Jayant Patel. For this work he also received the Sir Keith Murdoch Award, a special accolade from News Corporation chairman Rupert Murdoch, as well as the 2005 Queensland Premier's Literary Awards for work advancing public debate.

Hedley Thomas lives in Brisbane with his wife, journalist Ruth Mathewson, and their two children.

SICK TO
DEATH

HEDLEY THOMAS

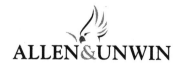

ALLEN&UNWIN

Lyrics from 'Sounds of Then' by Ganggajang are reproduced with the permission of the band.

First published in 2007

Allen & Unwin
83 Alexander Street
Crows Nest NSW 2065
Australia
Phone: (61 2) 8425 0100
Fax: (61 2) 9906 2218
Email: info@allenandunwin.com
Web: www.allenandunwin.com

National Library of Australia
Cataloguing-in-Publication entry:

Thomas, Hedley.
    Sick to death: a manipulative surgeon and a health system
    in crisis – a disaster waiting to happen.

    ISBN 978 1 74114 881 7.

    1. Patel, Jayant. 2. Queensland. Bundaberg Hospital
    Commission of Inquiry. 3. Queensland. Queensland Health.
    4. Bundaberg Base Hospital. 5. Physicians - Malpractice -
    Queensland. 6. Public health administration - Queensland.
    I. Title.

    610.92

Edited by Jo Jarrah
Cover design by Phil Campbell, based on a concept used by Jeff Young in *The Bulletin* 14/06/05
Text designed by Phil Campbell
Typeset by J&M Typesetting
Printed in Australia by Griffin Press

10 9 8 7 6 5 4 3 2 1

For Ruth, Alexander and Sarah.
Most of all, for Diana.
I miss you, Mum.

Contents

Foreword

AS Hedley Thomas accurately describes it, this is the story of the 'once in a lifetime scandal of Jayant Patel and the wider story of how political interference and bureaucratic incompetence conspired against a health system'. It is an absorbing account; even though I knew many, though by no means most, of the facts Mr Thomas relates, I found this book hard to put down. For those who find some of it hard to believe, I can say that, to the extent that it covers the evidence in my inquiry, it is an accurate account.

Moreover, whilst I may not agree with all of Mr Thomas's opinions, I believe that this book is a salutary warning to present and future governments, to the bureaucracy and to the public as to what can happen when problems are concealed. I hope that the warning is heeded.

There is one glaring omission in the book. Whilst Mr Thomas praises the roles of Ms Hoffman and Mr Messenger in bringing the scandal to light, he is unduly modest about his own contribution. This is part of what I said about him in my report:

'His investigative skill, persistence and undoubted authority as a respected journalist ensured that public notice and government action was taken, notwithstanding the apparent reluctance of hospital administrators and officers of Queensland Health to take appropriate action to permit the matter to be exposed.'

I went on later in the report to detail his important contribution to this.

The revelations of Mr Thomas and others, leading to my inquiry and report, have already resulted in a huge increase in the health budget and substantial worthwhile reforms. Beneficial consequences of those reforms may not emerge for some time. More importantly, these benefits will ultimately be lost unless government and the bureaucracy maintain the will to put patient care and openness ahead of economic rationalism. This compelling account will focus attention on that need.

The Hon Geoffrey Davies AO
Commissioner of the Queensland Public Hospitals Commission of Inquiry

Overview of the health system in Queensland

The hierarchy in any health system and the different titles and structures can be confusing. The following descriptions of the relevant parts of Queensland's health system pertain to the period of time covered in this book.

Queensland Health is the organisation empowered by the state government to administer public hospitals and the health system. It is one of the largest employers in the state with more than 60,000 staff.

The **Health Minister** is the political leader of the organisation. Between 1995 and 2007, there have been five health ministers and all are mentioned in this book: Mike Horan, Peter Beattie, Wendy Edmond, Gordon Nuttall and Stephen Robertson. Mr Horan was a health minister in a previous Coalition Government, whereas the other four have served as ministers in a Labor Government.

The **Director-General** is the administrative leader of the organisation. Dr Rob Stable served as Director-General from 1995 to 2003. When he resigned from the position, he was replaced by Dr Steve Buckland.

The **Chief Health Officer** has a statutory role to ensure independence and uphold standards of safety. Dr Gerry FitzGerald served as Chief Health Officer during Dr Jayant Patel's time in Australia.

The **District Manager** is the overall leader of a hospital and health facilities in a particular area. Peter Leck served as the District Manager for Bundaberg.

The **Zonal Manager** oversees the management of the hospitals and health facilities in several districts. Dan Bergin served as Zonal Manager with responsibility for Bundaberg.

The **Director of Medical Services** manages the clinical aspects of a hospital and answers to the District Manager. Dr Darren Keating served as Director of Medical Services and reported to Peter Leck.

The **Director of Surgery** manages the surgical work of a hospital and reports to the Director of Medical Services. In this book there were three: Dr Charles Nankivell, Dr Sam Baker and Dr Jayant Patel.

The **Director of Medicine** manages the medical and non-surgical work of a hospital. Dr Peter Miach, a renal specialist, served as Director of Medicine and reported to Dr Darren Keating.

The **Director of the Intensive Care Unit** has overall responsibility for the patients in this specialised area. Dr Martin Carter, an anaesthetist, served as Director of ICU and reported to Dr Darren Keating.

A **Visiting Medical Officer (VMO)** is a doctor and specialist in private practice with a contract to visit and consult part-time in public hospitals.

A **Senior Medical Officer (SMO)** is a doctor with extensive experience and is generally working under the supervision of a specialist in public hospitals.

A **Principal House Officer (PHO)** is a doctor in a third year of practical experience post graduate.

A **Senior House Officer (SHO)** is a doctor in a second year of practical experience post graduate.

A **Junior House Officer (JHO)** is a doctor in a first year of practical experience post graduate.

An **Intern** is a new graduate accepted into a hospital training program.

An **Overseas Trained Doctor** is a doctor who has graduated from a medical school outside Australia.

The **Health Rights Commission of Queensland** is a statutory body empowered to investigate and resolve complaints about health services.

The **Medical Board of Queensland** is a statutory body empowered to regulate and discipline health practitioners as part of a mandate to protect the public.

The **Health Practitioners' Tribunal** is a court in Queensland in which health care providers may be formally sanctioned and disciplined by a District Court judge after a formal review of evidence.

The **Australian Medical Association** is the peak membership body for doctors, who pay fees as if to a trade union. Membership is not compulsory. Each state has its own leader. In this book, the relevant leaders have been Dr Ingrid Tall, Dr David Molloy and Dr Steve Hambleton.

The **Local Medical Association** in Bundaberg comprised doctors who sought to promote better health in the district.

The children

Bundaberg Hospital, Queensland, January 1928

DOCTOR Ewing George Thomson held a little amber bottle in his large hands at the Bundaberg Hospital beside the Burnett River. One of 30 in a batch sent by rail from the Commonwealth Serum Laboratories in Melbourne to the Health Department in Brisbane, the rubber-capped bottle had been filled during a sterile process with precisely 100 millilitres of diphtheria toxin-antitoxin.

Unlike the bottles in a number of other batches, this one did not contain antiseptic. It had no safeguard to prevent the growth of micro-organisms if any were accidentally introduced to the mixture. Inexplicably, a notice warning of this omission was not forwarded from Brisbane to the thriving town of Bundaberg. Dr Thomson was hours away from becoming an unknowing killer in the community he served as a Medical Officer of Health.

Diphtheria bacteria, usually spread in droplets of moisture coughed into the air, was a major threat to youngsters. The symptoms almost always came on quickly. A sore throat, fever, rapid heart rate, nausea, vomiting, chills and a headache would develop as soon as 24 hours after the bacteria had begun to multiply near the tonsils and other parts of the throat. The toxins produced by the bacteria were relentless and lethal. They blocked airways, making it hard to breathe, and attacked the heart, brain, nerves and kidneys. Death was a common outcome for the youngest sufferers.

Dr Thomson was doing a public service. Many of the local children had been hit by diphtheria in the months before the inoculations arrived. The lucky ones had recovered only after spending up to a month in Bundaberg Hospital. With the arrival of the amber bottles, Dr Thomson held a lifesaving remedy. He must have wondered how many children would be saved from the ravages of diphtheria as a result of his efforts.

Over the course of a few days in late January, Dr Thomson soothed, cajoled and sought to protect from death a good number of the town's youngsters, including his own son.

The parents who went to Dr Thomson's surgery and to a makeshift medical centre at the Bundaberg Council Chambers, in a room previously occupied by the town's civil engineer, returned home feeling safely assured. The children giggled, resisted and some even shed a few tears as Dr Thomson punctured their delicate skin with the needle and firmly pushed the plunger to release the toxin-antitoxin. And so began a medical catastrophe. Eighteen of the 21 children became seriously ill within hours of the last round of inoculations. The staff of Bundaberg Hospital feared the worst as vomiting, semi-conscious children, some of whom could no longer recognise their parents, were carried in for urgent treatment.

'They were confronted by an emergency which taxed all their powers,' reported Dr Charles Kellaway, the chairman of the subsequent Royal Commission of Inquiry into the Fatalities at Bundaberg. 'The unavoidable absence of skilled specialist aid early on the 28th and the heavy strain on the resources of the hospital staff in the treatment of so many very sick children, naturally made the clinical records somewhat incomplete.'

Nine of the youngsters died in the hospital on 28 January as their parents wept and railed against the suspected killer, a mixture of turbid fluid that had been represented as a lifesaver. The treatment was basic: cold compresses to the head to comfort the children with fever, sips of water, bowel washouts and, during the severe convulsions of one child, chloroform.

A tenth fatality occurred in Dr Schmidt's surgery in town. The little boy, William Follitt, aged two, was in the best of spirits at 7 pm, three hours after his inoculation, and asleep by 9 pm. His mother was woken at 11 pm by the lad 'rattling his cot with the shivers'. He vomited for 15 minutes. His head was hot to touch. His body felt cold. Eventually he drifted off to sleep. But he never awoke. His parents discovered him unconscious at 7.30 am with a blotchy purple mottling of the skin, blue lips and eyelids and heavy breathing. Death followed soon afterwards.

The eleventh child died at the nearby St Vincent's Hospital. The twelfth, Guy Marsden Coates, seven, succumbed in his parents' arms at their home in nearby Kalkie.

Three brothers, Thomas Robinson, five, William, four, and Mervyn, 23 months, were lost within hours of each other. 'We did what we thought was in the best interests of the children themselves and for the city, when we decided to have them immunised against diphtheria,' said Mr Thomas Robinson, who had emigrated from England six years earlier. His wife, Ethel, was inconsolable. 'Immunisation had been a success in other cities, and we had every confidence in it. But apparently something has gone wrong, and our little darlings count among the victims. Two days ago the home was full of life, and look at it now.'

At 3 pm on this day of unprecedented tragedy in Bundaberg, a shaken Dr Hains, superintendent in charge of Bundaberg Hospital, told the local police chief of the sudden and unexpected death toll. Dr Schmidt performed eight autopsies in as many hours before the exhausted man refused to do any more without expert help. Bundaberg had no facility at its morgue to store bodies at a temperature below the summer highs.

On 30 January 1928, Bundaberg's *NewsMail* reported the 12 deaths with compassion and clarity while demanding an explanation from authorities. As the *NewsMail* reported:

> It was a never-to-be forgotten day for the hospital staff, what with children dying, others writhing in the throes of death and the sobbing of heartbroken parents, sisters and brothers, was a scene, only those who went through it can describe. There were many touching incidents in the ward. Mr & Mrs Sheppard had two of their children die simultaneously. Despite this heavy blow

they bore up with true fortitude in hopes of their other two boys pulling through, and at their bedsides a grief stricken father and mother maintain a silent vigil.

In the midst of their sorrow they have a kindly word for the other parents who have lost their dear ones, and each has also a kindly word to say for Dr Ewing Thomson, with whom in the unfortunate position the virulent serum has placed him there is widespread sympathy. He is naturally feeling the position acutely.

The investigators looked at the common symptoms in the most severe cases – extremely rapid pulse rate, diarrhoea, vomiting of blood-stained bile, loss of consciousness and widely dilated pupils. In their final minutes, the children suffered convulsions. There was, almost uniformly, a deep blotchy cyanosis, or discolouration of the skin – the result of a lack of oxygen in the blood.

Food poisoning as a probable cause was quickly ruled out, along with some other acute disease unrelated to the injection. Another possibility – that a tetanus toxin might have been produced in the bottle and caused rapid death – was also ruled out. Laboratory investigations into the remaining fluid in Dr Thomson's bottle isolated one organism. Named the Bundaberg Staphylococcus, it was found to be identical to the staphylococci isolated in pure culture from abscesses at the site of injection of five of the children who had survived.

But how did it get there? The source of the contamination was not the Commonwealth Serum Laboratories. All the unopened bottles from the same batch and other batches were examined. They were found to be sterile. When the little amber bottle in question reached Dr Thomson's surgery on 7 January, it was uncontaminated. He stored it in his cupboard until it was used for inoculations on 17 January and on four subsequent days culminating on the fateful day of 27 January. Contamination occurred on one of these occasions when the mixture was being removed from the bottle for injection into the children.

After thoroughly scrubbing his hands with soap and water, Dr Thomson had fixed the needle to the nozzle of the syringe – picking it out of sterile water with his fingers instead of carrying out the task with a pair of sterile forceps. His re-enactment and subsequent tests proved Dr Thomson himself had unwittingly introduced the bacteria before injecting it into the children. In 1928, Dr Thomson made a single mistake in procedures with immediate and tragic consequences. Did he die a broken man, haunted by his error of judgement?

Almost 80 years later, Bundaberg would experience another series of medical tragedies. How much more sinister were the actions of Dr Jayant Patel, Bundaberg Hospital's Director of Surgery, a man who deceived a lax regulatory regime, then bullied and undermined those who challenged him? The surgeon exploited a hear-no-evil, see-no-evil health system until his unmasking in 2005 as a dangerous fraud. His incompetence with a scalpel was to make him a killer. He will face a trial for manslaughter and other serious criminal charges.

This book is the true story of Dr Patel and the harm he caused. It is also the story of the efforts of a few people to expose his wrong-doing, despite the many obstacles placed in their way.

PART ONE

CHAOS

1

Happy days

January 2002

GERARD Neville put the last bag in the family car as his wife Lorraine urged the three children to hurry downstairs. A fit, middle-aged public health physician for Queensland Health, Gerard ran beside the Brisbane River most mornings, even in the subtropical humidity of summer, before going to work to plan policy for the well-being of a few million men, women and children. They were known, in accordance with the corporate vernacular, as clients.

The years had been kind to Gerard. He remained free of the stress of providing clinical care in an organisation starved of funds. While his friends, many of them fellow graduates of the University of Queensland's Medical School in the leafy grounds of Herston, had opted for careers in operating theatres with late-night call-outs, long hours and, eventually, private rooms as highly paid specialists, Gerard enjoyed a steady public service routine. He was adept at his office job, never shirking unpopular assignments such as telling his political masters the unpalatable reality about the effect of their policies. He would never reach the top of a highly politicised bureaucracy. Nor did he aspire to.

They made a handsome couple, Gerard and Lorraine. A tall and softly spoken teacher, she met Gerard when he was a rural GP, five years after his graduation. Their motto might have been permanence and stability. They were stylish, but not flashy. Professional, but not elitist. They were Catholic with middle-class values, healthy children, secure careers and a comfortable, newly renovated house on a hill in the Brisbane middle class suburb of Toowong.

Laura, 14, Elise, ten, and Michael, eight, needed little encouragement to leave their Brisbane home at the height of the summer heatwave. Across the city, thousands of people without air conditioning were seeking refuge in shopping centres and cinemas. Temperatures were about to soar into the high 30s with only limited relief from the scattered showers and afternoon storms. The Nevilles were going somewhere infinitely more appealing. In two hours they would arrive at Kings Beach in Caloundra for the start of an annual holiday ritual: exploring rock-pools, swimming in the surf, lazing around the pool and choosing from the dinner specials at nearby restaurants.

As Gerard nosed the car, one of the perks of his package with Queensland Health, down the neatly paved driveway and turned left onto Milton Road for the drive north, Lorraine felt uneasy. Usually, the Neville family would stay at Pandanus Court in Caloundra for the Christmas holidays. Their familiarity over the years with the old block of units closest to the beach was part of the fun. Returning to Pandanus was a bit like visiting a favourite aunty, notwithstanding her flaws. She was safe and would not produce any surprises.

When Lorraine had called months earlier to make the usual holiday booking, the woman at Henzell's Real Estate Agency explained Pandanus would not be available this time. The old block was being redeveloped and Aunty was to receive an overdue facelift. Instead, Lorraine was offered a unit in Monterey Lodge, a block not known to her.

The plan was to spend a week there, dash back to Brisbane the following Saturday, unload the car, water the garden, check the mail, feed the children, return calls, load the car again and drive across the city to catch the afternoon ferry from Cleveland to Stradbroke Island for a further seven days holidaying.

Lorraine's first impression of Unit 3 at Monterey Lodge confirmed her unease. The living space was long, dark and narrow. The floor throughout seemed to be hard concrete with a thin wood veneer surface. The place felt austere and uninviting. Before they had begun to unpack, before Lorraine could take in the natural beauty of the water beyond the buildings, she had regrets.

As Lorraine tried to bury her misgivings and put on a bright face, and Gerard carried the bags inside, Elise ran to the second bedroom and squealed with delight. As expected, there was a set of bunk beds. They were unspectacular: lightly-framed and well used, they stood exactly 1.43 metres high in one corner of the room. The top bunk had been promised days earlier to Elise, who excitedly told her friends and reminded Michael and Laura that she would soon be towering over them, morning and night. A bright girl with sparkling blue eyes, a cherubic face and a gift for bringing calm and laughter into awkward situations, Elise looked at the top bunk and beamed. She clambered up and bounced on the mattress.

A trundle bed had been stored under the lower bed. Lorraine dragged it out on the Saturday afternoon and put it against the wall, forming an L-shape with the bunks.

Lorraine frowned at the glass-topped table in the room. It was an accident waiting to happen. She carried it into the main bedroom where she and Gerard would be sleeping. Next she hauled a low set of wooden bedside drawers from the main bedroom to the children's room.

As Lorraine had feared, the unit was hot. Its bricks absorbed heat through the day. The windows missed the best of the sea breezes, and there were no ceiling fans. Lorraine put one of the electric fans she had brought from Brisbane on the bedside drawers. At least the children would be comfortable as they slept.

Lorraine took one more precaution before satisfying herself that she had made the best of things. She spread quilts and blankets along the floor below the bunk beds. Michael, who would be in the bottom bunk, was a restless sleeper though neither he nor Elise had any history of falling out of bed. But, just in case, the quilts might soften an unlikely accidental fall.

The family woke to a glorious Sunday morning and devoted it to the beach and the pool. Lorraine's worries eased. As the sun disappeared behind the Glasshouse Mountains, the family walked to Bulcock Beach for fish and chips at a sidewalk table. After they returned to the unit, Michael went to bed first. He was sleeping soundly by 9 pm when Lorraine checked on him. Elise, nestled beside her mother on the sofa, stayed contentedly reading her novel. From time to time she looked up at the TV.

An hour after Michael had turned in, Elise was ready for bed. She kissed her parents and smiled as Lorraine tucked her in for a second night in the top bunk.

Lorraine, who had made a point of picking the children's clutter off the floor to prevent a stumble in the dark, did not notice something amiss as she turned out the lights. The family had no experience with bunk beds. The safety rails that prevent a child rolling out were not there.

As they were on holidays, Laura was allowed to stay up with her parents until the late movie ended. Shortly before midnight they all went to bed and, within minutes, everyone was sleeping.

At 1.50 am Lorraine woke up suddenly. Gerard sat upright. They had both heard it, a loud noise. A heavy thud. In the seconds that followed, moaning noises drifted from the bedroom and, instantly, Lorraine guessed what had happened: 'Oh my God, Gerard, I think Elise has fallen out of bed!'

They hurried to the bedroom where Elise was lying, curled up, on her right side. She was on the quilt on the floor with her head towards the narrow shelf and doorless cupboard in the room. Lorraine frantically moved the small drawers with the fan on top so she and Gerard could both fit in the room more easily to tend their stricken child.

'Elise, are you okay? Can you move your arms and legs?' asked Lorraine, who needed immediate affirmation that Elise had not broken any limbs.

Elise could move her limbs, but Lorraine's relief was tempered by a new fear: Elise was in great pain.

'My head hurts,' she cried in the half-light.

Gerard tried to contain his own anxiety in the gloomy bedroom as Elise lay on the floor with her Winnie the Pooh teddy bear, rubbing her head and whimpering softly. He took charge. He was the doctor. He might not have practised medicine for 18 years but he knew something about head injury.

'Try and keep calm. I'll take her to our bed and have a look at her,' he said in as measured a tone as he could manage.

Gerard checked her limbs, neck, chest and stomach for breaks or pain. He carried Elise to the main bedroom and brought the mattress from her top bunk. They lay her down on it on the floor in their room. She continued moaning in obvious pain. 'My head hurts a lot, here,' she said, touching the left side.

Lorraine, shaking with worry and fear, wanted to rush Elise to hospital. She was becoming frantic. Gerard resisted. He doubted Elise had been unconscious after the fall. He persuaded Lorraine that they could safely watch her in the unit for the time being.

'Stop panicking, everything will be okay,' Gerard said.

Elise piped up, 'Yes, Mummy, don't panic. You're making me worried.'

'I'm sorry. Everything will be alright,' Lorraine replied.

'No, it won't, Mum. There's something really wrong.'

2

The shift

January 2002

ANDREW Doneman looked at the clock on the wall above one of the Caloundra Hospital ward beds. Almost 3 am. He sighed with relief. He wouldn't wish the graveyard shift on his worst enemy. He knew exactly how long he had been going without a rest. Having come on duty at 8 am the previous day, he was at the 19-hour mark of a 24-hour shift. Doneman, a father of two young children, was exhausted. He would never touch alcohol while at work, but the effect of his fatigue equated to a blood alcohol reading of .05 per cent.

Long-distance truck drivers could be forced off the road if found working dangerously long hours. Economic necessity and demanding bosses forced the drivers to stay awake with amphetamines as they hurtled down the country's highways. Airline operators had much more to lose. The repercussions from carnage caused by a Mack truck colliding with a family car were nothing compared with those that might follow a Boeing 747 ploughing into a mountain due to pilot fatigue. Australian pilots were permitted a maximum number of hours in the cockpit on long-haul flights after which strict regulations stipulated a lengthy rest in the bunks. Nurses, too, were banned from working excessive hours. Yet doctors like Doneman in Queensland's public hospitals were given no choice. At this time of year, when many of the senior doctors were holidaying with their own families, those on the bottom rung were in greater demand than usual.

The chronic shortage of doctors nationally was worse in Queensland, which had the lowest number of registered doctors per head of population of any state or territory. There were about 2500 more doctors in Victoria, a state with a similar population but without the challenges unique to Queensland of decentralisation, poor working conditions and remote and Indigenous communities.

Doneman had few complaints. He would do the hours, a rite of passage, and move up the ranks. He was not the most junior doctor in Queensland, but he was the least experienced doctor to be put in charge of the 80-bed Caloundra Hospital overnight. For the duration of this shift, he was the only doctor on duty. A quietly ambitious 37-year-old, Doneman did not look like a newcomer to medicine. But he only began studying medicine in his late 20s. His confidence and age sometimes made his patients suspect, wrongly, that he was experienced. Just two years after receiving his Bachelor of Medicine and Bachelor of Surgery from the University of Queensland, he was making clinical decisions without having to defer to senior colleagues.

Doneman had worked in hospitals known as God's waiting rooms because they catered to a large population of elderly retirees who had moved to the Sunshine Coast for its warm climate, beaches and lawn bowls. As a junior house officer – almost the lowest-ranking doctor on the scale – he had treated worn-out knees supporting the overweight and the sedentary. He had treated gynaecological issues common to elderly women who had borne children. During rotations in paediatrics, orthopaedics, anaesthetics, obstetrics, gynaecology and emergency medicine, he had seen dozens of bright-eyed babies at the start of life and the old and frail who were soon to depart. Maybe they sensed in his bedside manner a contagious energy and enthusiasm for medicine.

After driving taxis to pay his way through medical school, Doneman had large bills and a meagre salary but he was doing what he loved. His colleagues had noted the positive feedback from his patients.

Somewhere within the Queensland Health bureaucracy, a secret document – headed 'Review of Emergency Services, Sunshine Coast Health Service District' – flagged potential dangers at Caloundra Hospital. The review had been compiled by a small team of experts who had been investigating the resources, safety and performance of emergency departments along the coastal strip. It was conducted on a confidential basis. Its author, Dr William Rodgers, found that the

Caloundra Emergency Department needed a minimum of four principal house officers. Further, their responsibilities should not be stretched to looking after in-patients as well as those coming into the Emergency Department during normal working hours.

Doneman, who knew nothing of the three-month-old report and its unheeded recommendations, was two years away from being made a principal house officer when he began his fateful shift in early January. He had responsibility for the entire hospital.

The nurses in the Emergency Department, Beverly Duncan and Diane Forbes, who had come on duty at 10.45 pm, were taking a break after a busy few hours. The patients were presenting with relatively minor ailments, and certainly none with emergencies. Most simply sought free treatment.

Uniquely, with beds in short supply and resources strictly limited, the hospital also had a bizarre practice. It did not admit children.

3

We need help

January 2002

ELISE was talking a little as Lorraine held an ice-pack to her head. Around 3 am she became agitated, flailing her arms and crying out with the pain. Laura and Michael, who had woken in the frantic commotion after the fall, looked on helplessly. Elise vomited. It was the last sign Gerard needed. He knew then that she had to go to hospital urgently and would probably need a CT (Computerised Tomography) scan. With detailed two-dimensional computer-enhanced x-ray images, a CT scan could highlight any abnormalities such as bleeding in Elise's brain or a fracture in her skull.

He was about to tell Lorraine of his decision. She beat him to it as Elise moaned and complained about the yucky taste of vomit in her mouth.

'Right! We're going to the hospital now,' Lorraine said as they cleaned Elise's face and clothes and quickly got changed.

Gerard's appearance of calm had dissolved. Now he, too, was shaking. The fear was sensed by Laura and Michael, who huddled together on the trundle bed. They were frightened for Elise and worried about being in the unfamiliar unit alone.

Lorraine cradled Elise in the back seat of the car as her head rested on a pillow that had been snatched up on the way out. Gerard drove to the nearby Caloundra public hospital in West Terrace but later would not even remember the route he took. He jabbed the illuminated night bell outside the Emergency Department until Beverly Duncan answered through the intercom, then opened the door. Gerard quickly explained what had happened. A fall. A head striking a hard floor. Ongoing pain. Headache. Vomiting.

They were directed to a room in the Emergency Department where Elise lay, very quiet, on the bed during a brief examination by Duncan, a United Kingdom-trained nurse who scrawled details on a clipboard and peered at the frightened child's pupils while shining a torch. Elise's pulse rate measured 54, a low reading.

An oxymeter on her finger measured her oxygen saturation levels as Duncan made small talk with Gerard. He explained he was a non-practising doctor, one of the 60 000 staff of Queensland Health. They were colleagues.

Duncan noted a child who was quietly spoken and unhappy. 'Where does it hurt?' she asked.

'I'm aching all over, but mainly I've got a headache,' Elise replied.

Duncan found the 'aching all over' answer strange. There was no obvious deformity to any limbs, no swelling and no specific pain suggestive of a fracture.

Lorraine was asked to leave the room to fill in forms at the front counter. 'I can hardly write as I'm shaking so much,' she breathed. Duncan, it seemed to Lorraine, ignored her and walked away, leaving the distraught mother wondering what she had done to receive such a cold reception at 3.25 am with an injured child.

Lorraine returned to the assessment room to remark to Gerard the lack of empathy. She weighed their options. They were in an open, functioning Emergency Department staffed by health professionals. Complaining might be counterproductive. It could lead to Elise being ignored. The alternative of leaving to find other medical help seemed impossible. So they waited.

Dr Andrew Doneman was at a bench writing up his notes for another patient, a man in a wheelchair, when Duncan explained the basics: a ten-year-old girl on holidays. A fall from a top bunk. Generalised aches and pains. Vomiting. No loss of consciousness.

In the central area of the Emergency Department, Duncan, Doneman and Diane Forbes discussed Elise's vital signs.

The chitchat seemed interminable to Lorraine, who was near

breaking point. Sensing no urgency among the staff, she pleaded with Gerard, who still felt guilty for keeping Elise in the Monterey unit for the first hour, to beg for action.

'How long will the doctor be?' he asked Forbes, who was sitting back at the nursing station. 'Please, is anyone going to come and see my daughter? We are very worried. My wife is very concerned. Can you come now, at least for her sake?'

Forbes had heard the questions a thousand times before. Everyone wanted to be seen yesterday. It was as if nobody else mattered or even existed. The patients, emotional and sometimes abusive, had no idea how busy the staff were and knew nothing about the pressures of competing priorities like paperwork. No, there was no point in arguing.

'He is just there. He will be with you shortly,' Forbes said, nodding towards the bench where Doneman was writing notes.

As Doneman walked into the assessment room, time was running out for Elise. A drop or two of blood had already seeped into her left ear. The fall had fractured Elise's skull and damaged the middle meningeal artery in her brain. Without surgery to drain the blood, which might have been obvious during a thorough examination, the growing clot would force the soft tissue in Elise's brain against the immovable bones in her skull. If left untreated, her brain could herniate, causing catastrophic injury.

4

The nursing life

TONI Hoffman went to the thesaurus just to be sure. Maverick. She liked it. But as with many nicknames it could be misconstrued. What else might it mean? *Independent. Nonconformist. Individual.* Yes, Hoffman had to agree that she was something of a maverick.

The nickname had been given to her in circumstances that were moderately controversial. As the senior nurse in charge of Bundaberg Base Hospital's combined Intensive Care and Coronary Care Unit since her arrival in 2000, Hoffman made a strong case over unsafe hours being worked by her staff. Most of the 15 nurses in the ICU were exhausted. The fatigue which stemmed from their early morning starts and late finishes was affecting clinical care.

A tired nurse could be dangerous, particularly in the ICU where the critically ill patients had the most tenuous hold on life. The nurses were not meant to leave the bedside of patients being helped to breathe by ventilating equipment. It only took a short lapse in concentration or momentary inattention for a fatal mistake to be made. Without fuss or rancour Hoffman had argued a case for more nurses and safer hours. Glennis Goodman, the Director of Nursing at the hospital, took Hoffman's submission to the next level. Eventually, the logic and commonsense of the argument were accepted. More nurses were employed. The dangerous shifts were abolished. The patients in ICU did not know that a fundamental change to the nursing roster gave them better odds of survival. But the staff knew.

Hoffman won immediate and long-lasting respect from the other nurses for her willingness to back them as well as the patients. She was a rarity – a middle manager prepared to raise her head above the parapet and speak out against convention and systems that had been imposed by her superiors and grudgingly accepted by the staff. But in Queensland Health, an organisation run down by political interference and financial neglect, Hoffman's style of robust outspokenness was rarely rewarded. The mavericks who agitated for something outside the square were usually the first to be muzzled.

Rebel. Loner. Misfit. Although it pained Hoffman to admit it, she probably was a loner. Maybe even a misfit. She did not have a boyfriend, yet all her best friends were married. They spent every spare moment with their children, talking about their children or planning events around their children. Her younger sister, Maree, was run off her feet with her two kids. At times when the demands of parenthood seemed limitless, Hoffman felt fortunate to have avoided those responsibilities. When the challenges in the ICU were unrelenting, and the deadlines for her university assignments seemingly impossible, she consoled herself that her life's journey was as it should be. At least she had her freedom. At least she had the time after work to devote to study even if there were occasional bouts of loneliness. Still, pragmatism could not change the fact that Hoffman loved children and regretted not having her own.

Although several of her long-term boyfriends would have made her happy as partners for life, Hoffman had always hesitated when things became serious. Marriage frightened her. It seemed like the end of the world. As a girl growing up in Ingleburn, south-west of Sydney, she had missed her father, Warwick, during his long road trips, hauling freight in the truck owned by the family business W & M Hoffman Transport.

She was 15 when her father decided to try his hand at growing potatoes, pumpkins, tomatoes and cabbages. Hoffman briefly resented him for taking the family from the outskirts of Sydney to a little community halfway between Brisbane and Toowoomba where almost everyone had unusual European surnames and spoke with a strange accent.

On her first day at Lockyer Valley State High, one of the students assumed she was a child of itinerant fruit-pickers. 'Will you be staying just a little while?' he asked the newcomer.

'I hope so,' she sniffed. The class booed.

Her first instinct had always been to speak her mind. *Rebel. Renegade. Dissident.*

Over time, the open spaces, summer days spent swimming in the local waterholes and camping with her new boyfriend made her grateful for the move away from Sydney. At the end of Year 12, she chose nursing – it offered accommodation, study and a salary. Having been accepted by the three major public hospitals in Brisbane, she opted for the Princess Alexandra.

Hoffman hated nursing as a young woman. She missed her animals, her younger brothers Andrew and Matthew and her baby sister Maree. In the first six months she thought she had experienced the worst things a nurse might be expected to do – everything from changing the dressings on severed limbs to helping pack a deep abdominal wound in which the intestines could be seen glistening. She received another surprise when one of the nurse educators stood up and asked the class: 'How do you wipe a patient's bottom?' At the time, Hoffman knew little about what she was letting herself in for.

After three years of work and study, she travelled overseas for three months, then returned to nurse in Tasmania. By 1981 she had gone back to the United Kingdom to do midwifery at Taunton in Somerset. While she was there, Hoffman was woken by the telephone at 5.17 am one day. She snuggled deeper under the covers, hoping the telephone was ringing for one of the other nurses who shared the hospital's accommodation. A short while later, someone was turning the handle on her door. 'You need to ring home,' the supervisor told her in a grave tone.

Toni's mother, Marie, answered the telephone at the family farm. 'Andrew's dead. He had a motorbike accident.'

Toni's younger brother had been visiting wineries near Stanthorpe with friends when he struck a power pole while rounding a corner. He had suffered a major chest wound and died at the scene. Partly as a result of the accident, Hoffman realised she wanted to specialise in intensive care. Although the patients wheeled into the ICU were often near death, they had at least been stabilised. Unlike in the Emergency Department, where the doctors and nurses struggled with drugs and electric paddles to maintain life, the prognosis of patients in the ICU could be more accurately predicted. There was relative calm in the ICU, necessarily staffed by the best doctors and visited regularly by specialists. Hoffman took great satisfaction in standing beside patients as they stared death in the face, then seeing them return to their families.

She obtained her first qualification in intensive care at King's College Hospital in London and went on to work in the IC wards at the Harley Street Clinic in London. Later, she was to work at the Launceston General Hospital.

Wanderlust took her to Riyadh in Saudi Arabia where she was a senior nurse for six years. The children in the paediatric wards quickened the ticking of her biological clock. She was 30 and in a secret relationship with a Saudi man. If ever she was going to surprise her family and friends by marrying, it was then.

When Hoffman returned, alone again, from Saudi Arabia after the first Gulf War, she settled in Caloundra, a relaxed beachside town on the Sunshine Coast. She threw herself into her studies by correspondence, working towards gaining qualifications as a Bachelor of Nursing from Monash University. By the middle of 2000 when she pipped one other senior nurse on the short list to win the job as nurse manager of the ICU at Bundaberg Base Hospital, Hoffman had found a substitute for children and married life.

Happily, Hoffman had moved north to the sugar town of Bundaberg. It was home now. She spent most nights and weekends in her rented cottage in Grimstead Street, surrounded by textbooks and determined to graduate from Monash University with a Masters in Bioethics. She decided her thesis would examine how health professionals involved in treating critically ill patients were subjective in determining quality of life. In Hoffman's experience as a nurse, perceptions about quality of life too often depended on the individual values of the carers – the doctors and the nurses – instead of the patient. She believed that a young and fit doctor who ran marathons would be less likely to appreciate how an elderly cripple might have an acceptable quality of life merely watching grandchildren run around the yard.

Hoffman decided that decisions about quality of life were best left to the patients and their next of kin. She enjoyed excellent working relationships with the doctors, but she hated it when they justified poor care, leading to death, as a path to a better outcome. 'How would they know?' she asked. As far as Hoffman was concerned, every life was precious no matter how poorly compromised the patient's health. She believed that the best possible care should be provided until the patient drew a final breath.

The hospital on Bourbong Street beside the Burnett River had seemed backward when she first arrived. And in many ways it was. The medical staff was largely made up of Overseas Trained Doctors, some of whom could barely be understood because of their broad accents or their inadequate command of English.

The district manager, Peter Leck, had no clinical qualifications but knew the key to success for him was staying within budget. The strict financial parameters were well understood by administrators who were remote from the patients. The easiest way to deal with a problem was to dismiss it with the excuse there was no money to fix it. Leck's job was not necessarily a job for life. A budgetary blow-out or a failure to get on top of the surgery waiting lists could mean the sack.

On the other hand, the doctors and nurses were united in the belief that public hospitals were for the sick and injured. The unforgiving economic rationalism of Premier Peter Beattie's Labor Government, Health Minister Wendy Edmond and her top bureaucrats in Queensland Health headquarters in Brisbane was distressing. Staff who for years had been dedicated to the public system were giving up, preferring to work in the better-funded private sector. As more and more demoralised clinicians quit, those left behind were increasingly pressured by administrators. The hospitals were infused with business strategies. Where once the medical superintendent concentrated on patient outcomes, the new priority was cutting costs and increasing potential revenues.

Nowhere was this more obvious than at Bundaberg Base Hospital in the months leading up to the arrival of Jayant Patel. The administrators were measuring performance not by lives saved, but by dollars saved. The hospital had become a lean, mean business.

5

Grim

IN January 2002, before Dr Charles Nankivell walked away for the last time from the Bundaberg Hospital on Bourbong Street, he hoped that the crisis in health care he was witnessing and repeatedly warning his managers about, might still be corrected. If the administrators who controlled budgets and human resources truly valued their highly skilled and passionate Director of Surgery, now was the time to show it. He hoped someone from head office would ring and say: 'We hear you're leaving. We're sad about that. Would you like to talk to us?' But nobody called.

Nankivell had been pushed to the brink of a physical and nervous breakdown. Despite the excessive hours he had been working, the patients were suffering. They were waiting too long for surgery. Nankivell was regularly spending 14 hours a day at the hospital, then being woken at home and asked to come in for a critical case or unexpected emergency. The weekends offered no respite – Nankivell had to work most Saturdays and Sundays. As one of two hospital surgeons serving a growing and ageing population of almost 80 000 people, most of whom were not privately insured, Nankivell needed urgent back-up. He had pleaded his case with everyone from his district manager, Peter Leck, to the head of Queensland Health, Dr Rob Stable. As Nankivell told Stable in a confidential memo in late 2001:

> I had my resignation letter ready one year ago. As it turned out, the same day I signed my resignation Dr Anderson was stood down. So it was not handed in. I stayed on in Bundaberg an

extra 12 months to try to help the patients here and with hope that things might improve.

I suffered enormous physical and mental exhaustion and was operating on patients when I was totally unfit. I will not allow any other person to go through this. This very ugly episode is well known throughout Queensland and is a big turnoff for surgeons thinking of coming to Bundaberg.

Our clinicians' meetings with Q Health have identified the problems with the Department of Surgery as the No.1 problem affecting the Bundaberg Base Hospital for several years. There has been no effective response to our concerns.

This has flabbergasted the staff...we seem to have no effective communication with Q Health. Clearly identified issues are not addressed and we don't seem to get appropriate feedback on why not.

Nankivell warned of numerous examples of unnecessarily delayed diagnoses of cancer, massively overbooked clinics, an Emergency Department in a 'shambles' and an inability to meet guidelines for the surgical waiting lists. But it was to no avail. Instead, his letters and telephone calls branded Nankivell as a complaining clinician. There was no extra funding because nobody was prepared to insist that extra funds be provided.

Nankivell was livid whenever the quality assurance data arrived from the statisticians in the administration. They would dwell on statistics showing, for example, that his patients stayed an average of 4.3 days, when in Brisbane the average was slightly less. Constant pressure was exerted to move the patients through faster. Time is money. But Nankivell's priority was to make his patients better. If that meant a longer stay, so be it.

He should not have been surprised by his failure to achieve change. The culture of Queensland Health was being distorted by a management model that described patients as clients. It was a culture which nurtured the creation of committees. Rarely was anything resolved. Decisive action on even minor matters was frowned upon; clinicians were expected to prepare a submission or a business case.

The pointlessness of it all infuriated Nankivell. After careful consideration, he eventually decided not to follow through with a plan to tell all to the local newspaper, the Bundaberg *NewsMail*. 'If I tell the truth to the media, I get sacked, but if people in administration spin-doctor the media, they get promoted,' he said.

Nankivell had examined Queensland Health's Code of Conduct. In one part it states: 'All employees are reminded that irresponsible discussion of any matters regarding the health service facilities, staff, and, most importantly, the patients is regarded as an offence.' Nankivell regarded that statement as a gag. He dubbed the Code of Conduct the Code of Silence.

Dr John Youngman, the second most senior administrator in the Queensland Health organisation, responded to Nankivell's and Bundaberg's crisis with a brief letter which made scant mention of the unsafe working practices that Nankivell suspected would kill either him or a patient. When he received Youngman's letter, Nankivell decided the hospital was a lost cause. 'That's it, I'm finished. I'm out of here,' Nankivell said.

His immediate predecessor, Dr Pitre Anderson, had suffered a worse fate for being outspoken about life-threatening problems. Anderson and the Director of Medical Services, vascular surgeon Dr Brian Thiele, had built up a strong surgery department. Thiele had an almost magical touch. Even after major operations, his patients were always in relatively great shape when taken from theatre to the ICU. Toni Hoffman marvelled at their robust condition.

But the constant struggle against an administration they regarded as closed and secretive eventually wore both specialists down. They abandoned the hospital. When Anderson went public in the *NewsMail* to warn of the dangers posed by exhausted surgeons, he was subjected to a scathing attack by Health Minister Wendy Edmond in State Parliament. 'I can understand Dr Anderson's need to constantly criticise the Bundaberg Hospital administration since they are the ones who exposed his double dipping and disservice to the public patients whom he was employed to care for,' Edmond said.

It was a typical Queensland Health ploy: discredit the whistle-blower by raising untested claims; then, create a diversion from the fundamental problems plaguing the system; and make sure other staff who might have been thinking of going public know they will face public censure.

After the departures of Anderson and Nankivell, Dr Sam Baker took on the job as Director of Surgery. He, too, tried to ensure management understood how dangerous the hospital had become because of its focus on the bottom line instead of outcomes for patients. 'There is little direction from management with regards to strategic direction. They refuse to clearly define the hospital's operational role in delivery of services and the critical mass of medical staff required to meet this role. They appear more interested in making targets than delivery of quality health care,' he wrote in an internal assessment memo.

Dr Chris Jelliffe, an anaesthetist at the hospital, was deeply concerned for the well-being of the staff and the patients. He had seen Nankivell deteriorate to the point where he looked like a beaten man, broken by the punishing hours he had to work. Jelliffe was also in a bad way due to the demands. He was sure that his own decision-making processes were impaired. He could not sleep despite being exhausted. His appetite had waned. But the hospital's waiting lists for surgery were lengthening and management had little interest in 'excuses'.

Jelliffe decided over Easter 2002 that his fatigue and the lack of staff made it unsafe to continue operating and anaesthetising. He cancelled any surgery that could safely wait for a couple of days. He was told to come to Peter Leck's office.

Leck, who had the anaesthetist's personnel file on his desk, began the conversation with an unusual question: 'Chris, just by the way, remind me of your visa status.'

As a United Kingdom-trained doctor, Jelliffe's visa to live in Australia was tied to his contract as an Overseas Trained Doctor. Queensland Health had special leverage over the imports. They were also cheaper to employ.

Jelliffe felt threatened by the district manager. He was certain Leck had asked the odd question at the start of a meeting about the cancellations of surgery to warn Jelliffe that his livelihood and aspirations to live in Australia were now on the line. Under different circumstances, Jelliffe might have felt bound to go back to theatre notwithstanding his exhaustion. But as he had recently married his Australian girlfriend, a fact Leck was not aware of, Jelliffe no longer relied on Queensland Health as a visa sponsor.

He left the meeting and told Baker about how Leck had tried to intimidate him.

'Jesus Christ, that's a bit rough,' Baker said.

Jelliffe could not stomach it for much longer. He quit in late 2002.

After repeated but unheeded pleas to management for help, Baker, too, decided the hospital was unsalvageable. He moved on in November 2002.

On 13 February 2003 – some six weeks before Jayant Patel would arrive from the US to fill the newly vacated Director of Surgery position at Bundaberg Base Hospital – seven specialist surgeons on the local medical advisory committee wrote a memo. It condemned 'the dictatorial, unresponsive, myopic and inflexible approach of management who have little regard or respect for specialists, their needs or aspirations'.

6

My brilliant career

Portland, Oregon, USA, January 2002

AS thick snow blanketed the wide lawn fronting his two-storey house in Beaverton, a suburb of professionals and middle-class millionaires on the edge of Portland, Dr Jayant Mukundray Patel, 51 and newly unemployed, reflected on his troubled past.

It never snowed in Jamnagar. When the heavens above the dusty, overcrowded city in the far west of India's Gujarat province brought the seasonal monsoon rains, impoverished farmers celebrated their good fortune. There would be another harvest, food for the family and the prospect of money from the maize to buy essentials for the next crop. Too much rain and there would be floods, death and destruction on a massive scale. Hundreds, sometimes thousands, of lives would be swept away with the flimsy homes and ragged belongings of the province's poorest wretches. Their misery would feature prominently in the local media for a few days. Loved ones would mourn. There would be renewed calls from ambitious legislators and community leaders for an inquiry into lax building standards. Somebody might flag a new approach to shanty housing to keep the most disadvantaged out of harm's way. Ultimately, nothing would change. It just made everyone feel a little better in the teeth of tragedy before moving on. This was their fate.

Not only did Jamnagar never see snow, its doctors, some of the most privileged and respected citizens in the province, were never subject to the same accountability as the hoi polloi. Patel sometimes wondered whether he would not have been better off had he stayed in his homeland. His superior family name, caste, academic excellence and status as a specialist surgeon meant something among his own people there.

Colleagues at the MP Shah Medical College and Guru Govindsingh Hospital had never dared question his judgement or aptitude with a scalpel. The patients did not complain. Deaths and injuries were an inevitable consequence for the patients of every hardworking surgeon. What part of this unquestionable logic did the American regulators of medicine and surgery not understand? The latest gratuitous insult had cut him deeply. He knew it must have been a source of gossip among his friends and colleagues in the medical community.

At least the little *BME Report*, published twice a year by the Oregon Board of Medical Examiners for the benefit − or, in Patel's case, public shaming − of registered and paid-up practitioners, would not be read in Jamnagar, where he was still hailed as a genius. 'Statement of Purpose: The BME Report is published to help promote medical excellence by providing current information about laws and issues affecting medical licensure and practice in Oregon.' Dr Philip F Parshley had written the lead article, headlined 'Responsibility Rests with Surgeon'. It sounded ominous. 'In medicine, the physician is "captain of the ship", and the Board of Medical Examiners takes a strong position that doctors are responsible for the patients under their care, whether that care is rendered directly or delegated to others.'

There was another heading: 'Board Actions'. The first column contained six names. Each was attached to a paragraph of vilifying and unambiguous text. There he was, the third name down. Nobody could have missed the dishonourable mention of Jamnagar's finest in the professional journal of the medical regulatory body of Oregon.

'PATEL, Jayant M., MD15991, Portland, Or.' The entry disclosed an active order, made by the Board of Medical Examiners in late 2000, forbidding Patel from performing a wide range of surgery.

It could have been much worse. A dreadful toll of death and permanent, life-shortening injury suffered by patients of Patel in the years since he began practising in Portland in 1989 went unreported by the newsletter. But the carnage had been noted in small, disparate parts elsewhere. There were the findings of a confidential internal audit of the outcomes from surgery of 79 of Patel's patients. There were the

subsequent investigative files of the BME. There were the legal deposi-
tions of the walking wounded whose financial settlements gave Patel
the dubious distinction of being the most successfully sued physician of
his employer, the huge Kaiser Permanente healthcare group. There
were his colleagues who had expressed alarm at the lethal repercussions
of his work.

Impossibly complex procedures that should never have been
attempted had led to patients like Marie Mesecher, a retired restaurant
owner with pancreatic cancer, dying unnecessarily. Patel had cut a critical vein and artery while trying to reach her tumour, causing massive
blood loss. Mesecher needed transfusions of more than three times her
body's volume of blood as other doctors tried desperately to save her
life. Her blood, the post-mortem report said, 'was pooling off the bed
and onto the floor' before she died that afternoon. Later, when her
daughter Sandra Ickert asked Kaiser Permanente staff about Patel's
competence, she was reassured that he was an outstanding specialist.

Patel knew his surgical career in the US was finished when the
BME Report published a clue to the truth about his surgery. In the
months that followed, he came under mounting pressure to resign from
Kaiser Permanente to avoid further humiliation – dismissal. Jamnagar's
most arrogant medical export resolved to take his talents to a fresh pool
of admiring peers, wherever they might be. He regarded himself as a
stellar surgeon who had been grievously wronged. Before the snow
melted outside his Beaverton mansion, he began using the Internet to
look for opportunities abroad. The huge international demand for
experienced doctors had spawned dozens of recruitment companies
with sophisticated web-based forums, search fields and even online
application forms. It cost Patel nothing to start sowing the seeds for a
new start in a country which knew nothing of his background.

Patel read again the testimonials of some of his former colleagues,
mentors like Kaiser Permanente's Chief of Surgery (retired), Edward A
Ariniello: 'I feel that wherever he works or whomever he works for will
be the beneficiary of his excellent skills and knowledge and will be all the
better for it. He will be an asset to any group, hospital or organisation.'

Patel particularly liked that last line. He could not have put it more
succinctly himself.

7

The web

December 2002 to March 2003

JAYANT Patel knew little about New Zealand and even less about Kaitaia, a small township in the country's far north. Its hospital, a modest 28-bed public facility, needed a doctor for a relatively undemanding position. There would be no surgery. It was a massive step down from the senior surgical positions Patel had held in Portland, Oregon, until resigning in disgrace in 2001.

At Kaitaia, the successful candidate would be mostly involved in pre- and post-operative care of the patients. On rare occasions Patel may have been needed in the operating theatre – but only to assist a surgeon. 'This is exactly the position I am looking for, a responsible practice in a small community,' Patel wrote on 10 December 2002. His enthusiasm was obvious. Although the position involved a move to the other side of the world, Patel said he would be available to travel in just three weeks. 'Please call me if you can if there is any interest,' he added.

For months, Patel had been scouring the Internet looking for work. He was bored. He had been humiliated in the Oregon medical community. He needed to go somewhere foreign. A country and a hospital where he would be welcomed and pampered. Where the doctors and nurses had no knowledge of his past.

He had registered with an Australian medical recruitment company, Wavelength Consulting, which pledged in its mission statement: 'We will always provide our clients with first class candidates, our candidates with first class opportunities, and both with unbeatable service. We will do so ethically and with the best interests of the candidate, client and wider community in mind.' Its website was busy with job descriptions and easy to navigate. Its staff responded promptly to his emails and queries.

The company, which had a paid-up capital of $2, was owned by Dr John Bethell and Claire Ponsford in Sydney. They headhunted overseas health professionals and matched them with vacancies in hospitals and private clinics throughout Australia and New Zealand. The company earned a commission from each placement. A chronic shortage of doctors and the constant bidding up of salaries by increasingly desperate employers had created a lucrative market. Bethell found he could make more money from his Internet business than he could earn by practising medicine.

But the hospital at Kaitaia would have to make do without Patel. He was flattered when a Wavelength staff member told him he would be 'too senior for this post'. Instead, Bethell had something else up his sleeve: a position as the Senior Medical Officer at the Bundaberg Base Hospital had become available.

Patel was again brimming with enthusiasm. He spoke to Bethell on the telephone and followed up in writing. 'I had good training and experience with the majority aspect of general and pediatric surgery including laparoscopic procedures, trauma surgery including vascular emergencies,' he said. 'I have excellent surgical experience and am very comfortable with the responsibility. I am getting a few offers within the US, however, my first priority is overseas work.' Patel explained that he was near retirement and financially secure. With a daughter in medical school and his wife, Kishoree, still practising as a doctor, he told Bethell that he wanted an altogether different work and life experience. He wanted an adventure.

Bethell liked what he heard. Patel had held a position as a staff surgeon with the same major organisation in Oregon for 12 years and he had headed a surgery residency program which involved teaching and mentoring junior surgeons. A number of articles he wrote jointly with other surgeons had been published in journals. And unlike some of the doctors who promoted their skills through the website, Patel was not overly demanding. 'He would expect relocation expenses and accommodation but does not need a big house,' Bethell told Dr Kees

Nydam, Bundaberg Hospital's acting Director of Medical Services. 'He needs a place to get a good cup of coffee in the morning.'

Patel sent glowing references from three of his US referees, Dr Peter Feldman, Dr Bhawar Singh and Dr Nora Dantas. Each of the references was written on Kaiser Permanente letterhead.

Feldman: I have known Dr Jayant Patel ever since he came to work at Kaiser Permanente in Portland, Oregon. I have many good things to say about Dr Patel. He has been a wonderful colleague over the years and has been a very hard worker. In addition to having a very busy surgical practice he was very active on hospital committees and in other administrative forums. He has a well above average interest in his work, and a well above average knowledge of surgery.

Singh: As a former chief and staff anaesthesiologist I have had the opportunity of working with Dr Patel on numerous occasions, both in elective and emergency situations. His balanced judgment, surgical skills and decisive steps, especially in the management of high risk complex procedures, has always been appreciated by us anaesthesiologists and other members of the OR team.

Dr Patel's professional expertise, passion and energy for quality patient care coupled with ethical and best practices advocacy, won him the vote of his colleagues for a 'Distinguished Physician Award' in 1995. These qualities undoubtedly will be an integral part of Dr J. Patel's professional career, irrespective of the place of his practice.

Dantas: I worked with him closely at our intensive care unit and saw him care for the most difficult surgical cases at our hospital. I saw the good results. The nursing staff had good things to say about his surgical skills, his compassionate care and his relationship with the nursing and medical staff.

My countless patients that he took care off [sic] for the last 10 years were very satisfied of [sic] his results and his skills, and I can say categorically, that no one ever gave me a negative feedback about him which I always get as a primary care physician when patients come back to me.

Patel's other testimonials were also superb. Dr Edward Ariniello was Chief of Surgery at the Kaiser Permanente group's Bess Kaiser Hospital when he hired Patel in 1989. According to Ariniello:

> From the time he started he dove into the work with full vigour. He generally did about 120 cases of pediatric surgery per year in addition to a full load of general surgery. Dr Patel had excellent results with no serious problems or complications. As far as general surgery is concerned he took on the easy cases and, more often, the more difficult, challenging and risky cases. He achieved remarkable results and successes. Insofar as patients are concerned, they keep coming back to him. They trust him, and he delivers the best care he can.

When Bethell called Feldman and Singh, both doctors continued the praise. Neither mentioned the most relevant chapter in their former colleague's career – his record of botch-ups and disciplinary action, although Feldman gave a cryptic clue when he said Patel 'sometimes took on complex cases handed to him by colleagues and found it hard to say no'.

Bethell voiced one minor concern – Patel had not worked for almost 18 months, according to his curriculum vitae. In a subsequent CV sent by Patel, the date on which he claimed to have left Kaiser Permanente in Portland had been changed from 2001 to 2002. But it went unnoticed.

On Christmas Eve, Patel received an early present: a letter of appointment as Senior Medical Officer at Bundaberg Base Hospital. He promptly signed and returned the document. His starting date was confirmed as 1 April 2003. Before he farewelled his wife Kishoree, daughter and friends in Oregon, there was a pile of paperwork and red tape to be dealt with.

Patel needed a rubber stamp from the Medical Board of Queensland to say he was a properly credentialled doctor. Although the Board had a statutory duty to register doctors and protect the public from charlatans, its procedures were negligently lax. The Board performed no independent checks of the references or credentials of incoming doctors. Their fellow physicians were above suspicion. In Patel's case the Board simply required a document from the Oregon Board of Medical Examiners certifying he was properly registered and had not been disciplined.

'I will fax you the letter and put the original in the mail,' Patel told Suzy Tawse, one of the Wavelength staff handling his file, in January.

Tawse forwarded the documents from Patel to Ainslie McMullen, an officer with the Medical Board of Queensland. Neither Tawse nor McMullen noticed that the certificate from Oregon hinted at a potentially serious problem. In black and white it said: 'Standing: PUBLIC ORDER ON FILE. SEE ATTACHED.' But there was nothing attached. The document setting out the details of Patel's negligence and disciplinary history had been removed.

One of the Medical Board forms requires doctors to declare whether their registration overseas has been the subject of any condition, suspension, undertaking or cancellation. Patel in his response wrote 'No'.

McMullen processed the file, one of hundreds she had handled for the Board. Wavelength would receive $13 924 for its efforts in recruiting Patel.

His travel plans were locked in by the administrative staff at Bundaberg Hospital. Patel was scheduled to arrive in Brisbane on a Qantas flight on 31 March, go to a 12.30 pm meeting with a Medical Board representative at Forestry House in the city, then head back to the airport for a 3.30 pm flight to Bundaberg.

'I am looking forward to meeting all of you and having a very productive year,' he told the hospital's Lyn McKean, who was taking care of his travel and accommodation. She had booked him into one of the nicer beachside apartments in Miller Street, Bargara – a 15-minute drive from the hospital. It offered a superb view of sand, volcanic rocks and sea.

'We are also looking forward to your arrival and I know you will have an enjoyable year,' McKean replied.

8

Flashback: a vicious cycle

IT was May 1993 and Jayant Patel, smiling warmly, uttered his umpteenth self-serving sentence in the 20 minutes he and Dr Sally Ehlers had been seated together. 'Congratulations! You've got the job,' he told the attractive woman. 'I make my decisions quickly.'

At 29 and newly separated from her husband – the father of her four-year-old son – Ehlers found the interview disturbing. She had the job, but already she was concerned about the underlying ambitions of her new boss. Ehlers wanted the position as second-year resident in an integrated surgical residency program, run by Emanuel Hospital and Health Center and Kaiser Foundation hospitals in Portland, Oregon. She guessed that Patel, the program director, had hired her because of her appearance, age and gender, not because of the strength of her impressive curriculum vitae.

Driving home, Ehlers replayed in her mind the clues to Patel's less-than-subtle antics and she recalled his repeated references to his age – he had boasted several times that he was 'only 39'. He and his wife Kishoree, a competent physician, had bought a mansion in Beaverton, an expensive suburb in north-east Portland, two years earlier for US$420 000, but Patel's partner since medical college in India rarely came up in conversation.

His ego was colossal. Aside from himself, Patel had little to talk about. He stressed how much he had achieved and how clever he was. The young surgical residents who looked up to Patel had voted him Teacher of the Year in 1991 and 1992. He was determined to 'educate' Ehlers and school her in the intricacies of a wonderful subject –

himself. He boasted how he had embarked on an extraordinarily suc-cessful journey in surgery, and he was still 'so young'. He wanted Ehlers to nod and fawn in obsequious approval and flatter him with tributes to his stellar career. Patel, who shamelessly complimented himself, had turned a job interview into a flawless self-appraisal. And, Ehlers con-cluded, he wanted her to understand something else: their age difference was trivial. The ten years separating the chain-smoking and overweight surgeon from the fit understudy was no barrier to a relationship outside the operating theatre, he insisted. But it was another clumsy lie, another hopeless misrepresentation. At that time, Patel was not 39. He had just turned forty-three.

It would take another seven years for regulators in Portland to ban Patel from a wide range of surgery. But the number of patients who were dying or suffering in pain due to his negligence was growing even before Ehlers received her letter of appointment. Every time his scalpel slipped and nicked an artery or vein or vital organ, Patel lacerated the quality of life of a patient in Oregon. In at least a handful of cases – the ones that stood out for the glaring ineptitude or because the families demanded answers – his blade was an instrument of death. And some of his colleagues had begun to express disquiet.

But before Ehlers had seen him operate or surveyed the dreadful complications in the patients, she was busy discouraging his advances. 'You may never get to have drinks with your program director again,' he told her in the car park, a month after their first meeting. 'What you really need is a boyfriend.'

Ehlers replied: 'Well, Dr Patel, I have a boyfriend. And you know I do. You have met him.'

Ehlers had been seeing another doctor, Atul Thakker. Patel knew about their blossoming relationship because Ehlers had introduced them at an annual resident graduation dinner. Dr Thakker was ethnic Indian, although the similarities with Patel ended there. He had grown up in the United States. He had graduated from the medical school at University of California Los Angeles (UCLA) and was a resident at Oregon Health & Science University. He was popular. And he was younger. When Patel again tried to start a relationship with Ehlers, she told him Thakker was a serious boyfriend. Patel's demeanour changed immediately for the worse.

Other young female doctors felt uncomfortable around Patel. As participants in the Emanuel residency program, they lived in adjoining accommodation. Patel would barge into the women's area without knocking, surprising the residents in various states of undress after a shower or while changing clothes. He had no place being there.

For the next three years, Patel prevented Ehlers from performing complex and challenging surgery. In educational conferences he was hostile and shouted her down when she offered answers. He singled her out for nasty asides and made her feel inferior around the other resident surgeons. Those surgeons in Patel's good books, those he dominated and groomed for his clique, clamoured and competed for his attention, but Ehlers wanted none of it. She suspected that Patel would have been reasonable towards her if it were not for Thakker's ethnicity. The handsome younger Indian unwittingly highlighted Patel's shortcomings.

On 12 January 1995, Patel sent her a formal letter accusing her of being argumentative, alienating nursing staff, manipulating the people around her, resisting constructive criticism and having little insight into her conduct. It was classic self-projection. Ehlers had been highly regarded and received outstanding marks before and subsequent to her contact with Patel, but he had decided to teach her a lesson. The letter went on to state:

> Your performance in your surgical residency at Emanuel has remained unsatisfactory. This is primarily because of your attitude and behaviour. You are being perceived as argumentative, disrespectful, dogmatic and arrogant. Being disrespectful, especially to the attending staff, is an unacceptable behaviour in this surgical residency program. I am placing you on probation immediately. If you desire, we will be very happy to arrange for counselling. Depending on the evaluations at the end of your probationary term you will either be removed from probation and allowed to continue, or be subject to disciplinary actions including removal or repeat.

Patel should have been more worried about his own failures in theatre. The corridor gossip at the Bess Kaiser Medical Center was spreading like a virus, with several doctors outside Patel's influence questioning the competence of the staff surgeon. Patel's knowledge of surgery was good. He was clearly an intelligent man. But in many procedures, particularly those involving painstaking and tedious work over several hours, his sloppiness was remarkable.

Some of the doctors had a theory: they believed his addiction to smoking was a large part of the problem. Craving a cigarette, when he should have been meticulously manoeuvring his scalpel around delicate organs, he would, they suggested, lose focus and nerve. He would rush the procedures, take shortcuts, leave theatre before the job was done and stride outside to light up. Sometimes, his patients paid with their lives, or their organs. But still none of his colleagues who harboured these concerns went to the authorities.

By late 1995, a restructuring of the hospital set-up led to Patel being reassigned to work with more experienced surgeons for the first time. Until then he had been top of the heap. He thrived on conflict and had reinforced perceptions of his aggressive nature by chastising another surgeon and questioning his expertise. But now, better surgeons were seeing his handiwork.

ALTHOUGH Jayant Patel had made a lot of money for the Kaiser Permanente group, the legal actions brought by the victims of his incompetence were increasingly expensive.

Ronela Tepei, 18, was suffering abdominal pain and a family history of polyposis – a predisposition to colon cancer – when she went to see Patel. As her father and her uncle had died at an early age of colon cancer, Ronela was at similar risk. Despite knowing the family history, Patel ordered the wrong diagnostic test for the young woman. The limited scope of the test meant its results were inconclusive, and Patel assured Ronela that she was fine. The failure to examine her entire colon meant that polyps, already present, went undetected. Her death at 20, of colon cancer, devastated her young husband, who was left to raise an infant son. The only consolation was financial – Kaiser Permanente settled the case for US$1.4 million.

The hospital group also paid out to the family of Leatrice Fairchild, who died two months after Patel removed part of her stomach. The surgical wound collapsed in a hideous mess, leading to serious complications and death. Kaiser settled this one for US$375 000.

Throughout 1995, there were more deaths, injuries and payouts, and a trio of shocking cases: Gerald Tucker, who bled to death (US$900 000); Helen Brooks, whose ureter was accidentally cut (confidential settlement); and Susan Tomberlin, whose femoral vein was cut (confidential settlement).

One of the younger surgeons tasked with assisting Patel, Dr Sanjeev Sharma, would later tell Susan Goldsmith, a senior investigative journalist at the *Oregonian* newspaper, of his efforts in the operating room to help Helen Brooks by alerting Patel to his mistake. 'I tried very hard to get him to realise there was a problem after the surgery,' said Sharma. 'I spoke up about Mrs Brooks to Patel, and he said, "It's OK, it's OK".'

Tomberlin discovered how she had been unnecessarily injured when a nurse told her that the operation had gone terribly wrong. 'When I saw another doctor, he said I was a walking time-bomb from this. They said "this could kill you if a piece of this blood clot gets loose",' she said. 'When I mentioned that to Dr Patel, he screamed at me like I was a two-year-old and told me I wasn't to talk to anybody about what happened.'

The hospital's managers and lawyers elected to keep the litigation and the payouts a secret from Oregon's regulatory body, the Board of Medical Examiners.

In mid 1996, in the months after the closure of the Bess Kaiser Medical Center, Dr Sally Ehlers went to a weekly meeting of doctors at another hospital, Providence St Vincent, to compare notes on problem surgeries. Ehlers disclosed the case of Duane Feakin, whose large intestine was removed by Patel. It was the wrong decision. Feakin suffered a string of serious complications and needed several operations over a few years to rectify the damage. His wounds had also fallen apart.

Feakin's poor outcomes mortified Ehlers. At the age of 14, she had been diagnosed with Hodgkin's disease. She was a cancer survivor and doctors had told her incorrectly at 18 that she was infertile. Her experiences gave her a unique understanding of the mental and physical pain suffered by patients. Ehlers knew Patel, her former teacher, was dishonest and a predator. But she could not figure out why Patel had rushed Feakin into having the original operation. Feakin had not been afflicted with ulcerative colitis. The young man suffered Crohn's disease, a fact established from the pathology report. It was as if Patel, whose boastfulness was legendary, wanted to do the most complex procedures for his own benefit.

A distressed Ehlers had been to see Patel to discuss his invasive operations and the complications that had ruined Feakin's quality of life. 'I have seen the pathology report and it shows Crohn's disease,' she told Patel.

The senior surgeon shrugged it off. 'Oh, I'm going to talk to the pathologist. I will get that straightened out,' Patel told her.

When Ehlers, safely out of Patel's clutches, went to the morbidity and mortality meeting at Providence St Vincent in mid 1996 and described Feakin's clinical history, including his most recent major operation weeks earlier and an intra-abdominal abscess, the other surgeons were unusually sombre. They had been wary of Patel before Ehlers spoke, but now – after hearing about the pointlessness of Feakin's misery – they were worried. Dr Roger Alberty, Chief of Surgery at the Providence St Vincent Medical Center, found that other surgeons doing the same surgery as Patel were having much better outcomes.

In the same year, Patel was threatened with disciplinary action by the regulatory authority in Washington State for seeking registration there and lying to conceal an earlier chapter in his disciplinary history.

By late 1997, several other surgeons employed by the Kaiser Permanente group were voicing concern. When the group's chiefs ordered a clinical audit of 79 of his operations, the findings were worse than they had feared. Several patients had bled to death because veins or arteries or organs were nicked in surgery and a worryingly high number of patients had suffered dehiscence – their wounds literally fell apart due to negligent technique.

In 1998, when the results of the clinical audit were in, Kaiser Permanente managers filed a confidential adverse action report with the US National Practitioner Databank. The patients Patel had operated on for the preceding decade remained unaware of the serious and adverse findings regarding his competence.

Patel's surgical work in hospitals operated by the Kaiser Permanente group was severely restricted for the first time in late June 1998. A new regimen established uniquely for him required 'mandatory second opinions before undertaking all complicated surgical cases, chart reviews, proctoring, attendance of surgical meetings...'

In the two years between Ehlers first voicing her long-held concerns in 1996 and the conclusion of the clinical audit in 1998, at least four patients died in circumstances where death should not have occurred. Numerous others were unnecessarily injured.

After hearing, finally, of the Patel cases, the Oregon Board of Medical Examiners, which registers practitioners to work and decides on disciplinary or regulatory action where the public may be at risk, held its own investigation. On 22 September 1998, Patel admitted to the Board's investigative committee that he had made serious surgical errors. Patel agreed to a range of formal restrictions on his surgery and he undertook to obtain second opinions before considering operations that were not straightforward.

It took two more years for the Board's restrictions and the formal finding of 'gross or repeated acts of negligence' to become a matter of public record. By 2001, as gossip and revelations about Patel's negligence went around Oregon's medical community, the surgeon had become a public embarrassment to the Kaiser Permanente group. His colleagues had presented him with an award in 1995, naming him Distinguished Physician of the Year. In June 2001, he resigned to avoid being fired. In the same year, he was also struck off the roll of practitioners in New York State, having also lied to the medical authorities there about his disciplinary history. Patel, desperate to return to the operating theatre, was being thwarted at every turn.

He was incompetent when he came to Bundaberg, but his incompetence was compounded by another factor. By April 2003, he had not picked up a scalpel for several years. He was much more deadly than he had ever been.

9

A new career

March to June 2003

JAYANT Patel was keen to see his new workplace after the Qantas flight from Brisbane touched down late in the afternoon of 31 March. Although tired from the travel, he was also excited. His charm and effusive friendliness rubbed off on Dr Kees Nydam, the acting Director of Medical Services, who showed him around the Bundaberg Hospital on Bourbong Street. Patel made light of his long journey as he cut a swathe through the administration offices, shaking hands with senior and junior staff. He read the Queensland Health Code of Conduct and provided a signature sample for the official registry.

Hours earlier in Brisbane he had been to the offices of the Medical Board and met one of its members, Dr John Waller. It involved little more than a friendly greeting and a glance at the file. Waller, overlooking the clue to the disciplinary action in Oregon, marked 'Yes' next to the criterion of Certificate of Good Standing.

The next morning when Patel arrived at Bundaberg Hospital for the start of his first working day as a Senior Medical Officer (SMO), the town was having a collective laugh. It was April Fool's Day. Patients, nurses and doctors at the hospital indulged each other with practical jokes and harmless gags. The Bundaberg *NewsMail* was in on the fun, reporting how rail lines at Quay Street had suddenly been removed. One reader failed to see the funny side after going to inspect the public works, only to find nothing had changed.

On that day, Patel was formally endorsed by the Medical Board. It granted him Registration Certificate Number 1030450 providing authorisation: 'To practise as a Senior Medical Officer in surgery at

Bundaberg Base Hospital or any other public hospital authorised by the Medical Superintendent on a temporary basis.'

The 'Dear Dr Patel' letter sent by the regulator on 1 April states in bold font: 'It is advised that you are not registered as a specialist.' This meant he had to be supervised. As Patel had come to Bundaberg to perform surgery, the Medical Board carelessly assumed the hospital already had a Director of Surgery – in other words, a highly qualified specialist who had been vetted and credentialled by the Royal Australasian College of Surgeons – to scrutinise his work and identify any problems. There was only one hitch. The last Director of Surgery, Dr Sam Baker, had quit in disgust months earlier.

Nydam, overawed by Patel, was embarrassed that a senior American surgeon with apparently immaculate qualifications was a mere SMO in a regional Queensland hospital. A week later, Dr Nydam, temporarily in charge of the hospital where he had done his internship a quarter-century earlier, made an executive decision to promote Patel to the position of Director of Surgery. Nydam was breaking the rules with his premature move to flatter and elevate an untested surgeon he barely knew. It was the worst decision he had made in his professional life.

In the year he had reluctantly been in charge of the hospital, Nydam felt like a military chief who, when he asked for generals, had been given majors. Now that he had a bona fide general when all he had asked for was a major, Nydam wanted to look after him. Nydam had long taken the view that people who worked in public health were either missionaries or idiots. He put Patel in the former category.

'Are we paying Jay Patel a director's allowance?' Nydam asked Georgie Rose, the hospital's Human Resources manager. 'If not, could we do so, please, as he is the Director of Surgery.'

When Jenny White, the senior nurse in charge of the operating theatres, met Patel, he laughed as he told her he had been given the director position. White was surprised. Nobody had assessed Patel's surgical technique. If it was anything like his personality – hot and cold, ranging from brash, domineering and rough to charming and obse-quious – the staff and patients were in for a wild ride.

Another American surgeon, Dr Jim Gaffield, was due to start at the hospital by the end of the month. White wondered why he had not been considered for the position of Director of Surgery. 'Well, it must be because I got here first,' said Patel.

In mid April Bundaberg Hospital greeted Dr Darren Keating as the new Director of Medical Services, to occupy on a permanent basis the position Nydam had been unhappily filling. Patel, already well ensconced, warmed to the reserved former Australian Defence Force doctor who arrived with his young family from a small regional public hospital in Western Australia. Keating had never managed a hospital. He displayed unusual traits for an executive. When staff came to see him in his office, he would invariably continue writing whatever letter or report he had in front of him. Sometimes he would not bother looking up. Doctors and nurses would leave his office shaking their head at his manner. Keating chose to remain isolated from most of the staff. He was rarely seen in the Intensive Care Unit, the wards or in medical meetings.

Keating was aloof. It came across as arrogance, but it could have been shyness and a lack of confidence. His limited and general clinical experience meant he was hopelessly out of his depth around specialists. Dr Martin Strahan, a Visiting Medical Officer, decided that Keating preferred to remain 'bunkered' in his office lest he encounter complaints. And Kees Nydam would later conclude: 'If he was standing against a grey wall you wouldn't even know that he was there.'

But right from the start Keating gave undivided attention to Jayant Patel. If it were not for Patel's remarkable gusto and his enthusiasm for surgery, the hospital's waiting lists would lengthen. And that would invite closer scrutiny of Keating's management from more senior bureaucrats in Brisbane.

Before anyone unnecessarily began to die or suffer injury at Bundaberg Hospital there were red flags – warnings that Patel's competence did not equal his confidence. He was too eager to operate. Too gung-ho. His judgement was questionable. When surgical errors were made, he fought to prevent patients being rushed to better-equipped hospitals in Brisbane, even when their complications were life-threatening and beyond the capacity of the regional hospital. 'It always looks right if we do the procedures where we also are capable of dealing with the complications,' Patel told management. It was a theme Patel hammered relentlessly at Bundaberg.

In the beginning the nurses put it down to his US training. But there were too many mishaps. There were too many squandered chances to improve a patient's prospects. It took a while for Patel's other motive in obstructing transfers to dawn on the nurses. He opposed the transfers because the damage he had caused to the patients could be identified by other surgeons.

WITH cancer on the inside upper section of his ear, Peter Dalgleish spoke to Patel in April about having it removed. Patel was shown the position and had the added benefit of the notes of the family doctor. On 20 May, Patel confidently went to work on the ear and declared the procedure a success. He had operated on the wrong part of the ear.

'Have you ever had your ear operated on? Let alone in the wrong place altogether?' Dalgleish asked Peter Leck, the hospital's manager. 'To say it is painful would be an understatement indeed. The cancer is still there.'

Dr Darren Keating spoke to Patel, who refused to accept that he had removed healthy tissue and overlooked the cancerous part.

Paul Jones went in for a procedure on his right scrotum, known as an epididymectomy. It was to have been performed under a general anaesthetic. To his great surprise, Jones received an entirely different procedure. Instead of examining Jones's private parts, Patel performed a gastroscopy. He pushed a scope down Jones's throat and oesophagus to investigate his stomach.

Jenny White witnessed an episode she likened to something out of the *M*A*S*H* comedy series set in a field hospital during the Korean War. There had been a traffic accident about 15 kilometres from the hospital. White received a frantic phone call from Patel, who was in a panic. 'I have got to go out to this accident site and I am going to need equipment to amputate limbs,' he told her.

White was already wary of Patel. 'What's he going to do?' she wondered. She collected equipment he would need: a battery operated power source, a large plastic container of blades and saws, and packs full of swabs and sutures.

Shortly afterwards the lift doors opened and she watched Patel rush out with two principal house officers, two interns and two medical students in tow. All were in their surgical scrubs. Patel was still frantic. 'Where's the equipment?' he shouted. 'Where's the equipment!'

'Look, I have it all here in a trolley,' White replied. The entourage swarmed back into the lift.

'You are in the wrong lift,' she yelled after them. One lift was programmed to go up and the other to go down. Patel was shouting at the staff and urging them to hurry while White was yelling: 'Dr Patel, Dr Patel! You are in the wrong lift.' He ignored the nurse and she watched the doors close. The lift ascended and then descended so they could pile out and get in the right lift.

As it turned out, Patel had no role to play in the accident. The passengers were freed by ambulance officers without the need to cut off limbs. When White reflected on the incident afterward she realised that Patel had not even notified an anaesthetist to provide pain relief for the victims should amputation be needed.

From the moment he arrived in Bundaberg, Patel strived to make himself invaluable to his new employer, Queensland Health, and the managers of the hospital in Bourbong Street. Nobody in Australia knew about the bloodletting in Oregon. Nor, Patel decided, did anyone need to know. Instead, Patel had discovered something about the Queensland public healthcare system. He planned to turn it to his advantage. By working hard and performing as many operations as humanly possible, he would cut the waiting lists for surgery. The waiting lists were held up by the media, the politicians and the patients as proof of either maladministration or well-oiled efficiency. By meeting the targets in surgery, he would make the hospital look good. He would give Peter Leck an opportunity to be lauded rather than lambasted by his bosses in Brisbane and by the Labor Party's local parliamentarian, Nita Cunningham.

In turn, Patel would make himself the most valued clinician in the district. With hard work, he could be so prolific the hospital's new Director of Medical Services would come to view him as indispensable.

Their success would be tied to him. They would come to need him more than he needed them.

Patel also knew that his zeal would be financially attractive to the hospital. In the end it always came down to money. The formula used by Queensland Health to fund the hospitals was deliberately structured to reward volume and complexity of operations. The more, the merrier. The riskier, the better. The cash flow depended on numbers, not outcomes. And when the hospitals did not meet the numbers, their funding shrank.

By doing more operations, and more complex operations, Patel would generate rivers of cash for the hospital. He would also generate rivers of blood from the patients. In the process, Patel would set out to prove he really could perform brilliant surgery. He wanted to recredential himself. He looked forward to complex operations such as oesophagectomies. Operations his United States peers had forbidden him from ever trying again.

10

Life and death

April to June 2003

JAMES Edward Phillips, 46, signed his life away on 10 May 2003, next to a handwritten asterisk on a consent form. It also bore the name and signature of the man who escorted him to a premature death. On the day he signed, Phillips brimmed with optimism and hope. He liked the look and confidence of Bundaberg Hospital's new Director of Surgery, Dr Jayant Patel, even if the operation being proposed was difficult to pronounce and harder to spell.

Oesophagectomy. An operation so complicated and risky, it should only be attempted at major hospitals by the most adept specialists, preferably gastroenterologists. To maintain proficiency, a surgeon had to perform a minimum of 30 such operations a year. It is an operation needing specialised and well-resourced Intensive Care Unit back-up. There is only one certainty after an oesophagectomy – the patient will need close monitoring for a long time in a well-equipped hospital. Oesophagectomies were well beyond the limited scope of the operating theatre and the adjacent ICU on the first floor of Bundaberg Hospital.

The operations were also hopelessly outside the expertise of Patel. His lamentable skills were at their negligent best when he was regularly performing far less complicated operations in hospitals in Portland, Oregon. There, his recklessness, rough handling, clumsy techniques and poor judgement had cost his employer millions of dollars in confidential settlements for wrongful death and wrongful harm.

James Phillips knew none of these additional risks when he signed on for an operation he hoped would cut out a small lesion in his oesophagus, the tube linking his throat with his stomach. The lesion was blocking part of Phillips's oesophagus and making it difficult for him to swallow food. Under Patel's plan it would be removed. He hoped it would prolong his life by several years.

The generic consent form required patients to acknowledge:

The doctor has explained my medical condition and the proposed procedure. I understand the risks of the procedure, including the risks that are specific to me, and the likely outcomes. The doctor has explained my prognosis and the risks of not having the procedure. I understand that no guarantee has been made that the procedure will improve the condition, and that the procedure may make my condition worse. On the basis of the above statements, I request to have the procedure.

On the same form Patel set out his planned strategy. He would make an incision in the abdomen. He would also make an incision on either the left side of the neck or the left side of the chest. He would slice through the tissue of the upper part of the stomach and the lower part of the oesophagus. It was a difficult manoeuvre but what came next was even harder. Patel would need literally to pull Phillips's stomach up and attempt a connection to whatever was left of his oesophagus.

A fortnight earlier, Phillips, whose serious kidney problems requiring constant dialysis made him a regular visitor to the hospital, had seen Dr Mark Appleyard for an examination of his oesophagus. Dr Appleyard put a flexible viewing tube into Phillips's mouth and carefully inserted it all the way to the duodenum, the first stage of the small intestine. Appleyard located a nodule which he noted had a 'concerning appearance'. It crumbled easily. It also bled easily on touching. 'I am concerned about the oesophageal nodule,' Appleyard wrote in the patient's notes.

Fortunately for Phillips, he had been in the safe hands of Dr Peter Miach, a highly regarded renal specialist in charge of the Renal Unit, who was also the Director of Medicine. He had supervised the ongoing dialysis. Phillips was a favourite patient of nurses in the Renal Unit. He rarely complained despite his serious kidney issues, constant dialysis and poor overall health.

The biopsy results after Appleyard's examination were discouraging. When the five pieces of pale tan and brownish tissue measuring up to 4 millimetres were analysed, they showed evidence of 'invasive adenocarcinoma'. In other words, a cancer in cells lining the walls of his oesophagus. Miach had asked Patel for an opinion. The surgeon recommended an oesophagectomy. Miach was against it. He believed Phillips was much too frail. Major surgery would be extremely dangerous in someone as ill as Phillips. Miach worried the man would die on the operating table.

On 19 May, Patel fast-tracked Phillips into theatre without Miach's knowledge. A little after 10 am, Patel began to make the incisions. He cut and removed the diseased tissue and pulled up the stomach. Phillips, still under a general anaesthetic, went downhill fast. His vital signs were rapidly deteriorating. For the last 45 minutes of his operation, there was no recordable blood pressure. To keep him alive and his blood circulating, he received massive doses of inotropic drugs to make his heart beat more strongly. Even the adrenaline in the drugs was of little benefit.

By mid afternoon, Patel had put down his instruments and Phillips was wheeled into the Intensive Care Unit in an extremely unstable condition. His pupils were fixed and dilated, indicating brain death. A renal vein, used to take blood away from the kidney, had become blocked. The blockage was almost inevitable: the charts for Phillips, who had not been offered an oesophagectomy by specialists in Brisbane despite their greater expertise, showed the artery was functioning at just 70 per cent. An oesophagectomy would almost guarantee thrombosis. And it did.

For much of the operation, Phillips was in the operating theatre with no dialysis access and a soaring potassium level, a precursor to cardiac arrest. While Patel cut, pulled and stitched, Phillips's heart had given up. His brain was starved of oxygen.

At bed 5 near the window of the ICU, its most senior nurse, Toni Hoffman, ensured that everything possible was being done for Phillips. During the wait for his arrival at the ICU, she'd been told by one of the nurses that the operation had gone badly. When she saw him, lying on his back in a white gown with a covering blanket shortly after 3 pm, Hoffman knew instinctively that he was highly unlikely to survive. 'It's an expensive way to die,' Dr Alison McCready, the anaesthetist who had been in theatre with Patel, told Hoffman as they checked the ventilating equipment to ensure it was inflating the man's lungs.

At this early stage, Hoffman knew little about the brash Director of Surgery. She had been on holidays when he toured the hospital and met the key staff on his first working day, 1 April. Already, seven weeks into his contract, there was gossip on the wards about his flirtatious behaviour with younger nurses. Hoffman was broad-minded. After nursing for more than 20 years in hospitals in Australia, Saudi Arabia and London, she was no longer surprised by the delusions of some doctors who assumed they were God's gift to the nurses. Or perhaps that the nurses were God's gift to them.

She also knew from experience in much larger hospitals that oesophagectomies challenged everyone – the patient, the surgical team and ICU staff. She wondered why such an ill patient had been subjected to the operation.

Hoffman was in good company. Miach, the doctor most familiar with the multiple health problems plaguing Phillips, agreed. 'I do not believe that this man should have ever gone to theatre,' said Miach. 'There was no urgency about it. There was no immediate, acute problem in this man – there was the major problem with his cancer of the oesophagus – but there was nothing acute that demanded that he be operated on straight away.'

As Hoffman watched the monitors, she questioned why Patel had been allowed to attempt it – and why he had risked it with a patient as weak as Phillips.

The nurses from the renal unit were distressed. Their bond with Phillips included his mum, who waited anxiously in the ICU relatives' room and the downstairs cafeteria for any news. When the nurses told her that Phillips's condition was very poor, his mother went to see Patel. Up to that point he had been telling her the exact opposite. Furious at being questioned, he stormed into the ICU to confront Hoffman and let rip with a furious tirade. 'It's embarrassing for this to happen,' he yelled. 'You should have notified me first about the patient's condition getting worse.'

She found the criticisms confusing. Phillips was at death's door – that much had been obvious before he went to the ICU. His perilous condition had not changed. Drugs were keeping him alive. Yet Patel insisted he was doing fine.

'The patient was not stable and we're not going to lie to the relatives. I don't see how you can say he is stable,' Hoffman said.

Patel took his complaint up with Dr Darren Keating, who had arrived to be the new Director of Medical Services a fortnight after Patel started. After Hoffman and the Director of Nursing, Glennis Goodman, met Keating to talk about the problems, he tried to mediate the conflict. Keating suggested to Hoffman that she sit down with Patel to explain the ICU's constraints 'and the need to work together as a team'. Hoffman wondered at the time why it was up to her to explain such fundamental issues to the hospital's most senior practising clinician. Surely, this was a task for Keating.

Soon afterwards, Hoffman and Patel spoke in her office about the dispute. She tried to explain the staffing and equipment limitations of Bundaberg's ICU. 'We can't keep patients for more than 48 hours. The patients need to be transferred to the larger hospitals in Brisbane,' she told him.

Patel bridled at the idea of losing his patients to a larger hospital where they would come under the care of specialists. 'I refuse to practise medicine like that. I will refuse to transfer my patients out,' Patel defiantly told her. He refused to speak to Hoffman again.

James Edward Phillips passed away at 10.15 pm on 21 May 2003, in his bed at the ICU. He had never regained consciousness. Patel had tackled a challenging, trouble-prone oesophagectomy which other surgeons would not have contemplated. It should have been no surprise to him when Phillips succumbed.

11

Memory lane

ONE evening in September 1981, Dr William L Craver, Chief of Surgery at the Genesee Hospital in upstate New York, received a worrying telephone call. He was accustomed to receiving calls outside normal working hours. He dealt with trauma. Patients ripped apart with gunshot wounds. Patients mutilated in serious car accidents.

The call he received on this particular evening was from a senior nurse. She had an unusual problem involving one of the young doctors. 'She was concerned because she had been called by the floor nurse who had been caring for a patient admitted that afternoon for an operation the next morning,' Dr Craver, now retired, told me from his home in the town of Canandaigua, near Rochester. 'Dr Patel was one of the surgical residents who rotated through our hospital from the University of Rochester. We were affiliated with the university.'

The patient had complained to the nurse that she was extremely tired. 'I really would like to get to sleep,' she told her. 'I know the house officer [doctor] is supposed to examine me first and I wish he would hurry up.'

The nurse looked at the patient's charts. 'She saw that there was a complete write-up and work-up and record of a physical examination by Dr Patel of the patient but he had never examined her,' recalled Craver. 'He had not been to her room. He had made it all up based on the notes of the attending surgeon. I went there and talked to the woman. The charts described a complete examination, including an examination of her breasts.'

Craver has a vivid memory of questioning the woman about these examinations and her answers. A nurse herself, she was adamant. 'I know when my breasts have been examined,' she told him.

'I called Dr Patel to my office to talk to him about it. He denied doing anything wrong. He was upset that anyone would question his judgement,' said Craver.

When Craver talked to surgeons and supervisors in other hospitals affiliated with the University of Rochester, he discovered that Patel had been the subject of several similar complaints. Craver decided that Patel was untrustworthy. A bad apple. He did not want him having any contact with the patients. Craver recommended he be fired from the program. The president of the university agreed.

'I was calling it the way it should be called,' said Craver. 'In surgery you are supposed to be honest and trustworthy with total integrity. He showed a total lack of integrity. Dr Patel had been working at our hospital for a couple of months at that point. Until then he had a good reputation. He was considered a good trainee. But the evidence against him held up. We were not making it up. I had no personal reason to be against Dr Patel.'

Official files document Patel's difficulties with regulatory authorities in New York State between 1981 and 1983, two decades before he ventured to Bundaberg. The files and the record of disciplinary action are matters of public record and have always been available from both the New York State Department of Health and the State Board for Professional Medical Conduct. They corroborate the recollections of Craver, who had not seen the material since the early 1980s.

The documents show that the floor nurse was Mary K Jackson. They show Patel had diligently written a history, physical examination, progress notes and admission orders into the medical record of the woman patient. They show that she was deeply distressed. Her surgeon, Dr Rene Menguy, recorded her comments.

On the same day, Patel had made similar entries in the medical records of two other women without personally having examined either of them. He concocted similar lies in the medical records of a further two patients. He had concocted the examination records to cover himself while he worked a second job at the nearby Rochester

Psychiatric Center when he was rostered to be available to respond to emergencies and calls at the Genesee Hospital, a sprawling 120-year-old institution on Alexander Street. After realising that both nurse Jackson and the surgeon, Menguy, were taking the complaints seriously and talking to the patients, Patel turned on one of the patients. She broke down crying when Patel accused her of trying to ruin his career. Patel told the woman her complaint would put his job and schooling in jeopardy.

A rigorous year-long investigation into Patel's antics by the Office of Professional Discipline, the investigative body which compiles evidence for the Board, produced more than 30 statements and exhibits. After the fifth and final day of hearings on 10 May 1983, in rooms at the Holiday Inn at Rochester Airport, the evidence filled more than 700 pages of transcript. Three medical practitioners (Dr Menguy, Dr Raymond F Shamos and Dr Craver), two nurses (Mary K Jackson and Gary W Nelson) and four patients testified on behalf of the prosecuting Department of Health.

Patel, testifying on his own behalf, was supported by the character references of four medical practitioners: Dr James S Williams, Dr Marguerite Dynski, Dr William G Farlow and Dr J Raymond Hinshaw.

As four members (three of whom were doctors) of the Hearing Committee of the State Board for Professional Medical Conduct weighed the evidence, they had to determine if Patel's fabrication of the history of patients demonstrated a 'moral unfitness to practise medicine'.

The charges included 'practicing the profession of medicine fraudulently by entering items in various patients' medical records without personally examining the patient'; as well as gross negligence and incompetence on more than one occasion. There was a charge of 'abandoning or neglecting a patient in need of immediate professional care without making reasonable arrangements'. Patel had also 'harassed, abused and intimidated [the first patient] in an effort to coerce her not to co-operate with an official hospital investigation'.

When most of the charges were proved, Patel's career hung by a thread. The matters were serious, involving gross and repeated acts of deception and grave breaches of trust. His conduct was analogous to a lawyer strapped for time, fabricating a series of statements on behalf of five clients. But a fictitious medical examination could have more serious repercussions.

The committee's members were influenced by the glowing references and laudatory testimony from medical colleagues on Patel's side. Patel's lawyer, John T Frizzell, from a law firm in Buffalo where Patel was then living, emphasised his client's talents and abilities.

Dr Williams called him 'an excellent clinician and very thorough, extremely dedicated'. In one prescient moment, he suggested Patel's 'ultimate contribution to the medical profession will be exceptional'.

Dr Dynski described Patel as one of the best resident doctors she had had contact with in her capacity as a chief resident. He was, she suggested, 'a person of high integrity who had made a mistake'.

Dr Hinshaw, equally effusive, described Patel as 'technically very gifted'. He rated his skills among the top three of the 200 residents he had worked with.

And although Menguy was a witness for the prosecuting authority, he had written in a 20 July 1981 letter that Patel was 'by far the best resident who has rotated with me'.

At the end of the hearings, the committee's chairman, Dr Paul M DeLuca, decided not to 'crush' Patel. He was censured and reprimanded. Instead of penalising him with an immediate fine, in July 1983 the committee put him on probation for three years. If he misbehaved again, he would be fined $5000.

Two months later, Dr David Axelrod, Commissioner of Health in the State of New York, reviewed the decision and decided that the hearing committee had been too lenient. He rejected the committee's findings where Patel was given the benefit of the doubt. 'The failure to examine patients prior to surgery evidences a disregard for and indifference to the results that may follow such failure, and thus constitutes gross negligence,' Axelrod ruled. He decided Patel had clearly demonstrated 'his moral unfitness to practice medicine'. Patel's wrongdoing, according to Axelrod, was 'a serious failure and should be punished by more than a censure and reprimand'.

The effect of the tougher line was negligible. All it meant was that Patel had to pay the $5000 fine. He was free to return to work. And he had a set of wonderful references from four respected doctors. Those doctors and their references would open new doors. Although fired from the Genesee Hospital where he had been doing his residency program, Patel had a springboard to a new job working with Hinshaw as his research associate. He entered the residency program of the University of Buffalo where he completed his general surgery training.

In 1988, Hinshaw helped Patel again. Wanting to put his New York troubles a long way behind him, he applied to work for the Kaiser Permanente healthcare group on the other side of the country, in Portland, Oregon. A laudatory letter dated 29 November 1988 from Hinshaw, then Chief of Surgery at Rochester General Hospital, to the Board of Medical Examiners in Oregon avoided any reference to the serious convictions against Patel. 'When Dr Patel was a member of our residency program he showed technical and professional brilliance. When I operated on the Chief of one of our specialty sections the doctor requested specifically the [sic] he be my assistant. That, in my experience is unique,' Hinshaw wrote.

On 23 January 1989, Hinshaw, whose distinguished 40-year surgical career at the University of Rochester was drawing to a close, received a letter from the Board. The Board's licence administrator, Jan Baggenstros, had discovered something about Patel's dismissal from the University of Rochester's residency program. Baggenstros, curious about Hinshaw's failure to flag this important chapter in Patel's career, sought more information.

Hinshaw's reply on 3 February 1989, four months before his retirement, acknowledged the disciplinary action but insisted that Patel had been harshly treated. He maintained it was a case of the unfair 'harassment of a brilliant young surgeon'. His letter to Baggenstros says:

When I appeared before the State Health Department in Dr Patel's behalf I was asked if I believed the charges against Dr Patel. I gave my reasons why I did not believe them.

I was asked what I would think if it could indeed be shown that Dr Patel had written a physical examination without having examined the patient. I stated that such behaviour on his part would seem so bizarre to me from having worked very closely with him that I would do my best to find out what circumstances caused such an aberration of behaviour.

Hinshaw died, aged 69, in 1993. Craver did not know until years later about Hinshaw's misleading letters of support for Patel in his job quest. Craver believed Hinshaw's unwavering support of Patel during the earlier disciplinary process was inescapably wrong. Hinshaw's stand was a source of tension between the two senior surgeons for years afterwards.

'I will never understand why, in the face of all this evidence, he would have applauded Dr Patel. It has made me lose some respect for a man who was a very fine surgeon,' Craver told me.

12

A tussle

June and July 2003

IN the days after James Phillips passed away in the Intensive Care Unit, Toni Hoffman became increasingly confused. She could cope with Jayant Patel's bombastic and patronising attitude. She could tolerate his 'kiss up and kick down' approach to management and nursing staff. But she worried about his clinical judgement and expertise.

Patel had been telling the nurses ad nauseam how experienced he was in the United States. One day he was a gold standard trauma surgeon. The next he was a cardiothoracic surgeon. There was a different qualification every other day. He had been doing complex surgery for 25 years. The next day it was 30 years. Another day it was 20 years.

Hoffman feared something else in Patel's character. Megalomania. A boldness bordering on recklessness. He seemed to lack insight into the risks he created for the patients. Hoffman was also wondering about his knowledge of best-practice drugs for the patients. He was demanding drugs like dopamine and dobutamine that had been superseded years earlier. When other doctors used modern drugs such as adrenaline and noradrenaline, Patel told the nurses to change the medication back to the obsolete drugs. He thought so differently to the other doctors and Hoffman, it was as if, she confided to Dr Darren Keating, they were 'from two different planets'.

Her attempts to call a truce after the death of Phillips failed dismally. Hoffman knew Patel now saw her as an enemy. He started undermining her authority and credibility, criticising her and the ICU in talks with younger doctors and nurses. She realised the less experienced doctors, who relied on Patel to advance their own careers, lacked the knowledge to see his flaws. They would almost always back him. But Patel was now dividing the nursing staff to grow his support base and isolate her. Having seen through Patel's grandiose claims early on, Hoffman had also worked out that Patel was not everything he said he was. She became a major threat. She had to be discredited. Patel began denigrating the ICU as 'Third World'. He made it clear that he did not trust Hoffman and several of the nurses in the unit.

On 3 June he walked into the ICU to announce he would be performing another oesophagectomy. The patient this time would be James Grave, sixty-three. 'I'll be in the unit for the whole two days while my oesophagectomy [patient] is in here until he leaves the unit,' Patel said.

Nurse Kay Boisen recoiled as Patel continued running the unit down. He made it known that he needed to be in the ICU for the two days because he thought so little of Hoffman's professionalism. Patel knew she had voiced concerns about the death of James Phillips to Dr Keating and the Director of Nursing, Glennis Goodman.

The 6 June operation on Grave led to a string of complications. Patel had paralysed Grave's vocal cord, which made it difficult for him to clear his airway and breathe. In the days afterwards, his wound fell apart twice due to dehiscence. The nurses rarely saw instances of dehiscence, meaning 'to gape', but with Patel it was becoming common. There was also leakage where Patel had clumsily rejoined Grave's gut. Grave, increasingly weak, was wheeled in for three further operations by Patel on 12, 16 and 18 June. While the anaesthetist, Dr Jon Joiner, and the junior, Dr James Boyd, tried to arrange a bed for him in Brisbane, Patel stubbornly resisted the transfer.

The perilous condition of Grave was obvious as he was moved between the ICU, the surgical ward and the operating theatre. Hoffman could not understand why he had not been transferred out. His life hung by a thread. Even when there was a bed available in Brisbane on 18 June, Patel refused to talk to the surgeons in Brisbane, making transfer impossible. 'Why are you doing these big operations there when you can't care for these patients?' an incredulous doctor from one of the larger hospitals asked Hoffman.

In her long career Hoffman had never taken on a Director of Surgery, but she could see that Grave would die unless someone intervened. She sent a note to Glennis Goodman, explaining that doctors at the Princess Alexandra Hospital and the Royal Brisbane have 'expressed their concern at why such surgery was done here when we don't have an intensivist. Meanwhile the patient continues to deteriorate and we have no bed to transfer him to. I think before any more surgery of this type is done here we really have to examine whether we can offer the appropriate follow up care,' Hoffman said.

Some 24 hours later as Grave languished and Patel predicted he would make a miraculous recovery if left in Bundaberg, Hoffman went to Keating. She told him of Grave's complications and how he needed increasing amounts of adrenaline because his condition was so unstable. 'There remains unresolved issues with the behaviour of the surgeon which is confusing for the nursing staff,' Hoffman told Keating. 'I believe we are working outside our scope of practice for a level one Intensive Care Unit. The ongoing issues regarding the transfer of patients and the designated level of this ICU may need to be discussed in more detail at a later date. The behaviour of the surgeon in the ICU needs also to be discussed as certain very disturbing scenarios have occurred.'

Hoffman was perturbed that Patel had not recognised another worrying feature in Grave's condition. He had a chylothorax, a build-up of a milky fluid in the intercostal catheter in his chest. Dr Joiner was also worried. He had found a bed for Grave in Brisbane. But when Patel discovered the arrangement he was furious and immediately threatened to quit. He confronted Joiner in the corridor between the ICU and theatre and abused him.

Joiner regarded Patel as forceful, loud and at times intimidating. But Joiner also felt sure of his own position – he had read a recent article in the British *Journal of Anaesthesia* warning of high death rates for oesophagectomy patients in smaller hospitals. When Joiner took his concerns to Keating, there were more histrionics. Patel had a tantrum and again threatened to quit. He then agreed to a compromise.

Finally, on 20 June Grave went to the Mater, a leading Brisbane private hospital which also receives public patients. Its Director of Critical Care Services, Dr Peter Cook, was surprised at Grave's condition and shocked that an oesophagectomy had been attempted at

Bundaberg. Dr Cook, an intensive care and anaesthesia specialist, talked at length about the case to a surgeon colleague, who shared his concerns. They agreed that Patel's contemplation of such procedures in Bundaberg called into question his competence and judgement. The botching of the operation gave them even greater cause for concern.

There was another worry. The charts for Grave showed the cancer had spread to lymph nodes outside his oesophagus and stomach. A large tumour was outside his bowel. Because of the cancer's spread, the oesophagectomy was not only traumatic and potentially lethal, it was also fruitless. Cook felt strongly that the doomed man should have been at home comforted by loved ones instead of in acute pain and distress from a failed oesophagectomy which could only shorten his life.

On 1 July, unaware of Hoffman's efforts, he telephoned Keating and explained the rocky future for Grave and the risks for patients having oesophagectomies in Bundaberg. The risks and issues were identical to those already outlined by Hoffman. Keating gave an assurance that he would take the matter up with Patel.

Cook decided to document his concerns. He knew about the connection between public hospital funding and the frequency of operations. He regarded it as an unhealthy policy which rewarded surgical volume instead of patient outcomes. It produced a dreadful conflict of interest. He questioned if Bundaberg was trying to widen its clinical practice to boost coffers. 'Clearly, this is not appropriate surgery to be done at a centre with such a small level of support services, particularly ICU,' he wrote in a memo.

But Patel remained determined to carry on. 'You will do what I say or I will go to Darren Keating. I will go to Peter Leck,' he told the ICU staff. 'The executive will do what I want them to do because I'm making them so much money. I'll resign if they don't let me keep my patients here.'

It was all bluff. Patel had nothing to return to in the United States except shame. He had been reminded of it in a surprise telephone call from an investigator with the Oregon Board of Medical Examiners, who was doing a routine licence check of disciplined doctors. 'I'm retired and practising medicine on a volunteer basis only,' Patel lied.

Keating had Joiner, Cook and Hoffman in one ear telling him the oesophagectomies were dangerous, while the forceful Patel was angrily making a fierce case to keep his patients in Bundaberg, and continue doing oesophagectomies. The operations were so complex, they were generously rewarded in extra funds for the hospital. Keating backed his Director of Surgery.

Nurse Gail Doherty was also becoming worried about Patel's insistence on the complex surgery. When she questioned Dr Martin Carter, the Director of Anaesthetics who headed the Intensive Care Unit, he had no qualms: 'The patients are fit for anaesthetic, and Dr Patel said he could do them, so we can't say no,' Carter said.

MEANWHILE, Dorothy Bryen and Muriel Pancheri had fallen into Patel's hands.

On 9 June, Patel made a technical error, tearing Bryen's bowel while attempting to repair a hernia. Her faeces leaked internally, causing a serious contamination and contributing to her death on 30 June.

Pancheri was so disorientated she could not recall her date of birth. The elderly woman's confusion extended to ignorance about the procedure Patel had arranged for her, a colonoscopy which involved inserting a scope into her anus. He alarmed one of the doctors with his overly vigorous use of the device. He appeared to be inexperienced with the procedure and had a tendency to push too hard, resulting in severe pain and an over inflation of the bowel. Pancheri succumbed weeks later.

13

Wounded pride

FOR his first five weeks as the Director of Surgery, Jayant Patel was shadowed on patient rounds by Gail Aylmer. The senior nurse noticed an alarming pattern as she walked with Patel from bed to bed. Patel, sometimes with an entourage of young trainee doctors, was cheerfully removing bandages, handling different instruments and poking around wet and fresh wound sites. Aylmer had no doubts about his work ethic, but his refusal to wash his hands between patients or to wear gloves made her blood boil.

Despite tactfully prompting him over several days to adopt basic hygiene, Aylmer had achieved nothing. She spoke to him as firmly as she dared about the critical need for infection control techniques. He still refused to wear gloves or scrub the pathogens from his hands. Aylmer cringed every time she saw Patel handling the patients. She feared contact could be transferring bacteria and unnecessarily causing infection. It was madness. Apart from the risk to the patients, she worried the younger doctors whom Patel influenced would pick up the dangerous habit.

Her next strategy was to walk around behind him with a box of gloves. Each time he stopped at a bed, she removed a new sterile pair of gloves for him to use. 'I shouldn't have to be giving you these gloves. I'm concerned about your practices with hand washing between patients,' Aylmer said. It worked for a while, but Aylmer knew other nurses with less experience or confidence to push Patel would have no chance.

For the benefit of the other doctors but mostly for the benefit of Patel's patients, Aylmer asked Judy O'Connor, the Medical Education

Officer, to run a lunchtime briefing session on the latest hand-washing and infection control measures. The idea was to do a 'glitterbug test' – put some fluorescent cream on the doctors' hands, rub it in and then ask them to wash their hands. Under an ultraviolet light in a darkened room, the parts of the hands that had not been washed thoroughly would stand out. Patel walked out to make a phone call. He did not return.

Delicate tissue and organs can usually withstand gentle exploration, nudging and prodding in a surgical procedure. Some surgeons like Dr Brian Thiele are renowned as much for their soft touch as their technical prowess. Patel had a reputation for neither. He ripped tissue. He battered organs. When suturing the wounds he treated fragile tissue with disdain. His rough handling inevitably bruised the tissue and organs. As well as being fertile beds for infection, the wounds were less likely to heal after being harshly treated. Stitches would make little difference to a wound which was bruised, wet and angry. Inevitably, these wounds would fall apart like an old and bruised piece of fruit. Known as wound dehiscence, it had happened twice to James Phillips after his oesophagectomy. Before Patel's arrival, post-surgical injuries in Bundaberg had been extremely rare.

By early July 2003, Aylmer had encountered almost as many instances of wound dehiscence in the preceding months as she had seen in over 20 years of nursing. She suspected most of the abdominal wounds were falling apart due to poor surgical technique rather than infection. There was gossip on the wards that Patel had told some of the junior doctors not to make reference to dehiscence in the patients' charts. Aylmer wanted to ensure the nurses were picking it up even if occurrences were being misrepresented. In an email to senior nurses she wrote:

> I am (as I know you are as well) becoming increasingly concerned re the number of wound dehiscence that have occurred over the last 6–8 weeks.
>
> While it does not appear that the dehiscence is relating to infection, this needs to be investigated further to identify the cause/s.

Things to consider for example include – how frequently this is occurring? what type of surgery is involved? how many days post-op did the dehiscence occur? Who the surgeon, assistants, scrub nurses etc were? What theatre did the surgery occur in? What ward they were nursed on?

Four days later, Aylmer compiled a report with patient charts on 13 instances of wound dehiscence. She included patients such as James Phillips. She noted the dehiscence suffered by John Banks, whose bowel was visible through the staple line after a diseased part of his colon was cut out. One staple had become embedded in his bowel. There was the case of June Benn, whose greater omentum, an apron of tissue holding the bowel together, was protruding from her wound.

Aylmer's report went to Dr Darren Keating. Later that day, she had an unexpected visit from Patel. He stood over her and explained why most of the 13 cases required no further analysis. He gave a variety of excuses and explanations. 'This is right, this is right, this is all accounted for,' he told her. Patel acknowledged in two cases that technique might have been to blame, although he did not accept personal responsibility. Junior doctors who worked alongside him in theatre copped the blame. 'If you do a lot of operations, you will have an increased likelihood of wound dehiscence,' Patel said.

Out of her depth and surprised that Patel rather than Keating had been to see her, Aylmer felt she had nowhere to turn and no way of being sure of her ground. She had expected the issues to be resolved by Keating after careful analysis. It was why she gave him the report. It was not her place to argue with the Director of Surgery about his clinical skills.

She was hearing disturbing feedback from others in the hospital. Jenny White told her that Patel 'did not seem to know his instruments well, using the wrong clamp for frail tissue, and his technique was rough'. White, who had witnessed Patel's anger when the issue of wound dehiscence was raised, was reluctant to document her concerns. Aylmer brought it up with the Director of Anaesthetics, Dr Martin Carter. She asked him whether Patel was a good surgeon.

'I wouldn't let him operate on me,' Carter replied. On another occasion when she was in the ICU staffroom, Aylmer overheard Carter refer to Patel as 'Dr Death'.

Meanwhile, Hoffman felt she had been let down by Carter. She had wanted him to stand up to Patel in the beginning. If Carter had bluntly told Patel 'this is how this intensive care unit runs', Aylmer would not have been in conflict with anyone. Patel might have got the message.

Disillusioned by the handling of the wound dehiscence report, Aylmer wondered why she bothered escalating such issues. Management did not want to hear about problems. She believed the hospital's executives took the view: 'If you're not going to deliver me good news, I don't want to know any news.'

Theatre nurse Damien Gaddes was similarly frustrated. A thoughtful and gentle carer with a reputation for putting the patients' interests first, Gaddes was shocked at Patel's techniques in major operations. When it came to routine surgery – procedures such as hernia repairs – Gaddes had few qualms about Patel's proficiency. But for more complex operations such as bowel resections, it was a different story. Gaddes had watched dozens of surgeons do the same procedure hundreds of times. When a bowel is resected or the end of the intestine is cut, the surgeon should assume they are contaminated. They should be held outside the abdominal cavity or swabbed with Aquacel Betadine to minimise contamination risks. But Gaddes had often seen Patel leave the end of a bowel freely clamped and the other end flopping around inside the abdominal cavity, raising the infection risk.

Patel had extensive dermatitis with small sores covering his arms. Gaddes watched Patel's haphazard gowning and gloving technique closely and concluded that contamination was often inevitable.

In the past when Gaddes had raised an issue about a pethidine-addicted doctor who was stealing drugs from the hospital's stores, a supervisor had threatened Gaddes with dismissal. He had no doubt that if a nurse had been discovered with empty ampoules of pethidine and classic symptoms of addiction, there would have been immediate suspension.

Gaddes resented the double standards. It seemed to him that doctors in hospitals were a protected species. He raised his concerns about Patel with Jenny White, the theatre nurse in charge.

'What do you expect me to do? You can't expect me to tell a surgeon what to do,' she said.

PATIENT Ian Fleming, a father of four and a former police officer, had hit it off with Patel when they first met in May 2003. Fleming put it down to Patel's friendly charm. They also shared a love of cricket. When Fleming asked him about India's youngest Test wicket-keeper, 18-year-old Parthiv Patel, who was on the tour of Australia, Patel lit up. 'He's my nephew,' Patel told him.

Fleming liked his easy manner. He did not know that Patel was one of the most common surnames in India. Tens of millions of people shared the name.

For months Fleming had been in pain with multiple growths, known as diverticulitis, in part of his large intestine. When an attack came on he would double up in agony. It took three attacks for Fleming to decide that surgery would be better than the pain.

Patel showed Fleming his chart and explained how he would cut out the growths. On 19 May while Fleming was under a general anaesthetic, his abdomen was cut from the navel to the groin. At home three days later, his stomach swelled and turned a bright angry red. The pain was excruciating. Fleming could not eat, sleep or walk properly. On 28 May when he returned to the hospital for treatment, Patel told him it was all in his head and that he was acting. 'Go home, give the wife and kids a kiss and have a great life,' he said.

Fleming did as he was told. At 9.30 pm the next night he was sitting on the sofa at home when a hole in his wound blew out. Blood and pus poured from the gaping opening. His wife had to use a sanitary napkin to cover it as they rushed to the Emergency Department. Fleming needed further surgery to correct the problem and was in hospital for a week with large doses of antibiotics for the infection. The nurses wrote on Fleming's chart that the wound was 'sucking and blowing bubbles'.

When he next saw Patel, the friendly rapport was gone. The surgeon seemed angry about Fleming's complications. Fleming believed that the nurses were more concerned than Patel about his welfare. They suggested a suction pump to drain fluid from his wound site, but Patel angrily refused. He was hostile to the nurses' suggestions that a different type of bandage be used. Fleming's wound dehiscence was noted by the nurses in his charts.

In October when Fleming complained to the hospital about Patel's handling of his case, Keating rang back and told him: 'I hear you have lodged a complaint against Dr Patel. I must tell you that he is a fine surgeon with impeccable credentials and we are lucky to have him here in Bundaberg. I understand you are bleeding internally since the operation but this can be caused by many factors.'

Back in the ICU, Hoffman was trying to look after a homeless man, John Breed, who had been living rough in parks around Bundaberg. When he reached the hospital in early July, he had a bleeding stomach ulcer and was in very poor condition. After Patel's operation, Hoffman could see that Breed's red and swollen stomach wound was clearly infected. He had no bowel sounds and his condition was steadily worsening. Hoffman believed he was showing classic signs of post-operative sepsis – the infection had spread through his bloodstream to the rest of his body.

Patel refused to acknowledge there was any sign of stomach infection. He put the problems down to a chest infection – an occurrence not uncommon for patients on ventilating equipment in an ICU.

'I can't believe it – what's he talking about?' Hoffman thought. Adamant there was no evidence of any chest infection, she knew that Breed should have been receiving intensive care in Brisbane. For a week Patel refused to let the man go.

Hoffman had correctly identified Breed's stomach infection, arising from Patel's surgery, as the problem. She heard nothing back from Patel. They were no longer on speaking terms.

After the eventual transfer of Breed to Brisbane, the nurses were told he had died. They collected his personal effects – clothes, dentures and spectacles.

The spectacles were added to a collection for a worthy cause. Days later, the nurses were relieved to discover he had survived. And for a few hours, there was a frantic search to recover his only spectacles.

14

Sex, lies and Dr Qureshi

August to December 2003

IN late August Annette Arrowsmith went to Bundaberg Hospital suffering pain in her left breast. She hoped a doctor would put her mind at ease – perhaps recommend medication for the pain and some tests to exclude cancer. Instead she was fondled for 90 minutes by a swarthy man with a moustache. He played with her breasts and asked if he could also examine the lower part of her body. Arrowsmith refused. She suspected Dr Tariq Qureshi, an Overseas Trained Doctor from Pakistan, was not interested in clinical care. She noticed his pants were wet.

In just two months since starting at the hospital with minimal supervision and orientation, Qureshi's complete lack of basic clinical knowledge had raised eyebrows around the hospital. He was regarded by Dr Peter Miach as 'unbelievably incompetent'. Miach, who could not understand how someone as ignorant about medicine could have been employed, doubted Qureshi had ever been trained as a doctor.

'I don't want this chap to work here. He's totally useless,' Miach told Dr Darren Keating. 'Look, if you want to pay him, put him in the library and get him to read a book but he's of no use to me.'

Qureshi was also unwelcome in the ICU. Dr Martin Carter did not want him to have anything to do with the patients. The nurses were wary of Qureshi for different reasons. He kept 'bumping' into them and squashing against their bodies.

Arrowsmith's formal complaint went to Keating, who made a detailed note of the circumstances and Qureshi's denial of anything untoward.

Several weeks later Karen McInnes came into the hospital for a deep vein thrombosis in her right calf. She said of her experience:

> Dr Qureshi came to examine my leg. After doing this he started rubbing my inner thigh down to my knee in a way that made me feel very uneasy.
>
> As I put my legs back under the blankets, he asked to listen to my chest. I lifted my top to just under my breast. He listened for a few minutes and then he pulled my top above my breasts and started moving the left one in every direction he could. I've never had a doctor do this to me before.

The examination made her skin crawl. McInnes wished she could 'curl up and go away'.

Keating told Qureshi he faced dismissal if he did not have a chaperone in future consultations with female patients. On 22 October Keating told the Medical Board of Queensland about the complaints. One of the staff later wrote back to say that an investigation might be mounted by September the following year.

The third complaint was more poignant. Amanda Bulley, undergoing neurological observations after seizures, became teary when Qureshi came into the cubicle. When the nurse, Daniela Tarlington, asked why she was so upset, Bulley explained that Qureshi had been in previously while she was having a seizure. Bulley could feel him kissing her face and putting his hand down her shirt to touch her breasts while she was having convulsions. Although able to see and feel the assault, she could not respond.

Qureshi continued to work at the hospital for seven months after the first complaint of a sexual nature, and some nine months after he had been rated as utterly incompetent by Dr Miach. The failure of management and the Medical Board to suspend him immediately reinforced a perception among nurses and doctors that serious complaints were not dealt with appropriately. Qureshi disappeared overseas in March 2004 when police began to look for him to ask questions about an unrelated petty crime. His destination was unknown.

Patel faced a less serious claim of sexual harassment. He had asked nurse Petrea Aslett for her home telephone number over the bed of a patient in surgery, then called her at all hours seeking a relationship. Aslett immediately regretted giving him the number. No matter how many times she told Patel she was not interested, he persisted. The calls ended after Keating, tipped off by Hoffman, took him aside one day and had a chat to him about the nurses forming the wrong impression.

'You can't do anything in Australia without getting into trouble,' Patel said the next day. He made a joke of the episode.

Meanwhile, Hoffman had heard a disturbing rumour which might have explained the willingness of Dr Martin Carter, the Director of Anaesthetics, to accede to Patel's refusal to transfer the patients. 'I am told that Dr Patel and Martin Carter have come to an agreement by which Dr Patel will operate only if Martin Carter agrees to not transfer this patient,' she told Keating in a September email.

Hoffman believed the situation was dire. Another patient, Mervyn Smith, was in a bad way with major chest and spleen injuries and five broken ribs after a road accident. He had suffered a string of serious complications since surgery by Patel. He needed long term intensivist management and the support of a cardiothoracic team – options available in Brisbane, not Bundaberg.

Hoffman's latest email to Keating raised for the first time a possible explanation for Patel's immunity – the purported arrangement. The email reiterated her concerns about 'what type of surgery should be done here in relation to our follow-up care and the services we can provide'.

Although she had no reply from Keating, he spoke about the matters to Patel and Carter. They denied they had done a deal over the care of patients. And they strenuously defended the handling of Mervyn Smith.

15

Fortuitous

WE had just switched off the lights and settled into bed when the house shook with a series of bangs. It was 10.30 pm on 23 October 2002.

Outside, the dust from an eerie freak storm swirled across the city of Brisbane. But in our bedroom, tiny splinters of glass sprayed our hair, faces and sheets. Our daughter Sarah, then 18 months old, awoke screaming.

One of four .45 calibre bullets had exploded through the bedroom window, 30 cm above our heads. It continued through the bathroom wall, shattering plaster, tiles and a mirror. Another bullet ripped into the toy room close to the eye level of my son Alexander, then three. Another ricocheted off the top of the carport. The path of the fourth bullet was never established.

It took several minutes to comprehend what had happened. Our neighbours, Chris and Louise, had seen a car speeding off. I asked if a tree had fallen on the house in the storm. 'No Hedley, you've been shot at,' Chris replied. I ran back upstairs and called 000. Our sanctuary in a quiet street in a semi-rural enclave on the western outskirts of Brisbane was soon full of police, dogs and ballistics experts. And then the media came. We wrapped up the children, packed overnight bags, and left.

A shooting at an investigative journalist's home was, according to the media commentators, unprecedented in Australia. Police narrowed a long list of suspects down to those with a definite motive arising from a number of stories I had written in the *Courier-Mail* exposing various scams. For three weeks we remained in Tasmania – touring, talking about out future and trying to be rational about suspicious-looking people who drove too close to our hire car or looked at us strangely in the streets of Hobart, Launceston and Strahan.

I considered quitting journalism. We would grow vegetables instead, in a mountain village behind the Sunshine Coast. Or take up a safe PR-type job in a distant corner of Rupert Murdoch's News Corporation, perhaps in London or New York. We were grateful for the compassion of John Hartigan, the company's Sydney-based CEO, and Lachlan Murdoch, Rupert's son, both of whom pledged support when it seemed I was losing my way.

Ruth and I were appalled at the cowardly act of the shooting and I became angry with people who seemed oblivious to our pain. Days after the shooting, strangers emailed and telephoned to urge me to step up my work, to look at their particular issues, to solve their problems. The level of self interest disgusted me. Let them put themselves and their families in the line of fire.

Until that point, my career had been charmed. At the age of 22, I had worked in the company's London office. While my friends went backpacking on shoestring budgets, I was paid to travel through Europe and the Middle East, reporting momentous events including the fall of the Berlin Wall, the violent revolution in Romania, and the first Gulf War. I had covered epic sporting contests – Wimbledon, the British Open Golf, the French Open – and silly squabbles within the Royal Family.

The London assignment was followed by six years in Hong Kong. In 1999, after witnessing the handover of the British colony to China, Ruth and I had returned to Australia with our baby boy. We started raising a family in Queensland. In the three years before October 2002, I had been toiling as an investigative journalist at the *Courier-Mail*. Property scams, crooked lawyers, venal politicians, dangerous doctors – they were all grist for the mill. Some of these stories had made a difference.

But after the shooting, I doubted I would care as much again about any of it. Journalism had put my wife and children in peril. After much soul-searching and counselling, we decided to stay in Brisbane. We decided to stay in journalism. We would have lost more, we reasoned, by giving up our home and profession. I returned to reporting, but dreaded the constant reminders of our trauma.

'Did they ever catch the bastard who shot up your house?' Although those who asked were well intentioned, the question aggravated us all the same. It forced us to relive something that we did not want to revisit and to mumble, clumsily, a reply to the contacts, acquaintances and stickybeaks who believed they had a right to discuss it. The question forced me to fight the tears welling in my eyes. It forced both of us to face reality – that the police had got next to nowhere despite a heavily-promoted investigation and the personal overseeing of the Police Commissioner, Bob Atkinson.

Almost a year after the shooting, the newspaper's editor, David Fagan, asked me to start working on a major project – an investigation and series of articles about health and the public hospital system. As he briefed me on the project, I privately weighed the risk of reprisals. Low.

The assignment was actually a lucky break. In Brisbane, in the exquisitely-appointed L'Estrange Terrace office of Dr Ingrid Tall, the new head of the Australian Medical Association's Queensland branch, I explained the potential angles. Tall held ambitions to be a Liberal Party politician. Her role in the northern branch of one of Australia's most powerful trade unions was a stepping stone.

I used the meeting with Tall to stress the seriousness of the articles on health I was preparing. The major series I planned would not be possible without her cooperation. I wanted to examine public hospital waiting lists, abominable conditions in emergency departments, morale, a lack of funding and the vacuum of political leadership. There was much more, I suspected, hence my appeal to Tall to involve her colleagues in medical centres and hospitals throughout the state. They held knowledge that the government spin doctors would render themselves dizzy trying to control.

Near the end of our 1 pm meeting, Tall raised a new topic. 'There are also serious concerns about Overseas Trained Doctors,' she said.

My response was dismissive. The issue smacked of racism. To my knowledge it had not been raised publicly as a serious problem in the past.

Tall pressed her point. 'No, it is a serious issue. Some of our members have good information about it. I can put you in touch with Dr Marsh Godsall. He knows it better than anyone.'

Godsall, who practised in Central Queensland, knew my wife Ruth's father, Dr Iain Mathewson, who practised in Mackay. When I returned to my office in Bowen Hills , another family-related medical contact from Mackay promised to help me crack the waiting lists fiasco. 'Waiting lists are manipulated by administrators to put themselves in the best light,' he said. 'You have heard the saying, lies, damned lies and statistics.'

Over the weekend I researched the subject of medical negligence and extracted part of a judgement by Lord Denning, an eminent judge of the House of Lords in Britain, from a famous case, *Roe v Minister of Health*. The relevant passage read:

> It is so easy to be wise after the event and to condemn as negligence that which was only a misadventure. We ought always to be on our guard against it, especially in cases against hospitals and doctors. Medical science has conferred great benefits on mankind, but these benefits are attended by considerable risks.
>
> Every surgical operation is attended by risks. We cannot take the benefits without taking the risks. Every advance in technique is also attended by risks. Doctors, like the rest of us, have to learn by experience; and experience often teaches in a hard way.

After the weekend, Godsall contacted me to emphasise the concerns about Overseas Trained Doctors (OTDs). He told me that the single biggest issue in the public health system was Queensland's dependency on them. He continued:

> We are also concerned that appropriate qualifications, including language skills, are not being ensured. This means the public is potentially and increasingly at risk from doctors with less than the skills required to work here, though they may be adequate in the environment in which they were trained, and who do not have the communication ability which is expected from those

selected for Australian medical schools. This in turn means the public purse is exposed to litigation.

Godsall mentioned a report by Bob Birrell, a Melbourne academic, which I found on the Internet. The report was alarming. Having at first been less than enthusiastic, I knew now that an investigation of the OTD story had real potential. It might be the backbone of the series.

Godsall also hinted that Queensland Health knew all too well about the dangers. One of its senior advisers, Dr Denis Lennox, had produced an important report. Godsall suggested the report had been deliberately smothered. As my interest soared, I told Godsall the story would become a priority. I was determined to see the report by Lennox.

'I do not think many appreciate the situation or are aware of it,' said Godsall. 'For example, you seemed incredulous this morning when I told you of the lack of vetting of the skills and qualifications.'

Godsall kept giving. Over several days, he sent me emails and telephoned with new snippets of information. 'I send you this to help put things in perspective for you, as if you are not living with these things on a daily basis it is very easy to misinterpret or be misled,' he said. 'I am telling everybody they can speak to you on or off the record and you will respect their request. Those with QH positions feel threatened because of the retribution that can be their lot.'

He offered names and telephone numbers of other doctors with insight into the issue. He urged me to investigate a death at a hospital in Charters Towers. He suggested I talk to a pharmacist in Mackay. He mentioned a GP in Bundaberg who had employed doctors from overseas. And he hinted, again, at this explosive secret report, adding 'if QH try to snow you, it will be difficult to get people to speak because of the Code of Conduct'.

After interviewing two Overseas Trained Doctors, I could see the story being a potential blockbuster. These doctors were stunned at the lack of screening of their qualifications and competence. 'They reflect your concerns,' I told Godsall. 'No doubt the spin from Queensland Health will be that if the system is working so poorly, why are there no or few complaints and why no adverse outcomes? I think that if your contacts can point to some events in which an OTD's conduct has produced a bigger problem, it would lend more credibility to the issue.'

I tried to impress on Godsall that a story involving clinicians merely expressing concern would have little or no impact. If he and his colleagues wanted to change the situation, they needed to think about cause and effect. They needed to reveal cases involving negligent clinical conduct with adverse consequences for patients.

The word went around the medical community. After a few days, I was urged to talk to Dr Chris Blenkin, a leading orthopaedic surgeon and the president of the Australian Orthopaedics Association's Queensland branch. Although his brother, Max, was a senior journalist in Canberra, Blenkin's professional contact with journalists had been limited before he heard from me. But he spoke frankly and strongly.

He cited a crisis at the public hospital in Hervey Bay, about 300 kilometres north of Brisbane, involving two Fiji-trained doctors being held out as consultants in orthopaedic surgery. Neither had done the training demanded of Australian surgeons nor had they been assessed or accredited by peers. Since their arrival at the hospital they had not been properly supervised. Inevitably, their lack of competence had raised concerns.

In the medical field, orthopods, as they are known, are often the butt of jokes. If cardiac surgery is a fine art, orthopaedic surgery is roadside labouring. It can quite literally involve a hammer, nails and brute force.

When I pressed Blenkin on the Hervey Bay situation, he promised to check into it more thoroughly. He called me a few days later and said he was sincerely worried. The dangers at the hospital, he explained, were 'unacceptable'. He detailed two of the most recent adverse outcomes in Hervey Bay – a femur that 'exploded because the pin was nailed in wrongly' and a hip fractured on the operating table:

> You have to see it to believe it. It highlights the problems that
> occur when we drop standards. You are better off with no one
> than someone who is bad because it is possible to do so much

damage. The community expects a reasonable standard but the damage done far outweighs any benefit in providing a service. Who knows why the medical superintendent and the district manager have gone down this path – they probably think a doctor is a doctor.

I decided it was imperative I talk to a number of doctors in different fields and in different parts of Queensland. I did not want the story to lack credibility for a failure to gauge a variety of views. In Atherton, North Queensland, Dr Bruce Cameron told me that a large number of doctors coming from overseas were simply unsuitable 'without significant upskilling'. 'There may be some situations where no doctor is safer than a bad doctor,' he said.

Dr Drew Speight, a GP at Bundaberg's Burnett Medical Centre, described the need to introduce a 'formal program of screening and mentoring'. 'I don't want to sound racist,' he said. 'We welcome these people here in a situation where there is a shortage of Australian doctors, but we need to ensure they have the skills.'

Dr David Molloy, who would be the next AMA Queensland president, called for systems to measure the experience and skills of Overseas Trained Doctors:

As the health system tightens with the emphasis on meeting budgets, nobody is available to evaluate the doctors when they hit the hospitals. Our natural inclination is to protect the medical system, but the fact is where there are language problems, and people are asked to work above their level, the potential for adverse outcomes has to be so much greater. Everyone knew this was a bit of a powder-keg. I think we have been afraid to approach it because of a fear of being seen as elitist and racist.

Anxious for the two Fiji-trained doctors to have an opportunity to comment, I telephoned one. He rejected the concerns and told of the community's gratitude for their work. 'We are not specialists,' he said. 'We are not saying that our qualifications mean we should be recognised as specialists. I don't think I have a lack of experience.'

Within a few days of hearing for the first time about the issue, I received a fax from a confidential source. Somebody had sent me the July 2003 report by Dr Denis Lennox, the senior Queensland Health workforce adviser. It ran for 18 pages and seemed complete, but for a signature. I turned to the Executive Summary, which said what I already knew – a chronic shortage of Australian graduates had resulted in an increasingly heavy reliance on Overseas Trained Doctors. My faith in Godsall rose as I read the warnings: 'Evidence is increasing of increased risk of OTD recruits being insufficiently assessed and prepared for practice in Queensland under pressure of recruitment of such increasingly large numbers of OTDs…some recent experience of Overseas Trained Doctors without the competence or capability for medical practice in Queensland presages adverse outcomes for patients, employees, community and medical profession.'

Lennox had done his homework. He mapped out a 'Policy and Tactical Response' embracing a comprehensive assessment and management process, bridging courses for doctors not up to scratch, Australian Medical Council examinations, and fellowship of the relevant medical colleges. Lennox wrote that these options would ensure doctors from overseas were appropriately qualified. 'It also protects the community from incompetent medical practice and consequent adverse outcomes…'

The report was the smoking gun. It evinced evidence that Queensland Health knew of the concerns because they had been distilled and emphasised by one of its managers. I felt even more strongly about the seriousness of the story, but I decided not to show my hand too soon.

On 21 October I wrote to my former colleague from the *Courier-Mail*, Steve Rous, who managed communications for the then Health Minister Wendy Edmond. As a seasoned political reporter before crossing to 'the dark side', Rous was one of the better advisers in the Beattie Government's army of spinners. He was also my main point of contact for the series I had been asked to produce.

I explained to Rous some of the issues I wanted dealt with in interviews with Edmond and her Director-General, Dr Rob Stable. I sought information to address 'the claims of clinicians and patients that the waiting lists are misleading because they don't indicate the waiting time for the appointments for assessments for surgery'. I also flagged my interest in the bigger picture issues. 'For example, what the community might want or expect versus what it is prepared to pay for'; and the 'increasing tensions arising out of strife of interests with what clinicians would like to do for patients versus administrators responsible for the budgets'.

The secrecy issues being raised constantly by the doctors and nurses concerned me. I emailed Rous about it:

> A number of clinicians claim that when they identify serious issues relating to public health, the problems are denied or not addressed seriously. They claim, as the Cairns doctors claimed earlier this year, that only by speaking out can they alert the public to what is 'really going on', but they risk their jobs by doing so.
>
> They say this puts them in an impossible situation. Can you address this please, with reference to the code of conduct, why it restricts the doctors from whistle-blowing, and why, in Qld Health's view, the doctors are no different from any other public servant when it comes to highlighting internal issues.

On the matter of Overseas Trained Doctors, I decided not to disclose that I had already been leaked the sensitive Lennox report. Instead, I asked for information:

> ...that addresses the numbers of Overseas Trained Doctors in Qld in both the private and public sector; the extent to which the system relies on them; and the due diligence undertaken to ensure they're sufficiently skilled.
>
> Does the Minister believe the current arrangements are adequate or is she concerned that doctors without appropriate experience or skills are slipping into an undermanned sector because of the chronic shortage?'
>
> What can be done to ensure that adverse outcomes are minimised?

Rous confirmed my appointments with Director-General Dr Rob Stable, his probable successor, Dr Steve Buckland, and Minister Wendy Edmond for Monday 27 October. Files and folders stuffed with documents about Queensland Health covered the kitchen table as I worked the telephone and read again the Lennox report on overseas doctors. When it came time to go to the 19th floor of the Queensland Health building in Charlotte Street on the afternoon of 27 October, I was well prepared.

In just a few days, Rob Stable, who took most of the questions while Buckland listened and occasionally added something, would be out of the top job in Queensland Health. He was leaving for a new role in the private sector heading up Bond University on the Gold Coast. He told me:

> We have some very good Overseas Trained Doctors in this state. But we are finding that where we now need to recruit from, some don't have the same degree of language skills. The pool of Australian medicine has not kept pace with demand. The market has changed. And we do everything practical, interviewing them, checking references, giving clinical scenarios.
>
> We have this situation – we have to provide services, we have hurdles in place. It's been reported to us that their communication skills have not been very good. But we have noticed this ourselves with the applicants.
>
> This is a no win. The politicians don't accept that they can't have doctors. Is no service better than taking the risk that one or two cases per year of the 600 we get in the public system in Queensland are not up to scratch?

Dr Buckland seemed perplexed. 'We are not in the business of causing harm and seeing adverse outcomes,' he said.

My meeting with Edmond covered a range of topics. She downplayed the problems facing health generally. There would always be people, she told me, who were like 'Chicken Little', talking about the sky falling in. It was her way of saying that the public health system was in good shape despite the regular reports from clinicians and patients to the contrary.

A few hours after meeting Stable, Buckland and Edmond, I sent a note asking further questions about the situation at Hervey Bay. Was it the only public hospital at which the qualifications of Overseas Trained Doctors were not recognised by the respective colleges? 'Also, can you copy to me a report by Qld Health's Dr Denis Lennox earlier this year into issues arising from overseas doctors?'

Kate O'Donnell, who handled Queensland Health's official responses to some of our queries, told me: 'This report has no official status and was not accepted or endorsed by Queensland Health executive.' Buckland and the Medical Board had received Lennox's report. They had read it. And they had buried it.

Discredit

November 2003

THE last patient left Dr Ross Cartmill's waiting room on Wickham Terrace above the lights of the city's office buildings some time after 7 pm.

A urologist with a successful private practice, Cartmill was also a Visiting Medical Officer – meaning he gave some of his time for relatively minimal financial return to look after patients and mentor junior doctors in Brisbane's public hospitals. For many specialists like Cartmill, the motive for doing part-time work in the public system was altruistic: they were giving something back to hospitals which had been their training ground years earlier. But Cartmill was now gravely worried about the performance and sustainability of public health care. I took notes as he vented his spleen:

> The first fact the community needs to understand is that doctors are afraid they will be sacked if they talk openly about what is actually happening in public hospitals.
>
> The second fact is that if doctors could talk openly, Queenslanders would hear that their public health system is chronically underfunded and suffers from an acute lack of staff and beds. It means people who need surgery wait much longer than they should and some people never get operations that would change their lives.
>
> The doctors and medical staff are frustrated because they feel unable to tell the community the whole story. The culture prevents people from hearing about the deficiencies. The doctors

are told they must report their concerns internally, but we have reached the point where we believe that reporting upwards will not make any difference anymore. Every so often, when someone breaks ranks, there is a crackdown and severe reprimand.

I had been hearing similar complaints from some of the most senior clinicians in Queensland. Many were fearful that they might be seen meeting me. We went to unusual lengths to avoid detection as they told me about a corporate culture that stamped violently on whistleblowers. One of Queensland's top specialists wanted to provide evidence of a clinical disaster in a hospital but insisted on a secret rendezvous in a car in a back street.

Six months earlier, Health Minister Wendy Edmond had turned on doctors in the North Queensland city of Cairns after they protested publicly about cuts in the services at the hospital. 'There will always be some whingers and I will meet with the whingers and talk to them,' Edmond told State Parliament in May 2003. The doctors, who had funded advertisements in the *Cairns Post* to make their point, were threatened with disciplinary action and dismissal.

'If only half the concerns about the clinical standards of some of the overseas doctors imported into Australia in the past few years are true, it would have serious ramifications for patients and the profession,' I reported in the *Courier-Mail* on 3 November 2003, in one of a handful of stories about this particular problem. 'Senior medical specialists, rural GPs and doctors in the public hospital system believe the failure of registration boards and the state and federal governments in checking the competence of imported overseas doctors could end up costing the community dearly.'

Many health professionals were also angry that the Beattie Government continued to promote itself for supposedly reducing the waiting times for surgery in hospitals. As Edmond and Premier Peter Beattie lauded themselves for achieving their 'best ever results for elective surgery', the clinicians insisted that the claims were a gross misrepresentation of the truth. Doctors were convinced an independent audit of the results would prove that the public was being told lies.

I looked at the situation overseas and elsewhere in Australia. In the United Kingdom, the National Audit Office had identified 'deliberate manipulation or mis-statement of the figures' in public hospitals in nine major districts.

In New South Wales, the Independent Commission Against Corruption was bringing charges after the discovery that a number of major public hospitals had falsified and misrepresented waiting list data. I mentioned the concerns to Queensland's Auditor-General Len Scanlan and sent him data, but he showed little interest in investigating.

On 17 November the interview with Cartmill was published in the *Courier-Mail* with an article about the alleged manipulation by Queensland Health of waiting list data. In Queensland, documents taken to Cabinet remain exempt from disclosure for 30 years. This law has been routinely exploited by politicians who have thwarted Freedom of Information applications and concealed sensitive documents from public scrutiny by taking documents to Cabinet.

Health Minister Edmond had taken waiting list data to Cabinet, ensuring their concealment for 30 years. She sent me a statement: 'Queensland waiting times for elective surgery are not misleading.'

Another prominent article revealed how patients needing urgent surgery had been left disfigured by aggressive cancers after operations were cancelled because of a lack of intensive care beds in hospitals. The next day, I wrote about a leaked memo written by Dr Phil Kay, an emergency department head, who was furious that administrators had decided to close the gynaecology unit in one of Queensland's largest hospitals.

The articles, part of the *Courier-Mail*'s series on the health system, were causing top-level angst. Edmond's efforts to keep health off the front page had failed. Her staff feared the series might do significant harm to the image of the Beattie Government just a few months out from the February 2004 state election.

The *Courier-Mail*'s editor, David Fagan, received an angry letter from Hendrik Gout, Queensland Health's Executive Manager for Media and Communications. Gout began by expressing his 'sincere concern about the ethics and behaviour of Hedley Thomas over the past few days'. He described me as an 'unprincipled, unprofessional, unscrupulous journalist'. In the 18 November missive, Gout said, 'Either the Minister's office is lying, or one of your own reporters has a Pinocchio nose. Hedley is making a practice of this.'

After examining my actions and double-checking the facts of the stories, I realised that Cartmill and the other doctors were right. The culture of fear and loathing in Queensland Health was thriving. It was an organisation with serious fundamental shortcomings which were being camouflaged by glossy PR and aggressive shoot-the-messenger strategies. It was little wonder that many clinicians were afraid to tell the truth.

A number of the doctors, professional administrators and former health chiefs had made a persuasive public case that the health system was in crisis. They were adamant that the public was being conned into believing it had one of the finest systems in the world. In fact, spending on health in Queensland was the lowest per capita in Australia. The underfunding of more than $1 billion a year had produced huge gaps. Doctors and health professionals had little incentive to remain in a system which treated them and their patients so poorly. The drain of experienced professionals, cutbacks on beds in hospitals, rationing of care and the punishment of administrators who did not churn through waiting lists while making budget, had set Queensland Health up for a painful fall.

When Dr Steve Buckland sought the top job as Director-General a few months after the *Courier-Mail's* series, he wrote a confidential letter acknowledging that Queensland Health's focus on fiscal management had suppressed its ability. 'This has also resulted in a disaffected workforce, a lack of innovative problem solving, strained relationships with other government agencies and a lack of public confidence in the system's capability,' Buckland wrote in his job application.

Publicly, however, the message from Queensland Health and its political sponsors was the exact opposite.

Starting over

LONG before the first European explorers ventured almost 400 kilometres north of Brisbane to identify future settlements and farming opportunities, a local Aboriginal tribe known as the Bunda had the area to themselves. The government assistant surveyor, James Charles Burnett, visited in the 1840s but failed to appreciate the potential of the rich volcanic soil. The oversight meant the Bunda people were left alone for another two decades.

The first white settlers, brothers John and Gavin Steuart, arrived on Christmas Day 1866 and began to raze the hardwoods. They were followed by European migrants keen to exploit the fertile black soil and the readily available water source of the Burnett River. Their success attracted industry and commerce; the settlement started to thrive. As the German word for town was *burg*, the area was named Bundaberg.

It owed its burgeoning prosperity to sugarcane and the toil of outsiders – dark-skinned Kanakas brought to work as bonded slaves in the cane fields. For a meagre wage, a roof over their heads and food, they were indentured for three years to the plantation owners. The conditions were invariably dreadful. In 1881 when the general hospital opened beside the Burnett River, it comprised four rooms, a cottage and a separate ward for the Kanakas. The following year, dozens of Ceylonese labourers arrived in Bundaberg under work contracts, but the demand for cheap labour was still unmet. The Bundaberg and Districts Historical Museum reported that 'for the next 30 years, Melanesian and Polynesian islanders provided almost the complete field labour for cane plantations and farms. At one stage, 3000 lived in the district.'

Bundaberg is famous for its rum, a product of its sugarcane, and a record-breaking aviator, Bert Hinkler. In February 1928 he flew from England to Australia in 15 days, an extraordinary feat at the time. The son of a local mill worker, his achievement lifted the town's spirits, coming a few weeks after the deaths of the 12 children inadvertently killed by Dr Ewing Thomson's injections against diphtheria.

The sugarcane plantations were still thriving when Jayant Patel arrived in 2003, and Bundaberg still relied heavily on imported labour. But now the most valuable imports were Overseas Trained Doctors. A medical workforce crisis, serious throughout Australia but dire in regional Queensland due to inferior salaries and conditions, meant OTDs were the backbone of the public hospital on Bourbong Street. Although the doctors coming from Third World countries were financially better off in Australia, they were easily exploited. Their employers knew that the foreign doctors could be forced to return to their own countries if their working visas were not renewed. Unlike Australian doctors who could change jobs after a dispute with management, the Overseas Trained Doctors were at a distinct disadvantage. It made some of them more willing to follow orders. And less likely to ask difficult questions.

Jayant Patel had little time for Bundaberg's history and attractions – the outlying resort islands, beaches and the largest mainland turtle hatchery in Australia. Unlike his predecessors, Dr Charles Nankivell and Dr Sam Baker, Patel delighted in being overburdened with surgical work. He spent most of his time at the hospital. But whereas most of the other Overseas Trained Doctors were submissive, Patel displayed bravado. He worked hard and exerted his influence over management.

One of his confidantes was Pam Samra, whom he saw at least four times a week at her restaurant, the Indian Curry Bazaar near the Sugarland Shopping Centre in Takalvan Street. They chatted freely and often about his career, his life in the United States and his efforts at the hospital. She was alarmed to hear from him one day that he had not slept for 30 hours because of the continuous work.

'Those hours are ridiculous. You shouldn't be doing that. What are you working so hard for? Take a break,' she told him.

'There are no other doctors to do the work,' Patel said. 'I've been asking for back-up for months. Nobody listens to me. But then I've been paid $40 000 in bonuses for getting through the waiting lists.'

In truth Patel had been arriving at the hospital before the other doctors so that he could beat them to the patients. He was creating work for himself. If Dr Martin Carter arrived at 7.30 am, Patel would be there the next day at 7 am. If Carter responded by coming in at 7 am, Patel trumped him with a 6.30 am start. Carter gave up. At this rate he would have been lying in wait for the surgeon, and coming to work at midnight.

Patel was intrigued by the circumstances of Pam Samra and her husband, Jindy. In accordance with the custom and tradition of India's Punjab state, their marriage was arranged despite Pam having been born and raised in Australia. It was a happy and prosperous union.

'I have no kids. I've never been married,' lied Patel, the married father. 'The only woman in my life is my mother in India.'

He told how he visited the old woman at the ancestral home in Jamnagar as often as possible. He sent funds to make her privileged life more comfortable.

'Why doesn't she move to America?' asked Samra.

But Patel said his mother would be unhappy in the United States, away from her friends and relatives.

Patel dressed smartly, often in a suit and tie. He tipped generously, usually rounding a $35 bill for his takeaway meals to $50. He ordered only vegetarian dishes and told her he was vegetarian. Samra heard from others that he ate meat elsewhere. Although he was occasionally arrogant, Samra nevertheless enjoyed their chats. Nobody else in the town spent as much on food at the Curry Bazaar as Patel. He was their best customer.

At least once a week after work he would bring a group of nurses or student doctors to the upstairs dining area. He enjoyed the company of Dr Jim Gaffield, who had also arrived from the United States, and the young Dr Anthony Athanasiov, an Australian graduate. Patel usually paid for the groups he brought to the restaurant. Samra suspected he was lonely. She regarded him as a hopeless flirt; he often had a hand on the lower back of one of the nurses. But he didn't grope. Although he would make the occasional proposition, the physical contact was never so overt that it led to a rebuke. When he was not entertaining the medical and nursing staff, he wanted to talk to Samra about her life. She wondered if he was attracted to her.

Patel's two-bedroom apartment in Sapphire Lodge at Bargara was tidy but never clean. The cigarettes he chain-smoked had left a pungent smell. The bathroom and toilet were always filthy. On one occasion, Carol Elliott, the owner's sister, went to the apartment to do some cleaning as part of an ongoing arrangement. The sheets needed washing. She removed Patel's things from the machine to do another load.

He walked in and began screaming and abusing the shocked woman in front of her two grandchildren. Patel was enraged. His tirade could be heard up and down Miller Street. 'Who took my washing out of here?' he demanded, even though it was obvious that Elliott had removed a few towels. 'You have no business! I'm a very important doctor. I'm the head doctor at the base hospital. How dare you!'

'Don't worry about it, you just go to the hospital and I will make sure the towels go on the line to dry,' Elliott said.

The encounter had upset her grandson. Elliott was worried it would influence the boy's view of dark-skinned people. 'Why did that black man scream at you, Gran?' the boy asked.

'He's not a nice man. Not all people that colour are like him,' she said.

When Patel's wife Kishoree and daughter came to visit from the US, he kept them away from the restaurant. He had told others that he was single. Elliott felt sorry for Kishoree, a medical practitioner in Portland.

During a chance meeting, Patel introduced his daughter and beamed with pride as he praised her as the family's next doctor. She would be graduating soon from medical school. But Patel scarcely acknowledged his wife, the demure woman beside him. Elliott walked away wondering what made him tick.

18

Doctors' germs

Late 2003 to early 2004

JOANNE Turner hovered over the patients in the Renal Unit at Bundaberg Hospital and waited for a tube to visibly redden – a telltale sign of blood being drawn from the internal jugular, just above the heart's right atrium. Everything looked satisfactory: the catheters with tubes burrowing into the chest; the two patients whose blood needed regular cleansing; the haemodialysis machine which would return the blood with fewer impurities and provide the patients a lease of life.

Turner frowned. The catheters, which had been surgically implanted by Jayant Patel, were not working. They appeared to be blocked. Effective haemodialysis with a Permacath-type catheter required a blood flow rate of more than 200 millilitres a minute. But Turner could not obtain a drop.

Patel arrived in the Renal Unit within minutes of being paged. When Turner explained the difficulty she was experiencing, the surgeon erupted. 'Flush it, Sister! Just get in there and flush it,' he said angrily.

Turner was immediately uneasy. She knew it was unsafe to flush the catheter until the removal of the heparin lock – a dose of an anti-coagulant drug called heparin, which stops blood from clotting at the end of the catheter. A low pressure injection of saline from a syringe is used to flush a catheter, but only after the removal of the heparin lock.

She had set up two sterile trays – one for each patient. Patel had neither washed his hands nor put on sterile gloves when he took the bung from the end of the catheter connected to the first patient. He picked up the sterile syringe and tried unsuccessfully to take blood from the line. To Turner's alarm, he then moved with the same syringe to the other patient.

Turner had never seen anything like it. Strict infection control measures in hospitals were critical in the Renal Unit where the chronic disease suppressed the patients' immune systems. The catheters were perfect conduits for blood. They were also perfect conduits for bacteria.

'This is the patient's set-up,' she said, pointing to the other sterile tray. How did you tactfully tell the Director of Surgery that his modus operandi was wrong and might be lethal? Turner did her best. 'Aren't you going to wash your hands?' she asked Patel. She urged him to put on the sterile gloves.

'Sister, I don't have germs,' he replied. She thought at first that he was joking – nobody would seriously believe such a comment, least of all a doctor. But Patel neither smiled nor corrected himself. 'I'm doing you a favour,' he said. The look on his face told Turner that he was annoyed at her attempts to insist on the gloves. He performed the procedure on the second patient with his bare hands.

Lynette Yeoman, one of the other nurses working the early shift, watched dumbfounded. She wondered how someone with so much experience could fail to appreciate the serious risk he posed to the ill patients. A third nurse, Carolyn Waters, walked off in disgust.

At the end of the shift the nurses spoke to their manager, Robyn Pollock. When Patel first arrived at the hospital he had little to do with the Renal Unit, but this had changed when he started inserting catheters in August. During his regular stops in Pollock's office he invariably turned the conversation from the patients to her personal life. The visits were usually uncomfortable for Pollock. She asked her staff to telephone if Patel stayed in her office more than a few minutes. The ruse usually worked.

Pollock had another reason to feel uncomfortable. She had been concerned for some weeks about complications with catheters implanted by Patel. Four patients had had peritoneal dialysis catheters placed by Patel – one in August, two in September and one in October – and each had suffered unnecessarily. In three of the patients, there were chronic infections at the exit sites. The fourth patient, whose catheter did not drain or flow properly, needed surgical intervention. Some of the catheters had moved internally and ended up in the wrong position.

After the nurses explained the events of the morning and Patel's handling of the patients, Pollock was aghast. Fearing that a patient might die, she raised the issues with Gail Aylmer, the nurse responsible for infection control. Aylmer, who had previously tried to tackle the wound dehiscence problems, arranged a meeting with Dr Darren Keating two days later.

Lindsay Druce was also worried. The clinical nurse had returned from maternity leave to find a rash of problems in the Renal Unit. It seemed to Druce that many of the problems were due to Patel's positioning of the catheters. Every one was either facing up or sideways. This meant that when the patients showered and moved around, it was inevitable that fluids and grit would collect in the catheters. As the fluids and debris could not drain or fall away from the exit site, the risks of infection from organisms thriving in the moist, warm environment soared.

When Aylmer and Pollock went to see Keating on 27 November, he wanted facts and figures, not anecdotal feedback. They repeated Patel's bizarre comment about not having germs. Keating asked how often infections were occurring – and how many cases involved Patel. 'You know, if I really need to go further with this I need data to support what you're saying,' Keating told the nurses.

When he spoke to Patel after the meeting with the nurses, the surgeon was affronted. He denied that there had been problems. He told Keating the nurses were wrong. And he stopped coming by Pollock's office.

As far as Keating was concerned, the work ethic of Patel and the great strides he was already making in reducing the waiting lists for surgery made him indispensable. Despite the growing concerns of the staff who had been to Keating, he lauded Patel in a 2 December 2003 performance report: 'Dr Patel effectively utilises his broad knowledge, skills and experience in general surgery to provide high quality of patient care. He is a willing and enthusiastic leader. He also brings understanding of clinical management subjects to appropriate forums.'

Keating chose the heading 'Performance better than expected' to give Patel a tick in nine out of eleven areas, including his clinical skills, knowledge base, judgement, communication, teamwork and professional responsibility. After just eight months in the job, Patel had his boss wrapped around his little finger.

But Dr Peter Miach, the nephrologist in charge of the Renal Unit, was rapidly losing confidence in Patel by late 2003. The catheter problems coupled with several other factors – Patel's insistence that he could perform any procedure and the almost inevitable complications – had made Miach increasingly wary. Some of Patel's procedures were cruel.

When Phillip Noppe, a patient suffering kidney failure, needed an operation in August to draw fluid away from his heart, it was decided that Patel would do a pericardial window – a procedure that involved cutting a hole in the chest to insert a drain. The build-up of fluid threatened to squeeze Noppe's heart and cause it to fail. Although a fine needle had been used to draw the bloody fluid from the pericardial sac, Miach realised that it would take the removal of a little bit of the pericardium to eradicate the problem.

Miach hardly ever went to theatre, but he decided to watch Patel's handiwork on Noppe. Miach winced. Noppe was screaming and moaning, and clearly felt excruciating pain. Patel had elected to do the invasive operation without anaesthetic, contrary to normal practice.

When Miach tried to transfer his patients south, away from Patel, for the catheter procedures, he was told by a doctor at the Royal Brisbane Hospital: 'We are not going to do it here. We don't have the time. We don't have the capacity.'

He asked Dr Jim Gaffield, the plastic surgeon who had arrived from the United States soon after Patel, for help.

'Look, this is not the sort of thing I'm used to. I prefer not to do them,' Gaffield said.

Robyn Pollock had another idea. She reached out to Brian Graham, who worked for a company with a contract to supply renal products to the hospitals. The company, Baxter Healthcare, was offering programs to train staff. Pollock had told Graham about the run of complications with catheters implanted on Patel's patients. She knew Patel was not interested in hearing from the nurses. Perhaps he would respond to an offer from Graham to provide support or education on placement technique.

Graham met Patel in the Renal Unit and explained the program. Patel pounced. 'Well, you can fly me to Brisbane, you can wine me and dine me, you can put me up somewhere nice, and then I might listen to what you have to say,' he said. Graham decided Patel was a lost cause.

On 16 December, Eric Nagle returned to the hospital for surgery to correct a catheter placement Patel had bungled when inserting it the previous month. Because it had not been tunnelled correctly during the first operation, the catheter was facing sideways instead of downwards. Internally, it had 'flipped up' under Nagle's liver. An x-ray showed the internal part of the catheter had migrated, resulting in impeded drainage. For the much-needed haemodialysis to work, Nagle's old catheter needed to be removed and replaced with a new one.

Nagle and his wife, Linda, were reassured on the eve of surgery. They believed it would be a routine procedure, conducted under a general anaesthetic in the operating theatre. They knew nothing of the nurses' concerns over Patel. Nor did they know about Miach's misgivings.

Lindsay Druce watched Nagle wheeled off to theatre. It was the last time she saw him. A guide wire used by Patel poked a hole through the main blood vessel going to Nagle's heart. The bleeding took place inside his pericardial sac. Nagle's blood pressure dropped suddenly.

As Patel and Dr Martin Carter, the top anaesthetist, tried frantically to rectify the situation, Nagle suffered a heart attack. His thoracic vein was punctured. He bled to death. None of the distraught nurses in the Renal Unit could recall anyone else ever dying during the placement of a catheter.

When Nagle's widow returned days later for an explanation, anything that might help her understand why a supposedly routine procedure had killed her husband, the nurses were at a loss. For Miach, it was the last straw. He decided that Patel would not perform any more catheter operations on his patients. 'If I have to send them to Brisbane, so be it,' Miach said. Before going on extended leave in January, he told a replacement nephrologist, Dr Martin Knapp: 'Keep Dr Patel away from the renal patients.'

Druce completed her report on complications from catheter placements. It showed that Patel had a 100 per cent failure rate: six catheter placements and multiple complications. All of the patients were adversely affected. One was dead.

With Miach overseas and Brisbane refusing to receive Bundaberg's patients, Pollock became desperate. She had seen yet another complication arising from Patel's handiwork. She and Druce went to see Patrick Martin, the acting Director of Nursing, to explain the problems, the directive from Miach and the uncertain future for patients needing catheters. Martin had little time for Patel. There was something amiss; something about the surgeon's personality that made Martin wary. He took the nurses' concerns to Keating.

'If the nurses want to play with the big boys, then they need to provide the evidence and bring it on,' Keating said.

Eventually, Pollock, Druce and Miach found a way to bypass Patel. The patients from the Renal Unit who needed catheter placements would go to a nearby private hospital where another surgeon performed the operations. There were no more problems. But even this highly unusual arrangement, which began after the nurses were able to provide Keating with documentation showing all six catheter placements by Patel had led to complications, did not result in the surgeon's clinical expertise being reviewed or questioned by management.

Toni Hoffman went to see Bundaberg Hospital District Manager Peter Leck at the end of February 2004 to tell him about the concerns over Patel. 'I just want to make you aware,' she said. She gave Leck a document headed 'ICU Issues with Ventilated Patients', which dealt with the worries about oesophagectomies, the refusal of Patel to transfer his patients to larger and better equipped hospitals and the compromising of their care.

'On several occasions when Dr Patel's patients have been in the ICU, he has refused to transfer his patient to Brisbane, even when the patients have deteriorated and have been in ICU for much longer than 24 to 48 hours,' Hoffman warned. 'Dr Patel has repeatedly threatened to resign, not put any elective surgery in ICU…and go straight to Peter Leck "as I have earned him half a million dollars this year".'

Keating was short-tempered when Leck asked him about the issues. 'If this keeps going, Dr Patel will leave,' Keating said.

Peter Leck, who mislaid his copy of the document a short time later, told Hoffman that if she wanted to do something about it she would need to come and see him, lodge a formal complaint and let the matter be progressed through official channels. Hoffman asked Leck not to do anything about Patel just yet. She wanted another chance to resolve it with Dr Martin Carter's help.

The hospital administrators had become not just highly dependent on Patel; they were also saving money. Keating had encouraged him to apply for a half-time position as an associate professor in surgery at the University of Queensland's School of Medicine. The criteria called for: 'Demonstrated expert knowledge and clinical experience in one or more of the surgical disciplines.'

When Keating sat on the three-person selection panel with a physician, Dr Llew Davies, and a senior lecturer in surgery, Dr Peter Bore, the decision was unanimous. In late 2003, Patel was appointed and given the authority to teach full-time students. His salary and other benefits of more than $80 000 a year were remitted to the coffers of Bundaberg Hospital.

Keating and Leck congratulated themselves on their business and management acumen. The hospital was humming.

19

The messenger

18 March 2004

ROB Messenger wanted to start with a few home truths. He looked up and smiled at his supporters in the public gallery of State Parliament in George Street, Brisbane. It had been a hard slog to arrive in this place. He hoped it would be worth it.

Nobody had ever accused Messenger of being born with a silver spoon in his mouth. At 4.30 pm on 18 March 2004, as the National Party's new Member for Burnett prepared to deliver his first speech, he felt unbeatable. 'I have to confess my journey to this historic chamber was not planned. As a child and teenager playing in the red dirt cane fields of South Kolan, I never harboured dreams of becoming a politician, and I will be the first to admit that I am only standing here before you because of God's grace,' he said.

With a nod to the gallery, Messenger explained how he drew inspiration from his father, Des, when self-doubt and fatigue set in. Des had been a cane-cutter in Bundaberg. Like the Kanakas a century ago, he had the backbreaking job of cutting and loading tonnes of cane a day for a meagre $1.60 a tonne. Messenger still marvelled at how Des managed to feed, clothe and shelter him and his two brothers, Greg and Danny.

When Messenger was a teenager he danced and sang to the evocative lyrics of Australian band Ganggajang's anthem, 'Sounds of Then', about growing up in Bundaberg.

> Out on the patio we'd sit,
> And the humidity we'd breathe,

We'd watch the lightning crack over cane fields
Laugh and think, this is Australia.

He remembered his mother, Irene, laughing and joking with the other women of the district while they picked tomatoes in 35-degree tropical heat. Irene lived for Rob's regular visits to her bedside at Bundaberg Hospital in the weeks before she finally succumbed to a particularly aggressive bowel cancer in September 2002. Messenger watched his well-known mother die at the hospital after an 18-month battle. He came to know the doctors and nurses. Some of them began confiding a few secrets and worries.

The hospital was running on empty. It had been managed to a standstill and starved of funds as the District Manager, Peter Leck, enforced rigid budgetary controls. Specialists and the best doctors were leaving, disillusioned and distressed at the deteriorating levels of care. All the while, public announcements and press releases from Queensland Health's Brisbane headquarters spewed positive but wholly misleading guff about the hospital in which Messenger had been born.

Messenger used his first speech to underline what he knew from his months on the campaign trail: the hospital was sick. It was a diseased limb of a very sick body, whose staff had been cowed into silence. 'These dedicated professionals must be allowed to tell the truth while avoiding any possibility of placing their careers with Queensland Health in jeopardy,' he said. 'These workers' stories must be heard and acted on if the people of the Burnett are ever to enjoy the level of health care that they richly deserve.'

The parlous condition of the health system was a major feature of the State election campaign in early 2004. The Coalition had paid for hard-hitting advertisements depicting people who had waited years for straightforward surgery, while the Australian Medical Association ran a highly effective campaign to highlight secrecy and underfunding in the health system.

Stung by the constant stories and revelations from clinicians about how patients were suffering because the hospitals could not cope with demand, Premier Peter Beattie threw money at the problems. The waiting lists for surgery were a significant part of Beattie's electoral strategy. He pledged a $110 million injection of extra funds to pay for thousands of extra operations. 'This new initiative will be the biggest effort to reduce elective waiting lists that Queensland has ever seen,' Beattie said. 'People have made it clear to me over a period of time they want these lists tackled. We have done well, but clearly we can do better. We will be making health our number one priority.'

Wendy Edmond had retired from politics. Beattie had kept a straight face while commending her as the country's best health minister. Now, new Health Minister Gordon Nuttall was telling his executive team to put every public hospital on notice: the waiting lists were critical.

In the internal confidential briefing paper he received after being sworn in, Nuttall was warned that Queensland Health had become extremely reliant on Overseas Trained Doctors who comprised 30 per cent of the medical workforce: 'Employment of Overseas Trained Doctors provides a short-term solution to doctor shortages. However, this approach brings with it a range of skill and competence issues.'

Messenger hammered health issues as stubbornly and relentlessly as he had during his electoral campaign. He repeatedly called for an independent investigation into Bundaberg Hospital, its procedures and practices. The attempts by the Beattie Government to silence him became farcical. At one point, Messenger had said: 'Rather than pulling back from this issue, I intend to turn up the blow torch.' The metaphor was too much for Nuttall, who called for a formal investigation into whether Messenger planned to commit arson or burn alive any bureaucrats.

Messenger was industrious and highly effective. He uncovered figures showing the hospital had just 136 beds – 81 fewer than in 1989, despite the region's steady growth. The door of his electorate office at Bargara, near Jayant Patel's home apartment, was always open to hospital staff with stories of crises. Doctors came to tell him how they had been forced to work 24-hour shifts, compromising patient care through sheer exhaustion. The regular outpourings were embarrassing Nuttall and infuriating the new Director-General of Health, Dr Steve Buckland, who had angrily banged the desk and abused Messenger in one memorable meeting.

During a short stint as acting Director of Nursing, Toni Hoffman was surprised to see Peter Leck, who read the speeches on the parliamentary website as soon as they had been posted, furiously denouncing something Messenger had said. Leck and Darren Keating stood at the computer screen and ridiculed the politician. An unprecedented meeting of the executive staff was called by Leck to discuss what effect having a National Party member would have on the hospital. Leck expected Messenger to create 'trouble'. Leck wondered if the parliamentarian was upset about the hospital's treatment of his mother.

Hoffman realised Messenger had become a major thorn in their side. She liked his courage and stamina. He was like a dog with a bone in relentlessly exposing the hospital's ills. He spoke of patients dying unnecessarily due to a dangerous culture. Borrowing from one of the maxims of Anglo-Irish statesman, politician and philosopher Edmund Burke, a leading light in the House of Commons more than 200 years ago, Messenger spoke of evil prospering while good men remained silent.

Hoffman wondered if she might one day pluck up the courage to go to Messenger about Jayant Patel. Good men had done nothing. It might be left to a good woman.

20

The catalyst
July 2004

DES Bramich liked to stay busy. If a job was worth doing, he reckoned, it was worth doing straight away. He was the sort of bloke who would happily do a good deed for family and friends without expecting anything for himself.

A little after 4.30 pm on Sunday 25 July, Bramich, 56, was doing one of those good deeds. It had been a glorious day in Agnes Water, a sleepy seafront community about an hour and a half's drive from Bundaberg. Bramich, who ran an earthmoving business with his son Mark, was beneath a caravan. He was helping to remove one of its tyres for his youngest son, Luke, before the sun disappeared on one of the shortest days of the year.

Mark was walking back to the Land Rover to get some tools when the caravan fell from its supports. The muffled thud as the weight came down onto his father's chest sounded ominous. Mark looked back and saw his father conscious, but gasping. He was clearly having trouble breathing. Unknown at the time, two of his ribs were badly fractured. A pleural membrane lining the inside of the chest wall was torn on the right side. The upper part of his sternum was also fractured, probably damaging arteries running down either side of his breastbone.

Mark rushed to get a jack from the car to try to lift the caravan off his dad's crushed chest. In the panic and fading light on an afternoon that had become suddenly bleak and foreboding, he fumbled to grip and lift the heavy steel contraption. Thankfully, help arrived quickly. A local medic, Dr Sailasa Vueti, one of the town's Overseas Trained

Doctors, inserted a tube to help Bramich breathe. The ambulance rushed to the accident site to provide emergency back-up and transport; a rescue helicopter arrived to airlift him to Bundaberg Hospital.

'Pack your bags and go to the hospital, Tess! Dad has had an accident,' Mark exclaimed to his father's wife. Tess trembled with worry as her friend Agnes Smyth gunned the white Commodore, beating the helicopter by 15 minutes. Tess was told her husband had suffered severe internal injuries, but that the prognosis was good once he had been stabilised in the trauma room. There were tests and scans of his chest. Des was thirsty, and with a nurse's approval Tess gave him an ice cube to wet his mouth. One of the doctors told Tess there was no reason why a fit middle-aged man, a non-smoker and non-drinker, would not make it. She was greatly comforted by the reassuring words even as they transferred her husband to the Intensive Care Unit. She watched the nurses there hooking him up to machines to monitor and assist his heart and breathing. They gave him morphine intravenously and an oxygen mask.

Tess, who was born in the Philippines, and Des had wed a decade earlier. Tess was Des's third wife. They often joked about how, at 33, she was younger than Mark, even though she was step-grandmother to Mark's kids. Des and Tess had not looked back. The Bramich father-and-son business was doing well. The couple had great friends in the town where everybody knew each other. Their young daughter, Maria, a quiet beauty with Tess's brown skin and smouldering dark eyes, was a family treasure.

Now, at 1 am, Tess kept a vigil in the hospital. When Des suggested that she should leave to get some sleep, the staff agreed, although they were more concerned about his rest.

When Tess returned at 6 am and saw him smiling in bed with most of the colour returned to his face, her spirits rose. By 9 am some of his extended family were perched around his bed in the ICU. 'Don't cry, I'm alright,' he told Mark's visibly distressed wife, Fatima. He was making jokes at his own expense and wisecracking about being far too young to die. 'I'm like a cat – I have nine lives,' he said. After x-rays and a cup of tea, he spoke about the accident. His son beamed when Des said that had it not been for Mark, the crush from the caravan would have put him in a coffin.

Toni Hoffman was touched by the natural affection and love enveloping her patient, who exuded a cheerfulness she put down to genuine family contentment. She chatted freely to Des and Tess. Their daughter, ten-year-old Maria, gazing at her Dad with those liquid eyes, was gorgeous. Hoffman gave her a soft white toy, a seal that she kept in the bottom of the filing cabinet for young children who came into the unit. At times like this Hoffman regretted some of the choices she had made. She looked at Des Bramich as the easygoing patriarch of a happy and loving clan. Hoffman wished things had turned out differently with some of the men she had loved. Her career had been fulfilling, but at home after the shift ended she sometimes felt desperately lonely.

By the time Tess returned from lunch, the bed in the ICU was empty. She was immediately worried, but Des was fine. He was doing so well that he had been wheeled into the surgical ward. That afternoon, after he had been helped into the chair beside his bed, Tess stayed and chatted with him until evening.

When she returned early the next morning, 27 July, Des was in a bad way. 'Darl, I really didn't have a good sleep last night because I was in pain all night,' he said.

Tess was confused. She had been assured that the morphine trickling into his veins would deaden the pain. She examined the intravenous connection and saw it had become loose and was dripping. 'Could you just please fix that properly?' she asked a nurse. They waited impatiently for a junior doctor to come by and reattach the line.

Des was encouraged to walk around the hospital corridors with a physiotherapist and an assistant. He hobbled in pain as they supported him under his armpits, then returned to bed and spoke by telephone to his worried mother and sister.

When the Bundaberg *NewsMail*'s reporter arrived, Des recounted the accident. 'Mark is my hero,' he said.

Tess returned from lunch to discover that he had suddenly collapsed and been rushed back to the ICU.

Hoffman, shocked at how rapidly he had deteriorated, calmly organised her staff. The nurses rushed to save his life; Des could not breathe and his blood pressure had plummeted. His heart was racing and the pain in his chest had become unbearable. He was slipping in and out of consciousness. Dr Iftikhar Younis, one of the anaesthetists, was attempting to resuscitate him with the help of three nurses.

'If the patient is going to need blood products, he will need to be flown out,' said Dr Martin Carter, the anaesthetist in charge of the ICU. Carter decided that as Bramich might need thoracic surgery, long-term ventilatory support and access to a blood bank, he should be rushed to one of the larger hospitals in Brisbane. There were urgent efforts to find a bed in Brisbane – Prince Charles Hospital was full, but a bed might be available at Princess Alexandra Hospital. The Royal Flying Doctor Service was readied for the mercy mission.

Hoffman relayed the message from the bed coordinators in Brisbane to Carter, Dr Jim Gaffield and Dr James Boyd, a Principal House Officer working under Patel's supervision. 'They've got a bed,' she exclaimed. Hoffman was ecstatically relieved. She could see that Bramich needed to be in a hospital which practised thoracic surgery. Under no circumstances did she want to see Bramich fall into the hands of Jayant Patel. The Director of Surgery had been absent from the hospital for all of May and June – he had taken study leave and holidays to return to Jamnagar in India to see his mother and then to Portland in the United States to spend time with his family. The run of complications, the conflict in the wards and the fears of the staff had disappeared. Patel's holiday was a blessing for all. Hoffman recalled the plight of Una Connors, whom Patel operated on for cancer of the sigmoid colon in April. The woman had to be rushed back by ambulance after a complete evisceration of the wound and her intestines being almost fully exposed.

Hoffman had grown unusually fond of Des Bramich and his family in the few hours she had spent with them in the ICU. But his perilous condition was worsening. As Dr Younis tried to put in a central line to convey drugs, the gravely ill man experienced ventricular standstill – his heart was refusing to pump blood.

Gaffield asked Patel to look at the x-rays of his chest. Patel seized the offer and in his booming voice started undoing the plans to transfer Bramich from Bundaberg. 'The patient doesn't need to go to Brisbane, he isn't sick enough. If we can't care for such simple things as fractured ribs, there is no point in doing any sort of trauma surgery at the hospital,' said Patel.

Hoffman, stricken with fear, waited for Gaffield to take charge. Bramich was Gaffield's patient. Carter had already come to the view that the best course was urgent transfer. Younis agreed. Arrangements had been made. But Patel's dominant personality was assuming control.

'He doesn't need to be transferred. I've been a cardiothoracic surgeon for 20 years. If he needs anything, I can do it here,' Patel said. He repeated the confident boasts to members of Bramich's family as Hoffman quietly pleaded for the transfer to go ahead.

'Please, Dr Gaffield, send this man through to Brisbane. Even if you think he doesn't need a cardiothoracic surgeon, I'm really afraid that he's going to die.'

'No, that won't happen. He won't die,' Gaffield replied. He said he wanted to do a CT scan to provide definitive information for the handover to the surgeons in Brisbane.

Patel disappeared back into the operating theatre to perform a colonoscopy on a patient, but in the course of the procedure he perforated the bowel. He insisted his injured patient should have a CT scan of the bowel before the gravely ill Bramich. 'A perforated bowel takes precedence over a non-urgent CT scan at all times,' Patel yelled. The latest botch-up, a rarity for most doctors but a common occurrence for Patel, meant that another doctor was needed to help him repair the bowel.

Hoffman asked Carter, who was due to leave to give a lecture, to accompany Bramich for the CT scan. He agreed. By the time they returned to the ICU the scan showed three litres of blood pooling in Bramich's chest. As Hoffman left the ICU at 7.30 pm to go home, the Royal Flying Doctor aircraft was being readied for the trip to Bundaberg. Hoffman had stayed back for three hours to ensure Bramich would get away for the help he so desperately needed. She walked to the hospital car park confident that Bramich would survive in Brisbane. Despite his problems, Hoffman felt sure he would wake up in the morning, 370 kilometres from Patel.

The stabbing

Late July 2004

'OH, did Mr Bramich get off all right?'

Outside the hospital elevator at the start of her shift the morning after the frantic efforts to save his life and move him to Brisbane, Toni Hoffman had bumped into Dr Martin Carter. She popped the question after a quick exchange of pleasantries.

'No. He died,' replied Carter.

When the Flying Doctor had finally arrived after 10 pm with flight nurse Anita Carr and Dr Jacqui Butler, their patient was closer to death than he had ever been. Patel had remained in control and declared him to be too sick to be transferred. Des Bramich died a little after midnight despite frantic resuscitation efforts by Dr Iftikhar Younis. The nurses were in tears. The Flying Doctor staff wept. Tess, Maria and Mark huddled together, shocked, crying and wondering what had gone wrong.

Hoffman was devastated. She thought of the beautiful little girl who no longer had a father. She guessed immediately that Patel's decision to halt the transfer was all about Patel and his determination to flaunt himself. It had little do with the welfare of patients.

Despite mounting evidence of needless deaths and injuries, the Director of Surgery remained delusional about his own abilities. The death of Bramich was the turning point. Hoffman decided from that moment to do everything in her power to highlight Patel's lethal menace. 'We have to do something about this, we cannot let this happen any longer,' she told Carter. She went to her office and broke down in tears. The Bundaberg *NewsMail* that day had a bright picture story about Des Bramich's near-death experience. He was sitting up in the photograph, looking larger than life. 'I thought I was going to die because I couldn't get any air. It never hit me until the next morning the reality of it – that I was in the hands of the gods,' Bramich says in the article.

Dr Martin Strahan, a general physician in private practice who worked part-time as a Visiting Medical Officer at the hospital, saw Hoffman sobbing and gently asked what was wrong. She told him about the Bramich case and the circumstances of several other deaths, and recounted the startling rates of wound breakdowns and complications. She told him how Carter referred to Patel behind his back as Dr Death; how the nurses were distraught with worry for the patients; how in the Renal Unit he had flouted basic anti-contamination standards; and how the Director of Medicine, Dr Peter Miach, refused to let Patel anywhere near his patients.

Strahan promised to go away and talk to some of his colleagues about Patel and his competence. Two days later, he told her: 'There's widespread concern but nobody is willing to stick their neck out yet.'

The untimely death of Des Bramich galvanised the nurses. Several of those nurses who had witnessed the last agonising hours of his life – Karen Fox, Vivian Tapiolas, Daniel Aitken and Sandra Sharp – were appalled at the turn of events. The ICU staff mourned in the beginning and then became angry as they reflected on all the patients Patel had harmed since he came to the hospital. They did not know the extent of Bramich's internal injuries. It was probable these injuries were so severe he may have died even if he had been transferred. But they understood that he had been robbed of at least a fighting chance by a bombastic surgeon who threw his weight around to prevent a transfer. First, Patel had insisted that Bramich was not sick enough to go. Then he was too sick.

They understood that Patel had spoken callously to the family, telling Tess that she should start praying because her husband would surely die; telling Tess and her daughter to stop crying at the bedside; telling anyone who cared to listen how his experience in trauma surgery made him better qualified than anyone in Brisbane to manage the care. At one point another nurse, Sharon Cree, had to move away from Patel because he was talking so obnoxiously about his wealth of experience and expertise.

Karen Fox was tormented by the death. She could not erase from her mind an image of Patel stabbing Bramich with a large needle. For some unexplained reason, Patel had decided that Bramich's critical condition might be due to blood between the two layers of the pericardium, a protective sac around the heart. Although an ultrasound had already proved there was no fluid there, Patel had diagnosed a cardiac tamponade. He decided to perform a pericardiocentesis.

Using a wide bore needle, he wanted to puncture the sac to drain nonexistent blood. The invasive procedure requires skill and strength. Patel botched it. The needle is supposed to go in within a few attempts. Patel stabbed the needle violently and repeatedly into the semi-conscious Bramich's chest. After flailing away in a frenzy, Patel finally extracted a minuscule few millilitres of blood.

Fox had never seen anything like it. Dr Carter and Dr Iftikhar Younis were also confused. They knew the ultrasound results gave no indication of blood in the sac. There appeared to be no good reason to be adding to Bramich's distress and pain. Younis was angry about it. He suspected Patel might have punctured a coronary vessel with his repeated stabbing motions.

'During this procedure, Dr Patel was loudly making comments that the patient will die and does not need to go to Brisbane,' a distraught Fox told Hoffman. 'I asked Dr Patel to mind what he was saying as the family were in the hallway.'

Patel had told Fox that the family members needed to know the seriousness of the situation. 'They need to be told face to face, not overhearing what's being said behind the curtains,' Fox replied. Fox told Hoffman all the distressing details, including how Patel had inserted a chest drain and 'poked and prodded using his fingers through the incision'.

Hoffman was so frustrated and worried about the situation, she telephoned the acting Coroner, Neil Lavering, and explained the concerns over Patel's competence. She described the Bramich death and the interference by Patel.

'Well, that confirms some of the things I've been thinking about what has been going on at the hospital,' said Lavering, adding he would await the documentation.

Hoffman also telephoned the Bundaberg Police Station and was put through to a senior officer. He asked if the hospital held morbidity and mortality meetings or had any other mechanisms that would identify negligence causing deaths. Neither the Coroner's office nor the police followed up.

Hoffman next prepared a Sentinel Event report. This was a major step – according to the protocol, a Sentinel Event is rare, serious and requires prompt and in-depth investigation. Hoffman's accompanying memo to management described how Patel bullied staff, misused the ICU, compromised care and constantly threatened to quit because he did not want his patients transferred. She wrote:

> The Director of the Unit, Dr Carter, is usually supportive and proactive about transferring patients, except when Dr Patel's patients are concerned. Dr Patel creates such an atmosphere of fear and intimidation in the unit that his behaviour is rarely challenged.
>
> On several occasions when Dr Patel's patients have been in the ICU, he has refused to transfer his patient to Brisbane, even when the patients have deteriorated and have been in ICU for much longer than 24-48 hours.
>
> He has done this when a bed has already been obtained. This has on several occasions placed the patient in jeopardy as they have further deteriorated.

Hoffman repeated the concerns she had expressed more than 12 months earlier to Darren Keating about the dangers inherent in the oesophagectomy procedures Patel had been determined to perform.

She said Patel's interference in the care of Des Bramich may have led to his death. She ended the two page document by saying Patel 'actually endangers the lives of the patients'.

'Wow, love, that's all pretty heavy,' said the acting Director of Nursing, Patrick Martin, who perused the document. 'It's very good though. My experience with Darren is to stick to facts and figures and not to be emotive. He absolutely turns off emotive approaches. Quote percentages and figures to him and he responds much more favourably.'

Hoffman had lost confidence in her line manager, the new Director of Nursing, Linda Mulligan. She was a stickler for the memo and formal appointments for meetings. But when it came to ward rounds, Mulligan was rarely seen by the nurses. Mulligan operated very differently to Glennis Goodman, who had retired.

A few weeks earlier when Hoffman went to Mulligan to voice concerns about Patel, she left the executive office feeling more powerless than ever. Mulligan had given her a book called *Coping With Difficult People* by Dr Robert Branson, to take home to read. She had suggested Hoffman should consult a psychologist and undergo training in conflict resolution.

Justice for Elise

Late July 2004

THE files describing ten-year-old Elise Neville's final few hours moved me to tears in the public area of the District Court registry in George Street, Brisbane. As Toni Hoffman and the other nurses at Bundaberg Hospital seethed and grieved over the death of Des Bramich, I became absorbed in the story of a little girl who had rolled the wrong way in her sleep and fallen out of a bunk bed during a holiday with her family on the Sunshine Coast. Leaning over a large dossier laid out on a chipped counter, I read hundreds of pages of witness statements and medical reports that helped reconstruct 7 January 2002 and the ensuing 48 hours.

Although some of the accounts differed, they documented the seriousness of Elise's head injury when she was rushed to Caloundra Hospital shortly after 3 am, the deficiencies of Dr Andrew Doneman and nurse Beverley Duncan's examination in the Emergency Department, the inevitable brain injury, and the agony of Elise's parents, Gerard and Lorraine. There was something primal about Gerard's pain, on raw display as graphically as if he had spilled his own blood throughout the dossier. He wrote: 'We will pursue this while there is still breath in our bodies and blood flowing in our hearts. The whole episode is an absolute scandal, and there is no way that we will ever let them get away with it.' He believed he had failed in his duty as a father and as a doctor to protect his daughter from harm; and he blamed himself, the fatigued Dr Doneman, the nurses, the system and the hospital. Neville further wrote:

The doctor came probably about 15 minutes after we first arrived at the hospital. His name was Andrew, as we recall. We didn't catch his surname. He took a very brief history. I told him that I was medically trained but that I had not done clinical work for very many years. We soon began a discussion about the need for a CT (computerised tomography) scan. He said: 'You can't CT everyone who hits their head.'

We return to a discussion about going to Nambour [Hospital]. We ask how far it is and how long it will take to get there. He still hasn't really examined Elise and he says something like: 'Lots of kids hit their head. Nambour will probably send you home too.'

We say that Elise has vomited and he says: 'Lots of kids vomit at night.' We say that Elise rarely vomits. He keeps reassuring; we keep sending signals of worry and concern. The discussions have gone on for some time and we are at an impasse. He then says something along the lines of: 'Look, I will do a neurological examination if that would make you feel better.'

He gets a tendon hammer to go with his torch. Elise has her eyes closed and won't cooperate with him. She is in pain and acting nothing like her normal self. We tell him that she is not normally like this. He then says coldly, in front of Elise as well: 'She's a ten-year-old girl, it's late, she has had a disturbed night and she is pulling the wool over her parents' eyes.'

By this stage, we have a child with a head injury, a large contusion over her left temple, a history of vomiting, and developing uncooperation. He finishes with something like: 'I don't think there will be any problems in your case. You're a sensible father. Take her home and watch her. Even if she starts to have problems, there will be plenty of time to do what needs to be done.' We didn't want to go home, but we had nowhere else to go as he and the hospital had totally rejected us.

I kept checking Elise's pulse, eyes, breathing and movement as she lay next to me on our bed. She was restless and kept moaning, crying and complaining about her sore head. I kept trying to diagnose what might be going on but it was all a blur and nothing made any sense to me. I convinced myself that Elise must just have a minor concussion at the very worst and we would see how she was a bit later and probably get some more medical attention in the morning.

Eventually, it was now some time after 6 am, Elise seemed to finally settle. Thinking that Elise was finally sleeping, I started to doze on and off as I lay next to her. I was never actually asleep, more just lying next to her with my eyes closed and trying to calm down. It had been a harrowing night. I suddenly jolted up from my dozing when I felt something was very wrong with Elise. So did Lorraine at the very same time. I looked at Elise and screamed: 'Oh, my God! Oh, my God!' It looked like she had a rash down the left side of her body. I rolled Elise on her back and saw it there too. Elise's eyes looked like they were popping out. Her jaw looked like it was rigid. I thought Elise was dead. I yelled to Lorraine: 'Get an ambulance.' I was absolutely distraught from that moment.

Lorraine couldn't turn on our mobile phone so she ran to the next-door unit for help. I carried Elise from our room to the living room and then back to our bedroom. I didn't know what to do. At about 7.30 am the ambulance took Elise, Lorraine and me.

The first face I saw was the same doctor from earlier in the night. He saw me and said: 'What happened?' He was visibly shocked. He became very pale. I frantically said something like: 'She's gone right off. She needs a neurosurgeon.' At one stage he said – was it to himself or was it to us? – something like: 'I'm so sorry. It's all my fault. What have I done? Oh, fuck!'

Annette Thompson, one of the nurses who helped with the resuscitation, saw Lorraine Neville lying on a bed in a waiting area for relatives. Thompson recalled:

She was in a foetal position and was cuddling a stuffed toy, which I assumed to be Elise's. Her eyes were shut and her physical appearance suggested that she had totally withdrawn into herself.

Mrs Neville was making no sound, but responded to my questions in a quiet voice. She told me that Elise was a 'lovely girl' and 'things like this shouldn't happen to someone like her'. She approached Elise's bed and spoke in whispers to her. Dr Neville was very upset and cried loudly as the helicopter departed. Mrs Neville began crying as well.

From Doneman's account of events, starting with Elise's first presentation at 3.25 am, she had been lying on her side facing away from him when he started a physical examination.

I coaxed her two to three times to turn and face me so that I could look into her eyes. Elise then rolled over and opened her eyes freely. I examined Elise's pupils and noted that they were equal and reactive to light. I noticed some swelling and bruising lateral to her left eye. I felt the area of swelling and did not palpate a skull fracture. Elise then said words to the effect 'I want some sleep' and pulled her sheet up and rolled back onto her left-hand side.

I did not consider the swelling to the side of the head to be unusual as, in my experience, it is not uncommon for children to suffer bruising to the head even after a short fall onto a soft surface. Mr Neville and I had a conversation regarding the indications for performing a CT scan and whether Elise required a CT scan. I had treated a few children with vomiting and diarrhoea at Caloundra Hospital and had been told that the hospital did not admit children for observation; therefore, I was of the impression that Elise could not be admitted for observations and I explained this to Mr Neville.

I told Mr Neville to keep an eye on Elise for the next day or so. The Nevilles left the hospital amicably. Mr Neville carried Elise from hospital. After the Nevilles left the hospital, there were no further patients so I went to sleep. At about 0700 hours, I rose and got dressed and, literally as I walked out of the room, Mr Neville arrived in the Emergency Department in a very distressed state. He was followed by the ambulance officers with Elise on a trolley. I was shocked that Elise's condition had so radically deteriorated. Mr Neville was extremely distraught while resuscitation procedures were taking place. He said words to the effect of 'It's my fault, it's a curse [being a doctor] and I fell asleep' on two to three occasions. I assured Mr Neville that it was not his fault, but my fault. In saying this, I did not intend it as an admission of fault, but as a feeling of personal responsibility as the last doctor to have attended Elise.

I had first read something about Elise in the *Courier-Mail* in late 2003. The description of her parents' relentless efforts to force Queensland Health, the Medical Board, the Nursing Council and the Health Rights Commission into rigorous self-examination was a small part of a much larger story.

I spoke about the case to Dr David Molloy, who had taken over from Dr Ingrid Tall as head of the Australian Medical Association in Queensland. 'It is one of those tragic issues that brings everything to account – the system, the junior doctor at the end of a very long shift in a small hospital, the lack of supervision and the protocols,' Molloy told me. 'There is significant concern that, in any hearing of this case, the system itself will be under scrutiny and, if so, Queensland Health will have to take a good hard look at its systems.'

My earlier investigations into Queensland Health had made me deeply suspicious of its management and culture. In November 2003, after my stories were published on the concerns over the standards of Overseas Trained Doctors in Queensland and the lack of checking of their credentials and skills, Gerard Neville emailed me:

I am not seeking anything from you, but I certainly encourage you and the *Courier-Mail* to keep the heat up in regard to professional health standards. I have absolutely no doubt there are real issues in regard to the competence of some health professionals. These issues are not being given the attention required to protect the community. It's just part of the bigger picture about the effectiveness of the system of ensuring that health professionals, whether trained overseas or locally, are competent and not putting their patients' lives at risk.

Now we were in July 2004 and the Medical Board of Queensland had decided that Dr Andrew Doneman, who had treated Elise Neville at Caloundra Hospital, would be prosecuted for unprofessional conduct in the Health Practitioners Tribunal, a part of the District Court. Queensland Health's dangerous policies had forced Doneman to work a 24-hour shift on the day Elise was brought in to the hospital by her worried parents. Yet the same organisation was hanging Doneman out to dry, having refused to fund his legal defence.

The Director-General, Dr Steve Buckland, was silent on the stupidity of the 24-hour shifts and the hospital's policy not to admit children. Nowhere in the file, a public document at the courts registry, was the confidential and damning Queensland Health report by Dr William Rodgers about the need for several experienced doctors to staff the Emergency Department at Caloundra Hospital.

By late July 2004, there was enough material on the public record to write several balanced and detailed stories about the haphazard culture in Queensland Health and its devastating effect on one family.

An emergency helicopter had taken Elise from Caloundra Hospital to the paediatric Intensive Care Unit at the Royal Children's Hospital in Brisbane, but even the transfer was bungled – it took twice as long as a road-trip. In Elise Neville's chart at the RCH, Dr David Coman noted: 'Unstable day. Irretrievable brain injury, with brain death the most likely outcome. Not responding to voice or head/neck stimuli.'

Jennifer Rich, a social worker who had been counselling Elise's parents as well as her older sister, Laura, and younger brother, Michael, wrote: 'Father is experiencing a lot of guilt associated with the accident and given his profession.' Rich's last entry in the hospital's electronic diary reported the family's request that 'foot and hand prints as well as a lock of hair be taken for themselves'.

One of the treating doctors would later break down over the waste of young life. A police officer wrote out a receipt for Elise's property: blue hat, white socks, statue of Mary, Winnie the Pooh teddy bear, blue-and-white shorts, pink top, hair clips, hair bands and a white ribbon.

Gerard wrote: 'Later that day, Lorraine and I decided to turn off Elise's life support. Elise died at 5.45 pm on 9 January 2002. As she died, peace came to her tormented face and her spirit and beauty rained over us all. She showed us she had gone to somewhere nice and safe, where people care for each other. Wherever heaven might be, I know it is certainly not in Caloundra Hospital...a dangerous place that should be closed.'

Lorraine wrote: 'She shone with happiness and a beauty of nature and soul that are irreplaceable and which will continue to be our inspiration and guiding light.'

There was a report by Dr Michael Redmond, a neurosurgeon, who wrote: 'It is considered unacceptable for a patient, following head injury, to "talk and die". Elise Neville is one who "talked and died". In a responsible medical system such as we enjoy, with such access to hospitals of ascending levels of sophistication, it is tragic and unacceptable that an event such as this should occur.'

Dr Johannes Wenzel, a specialist in Emergency Medicine, wrote: 'I see it as a system problem that our public hospitals put junior doctors into positions where they have to deal with presentations beyond their expertise...combined with the fact that working long shifts reduces the decision-making ability to a similar level as a person with .05 per cent blood alcohol content.'

According to the independent medical experts who studied all the case notes and statements, Dr Doneman had made 'a tragic, wrong call'. He had done an incomplete examination of Elise, although he must have been fatigued after working 19 hours of a 24-hour shift. If he had thoroughly questioned and examined her or urged her parents to go to another hospital for a CT scan of her skull, its fracture and the haemorrhage would have been obvious. There still would have been time to relieve the pressure building from the accumulation of blood before her brain's soft tissue was crushed.

In his defence, Doneman wrote: 'I would sincerely hope that doctors are not rostered on for any longer than a 12-hour shift. Twenty-four-hour shifts without a break are excessive and dangerous and no patient or doctor should ever be put through the devastation that both the Nevilles and my family have had to endure.'

When I called Gerard Neville to tell him that I planned to write several lengthy stories about the case, he agreed to a meeting. Lorraine served tea and biscuits as we talked about Elise in the family home in Toowong, filled with her image and memory but cloaked in quiet sadness. Lorraine told me:

> We live with the ongoing trauma. We ask ourselves what could we have done, what did we miss, how could we have let this happen?
>
> It is so cruel for Gerard. He had the very best of intentions. Fate had something else in mind. We do not want to be seen to be vindictive and nasty to certain individuals in this. It is more about the bigger picture and how it can be improved. Elise was just as perfect a child as you could ever have. The last thing she would have remembered was putting her head on Daddy's shoulder as he carried her in from the car to the unit.

Gerard's grief was still angry. He looked like a man who had lost much of his will to live. He said:

> I know people look at me and say 'how did this happen, how did you let this happen?' Of course I have blamed myself. I'm a doctor and I'm a father. It's tragic. It's a cancer. It eats away at you. I don't trust Health at all. I don't respect Health and I work there. It's a terrible dilemma.
>
> Now I have a more important job to do. I'm trying to bring the Queensland health system into the 21st century. I want to see some honesty in the health system. If this can put pressure on the system to respond in a learning way, then it is worth it.
>
> Maybe I have been relentless but I'm going to stay that way because the truth leads to findings and they will lead to recommendations that can improve things. We will get comfort

knowing that something good will come out of this. I know for a fact that if we did nothing, nothing would change.

Elise and I have made up. We have worked it out. She's forgiven me. I know this sounds nuts, but one day when I sat next to her grave, I saw her and she was deliriously happy. But I still want her back. It shouldn't have happened. She wasn't given a chance.

The unfairness and emotion of it all made the stories difficult to write. I knew that Doneman, a father of young children himself, was in agony and had been punishing himself over Elise's death. I knew his sister Paula, a colleague at the *Courier-Mail*, was not in favour of me exposing her brother to public scrutiny, but I hoped she understood it was unavoidable. I talked over the angles with my wife, Ruth.

We pledged never to let our children, who yearned to know the story of the little girl, sleep in bunk beds. My daughter Sarah, three, came home from kindergarten with a drawing of Elise. She had been asking me to tell her bedtime stories about Elise for a week. Sarah told her teacher the story of the accident.

Before anything was published I spoke to Dr Steve Buckland, the Director-General of Queensland Health, in his office with his media manager Leisa Schultz. He did not appear overly concerned at the major systemic issues – the 24-hour shifts, the rostering of inexperienced doctors to take charge of emergency departments. It occurred to me that it was easier for Buckland and the regulatory system to punish Doneman than to look at glaring and fundamental flaws that would take honesty, courage and money to remedy. Before I went to see Buckland, he had a meeting with Gerard. 'He clearly does not have a positive outlook on Hedley Thomas or what his motives might be – says he is "a grub",' Gerard wrote in his diary that day.

After seeing the photographs of Elise at her parents' home, I asked Gerard and Lorraine for permission to publish one. They considered the request overnight and Gerard called me the next day to agree. 'I want every health professional in Queensland to stare into her eyes. Maybe it will cause them to search their conscience and appreciate what we are trying to do,' he said.

When the main feature and several accompanying stories were published prominently on Saturday 31 July, the reaction was immediate and overwhelming. Many doctors were furious at the punishment of Doneman. Staff and users of the health system were furious at its obvious shortcomings. Readers called me to say they wept for Elise and her parents. The Australian Medical Association demanded action by the Beattie Government to stop unsafe practices in the health system.

Toni Hoffman had never contacted a journalist before. She cried when she stared into the eyes of Elise Neville, and then she sat down to write an email.

> Dear Hedley, I read your article in this morning's *Courier-Mail* with dismay. I am one of the nurses who continues to work in the environment you describe. This week I stayed 3 hrs after my shift finished to try and ensure a patient was transferred to Brisbane from the provincial hospital where I work.
>
> One of the surgeons involved in the case insisted the patient did not need transfer despite the fact our hospital does not have the facilities to care for such a patient. Finally the retrieval team was on its way and I left. When I returned in the am I expected that the patient would have been transferred, only to find he had died 2 hrs after the team arrived.
>
> The intimidating, bullying surgeon of course was not wrong, he had delayed a transfer for several hours, despite the pleas of the nursing staff. There is no-one we can complain to.
>
> The hospital hierarchy believe this surgeon is doing a great job because he is making the hospital money and keeping the waiting lists down. If we complain we are in danger of losing our jobs. No-one will notice in the patient's notes the delay. It's not obvious except to those of us who were there.
>
> The nursing staff were so distraught the next day. We are told to follow the proper protocol to deal with such issues, only to find no-one supporting us. The poor family of the patient will believe all was done for this patient, when we know this is not the case.

Keep up the good work at examining what is going on in our hospital. How dare QLD Health make Dr Doneman the scapegoat for a system which does not work. There are so many good, kind and caring people out there trying to do the best they can. But it is not working.

Toni Hoffman.

Suspicious minds

Late July to October 2004

NURSE Michelle Hunter was seeing too many surgical disasters with a common feature. There were more wound breakdowns, infections and complications connected to the surgery of Jayant Patel than all the other doctors in the hospital. 'Is anyone looking at what's going on here?' she asked Di Jenkin, the manager of the Surgical Unit.

Hunter, back in Bundaberg after a stint in the vascular surgical ward of a large hospital in Bath in the United Kingdom, was stunned by some of Patel's decisions, such as when he ordered that a plaster be put on a man's amputated leg stump. After several days, she asked Patel to look at the wound. It had completely fallen apart. He casually told her to take out the stitches and remove the necrotic tissue as there was little he could do. The man died a few weeks later.

Patel's lack of hygiene appalled the nurse. 'I want you to go and wash your hands before you go to the next patient,' Hunter told him. But when Hunter was not around, Patel went back to his old habit of moving from bed to bed and touching wounds without once washing his hands.

Hunter, who was harbouring serious doubts about Patel's competence, wondered if the surgeon had been involved in any negligence cases in Oregon where, he often boasted, he had extensive experience. After a Google search linked her to the website for the Oregon Board of Medical Examiners, she put his name in the search field. The information that appeared was amazing. Dr Jayant Patel had been subjected to recent serious disciplinary action. He had been barred from performing a wide range of surgery because of his proven incompetence.

Although shocked, Hunter decided that information so easily discovered had to be known to the Medical Board of Queensland and the hospital's managers if indeed it related to the same Jayant Patel.

One evening Karen Stumer, a nurse in the ICU, received an unusual request from a theatre wardsman. He had rushed out of surgery and was in a state of mild panic. 'Can we have some mouth swabs? It's urgent!' he said.

Stumer wondered why they were needed in surgery. She went to the stockroom and removed a handful of the swabs, which were used in the ICU to clean patients' mouths, from a carton. 'What's the problem?' she asked.

'We need them because Dr Patel has flushed the bowel backwards. We have to clean out the patient's mouth before he wakes up.'

Stumer felt physically sick. Patel's bungled flushing technique meant the patient's faecal matter had gone the wrong way, instead of being washed out at the lower end.

By the end of July, amid serious disquiet among nurses and some of the doctors over Des Bramich's death, Patel had been the Director of Surgery for 16 months. Yet he had steadfastly refused to seek fellowship of the College of Surgeons, even though it would have given him formal specialist status, a hefty raise and more boasting rights. Patel kept making excuses. In truth, he must have known that fellowship would be granted only after a careful vetting and accreditation exercise. His United States bans would be discovered.

His managers, Dr Darren Keating and Peter Leck, did not twig. They were delighted Patel had made such a significant dent in the waiting lists. But as both Hoffman and Martin Carter had made known their worries about the Bramich case, Keating decided to look into it. He asked Patel, Carter, Jim Gaffield and Iftikhar Younis to supply reports on the care of Bramich. Their accounts were in conflict. When Patel saw the Sentinel Event report by Hoffman, he denounced it as 'based on misinformation, misrepresentation and personal bias'.

The email Hoffman had sent to me after reading the 31 July story about Elise Neville remained unopened until my return from a family holiday. The cabin we had booked into near Adaminaby, a 45-minute drive from the ski fields at Mount Selywn in New South Wales'

Kosciuszko National Park, was cosy, but when we saw the bunk beds for the children we again thought of Elise. We covered the top bunk with suitcases and organised the bedding to ensure Sarah and Alexander would sleep together on the bottom bunk.

On my return to work in mid August I emailed Hoffman: 'I'm very concerned by the situation you've described. How do you feel about me investigating it – in a way, of course, that does not affect you?' Hoffman replied:

> I would be very grateful on behalf of Queensland health patients if you would investigate the situation that currently exists in Queensland Health, especially in the provincial areas where we are very much at the mercy of third world doctors and management who do not support the grass roots and who consistently lie to cover up what is really going on.
>
> I have invested a lot of time, money and study in my career, but I am increasingly concerned about the state of affairs and just wish management would be accountable.

Hoffman had deliberately not disclosed the hospital or town in which she worked. She wanted to continue pressing her concerns about Patel through official channels. In relation to a patient's death she described, she said: 'The surgeon continues to operate, even though Queensland Health are doing a preliminary investigation. The Coroner is investigating. I really feel QH is out of control with protecting incompetent doctors regardless.'

The lack of feedback from management to Hoffman gave her little confidence. At the urging of other nurses, she pleaded for advice from Vicki Smyth and Kym Barry of the Queensland Nurses' Union.

Hoffman had been going back over the records, looking at deaths and complications in the ICU in the previous 16 months. She revealed how concerned she had become.

'You can't collect that sort of information and not act on it,' Barry said.

ANTOINE Gautray asked his friends and family to wish him well before going into the hospital in early September for a Whipple's procedure – an extremely complex operation to remove a tumour in the head of his pancreas. Although it was a procedure Patel had bungled in Portland with fatal consequences, resulting in him being specifically restricted from attempting it again, he decided to use Gautray as his guinea pig in a hospital ill-equipped for the post-operative care that would be needed.

Gautray was a seriously unwell man when he came out of theatre. The extent of his cancer was such that the operation would almost certainly kill him before the disease took his life. Few if any surgeons would have operated on Gautray in his perilous condition. In his trademark cocksure manner, Patel forged ahead.

Gautray died in late September after a stormy and prolonged stay in the Intensive Care Unit. His death certificate stated Klebsiella: towards the end, a dark brown and sticky sputum that Gautray had been coughing up caused pneumonia and pockets of pus in the lining of his lungs.

The week after Gautray's death, Patel operated on Ian Vowles, a cabinet-maker who had a polyp in the lining of his bowel. Instead of simply removing the fleshy growth, Patel opted for drastic action – removal of the entire bowel.

'Well, the cyst is attached to the wall of your bowel and I cannot see what's in behind it. Your bowel does not like your body. We will whip it out,' Patel told him. 'I've done a lot of these operations before. People, after they get well again, they go skiing. You'll have no worries whatsoever.'

The operation was entirely unnecessary. The polyp was benign. At the time Patel did the operation, there was nothing to suggest it might develop into cancer.

At 57, Vowles was fitted with an ileostomy bag. There were serious post-operative complications. His quality of life was never the same again.

GLENN Tathem usually tried to inject humour into his deadly serious talks for Queensland Health. A few jokes sprinkled here and there made the subject, ethical awareness, less foreboding for hospital staff.

A misconduct investigator based in Brisbane, Tathem went to Bundaberg Hospital to remind the staff of their obligations under the Code of Conduct.

'Some people think that people who complain are dobbers. Do you agree?' he asked.

Toni Hoffman and the other nurses were increasingly alarmed as they watched one part of Tathem's PowerPoint presentation, headed 'Breach of Confidentiality – The Small Town Scandal'. Another part related to whistleblowing about serious threats to safety. Tathem and the explanatory material warned that a whistleblower who disclosed information to a union representative, the media or a Member of Parliament could be sacked and even imprisoned for committing a criminal offence.

'I'm so glad you didn't do what you were going to do,' Gail Aylmer said to Hoffman.

The nurses were alarmed at the timing of the presentation and the consequences for staff who spoke outside the system, even though the system was not properly responding to complaints made internally.

Until Tathem's sobering warning, Hoffman had been ready to go to Brisbane with a union official to bring Jayant Patel to the Health Rights Commission's notice. Now she was scared. She wondered if the timing of the talk was more than a coincidence; and whether she might already be in trouble for confiding information to me and the union.

24

The outpouring

October to November 2004

TONI Hoffman finally lost patience with her smug and unresponsive managers. She had heard more than enough about the merits of mediation. She did not want psychological counselling. She felt patronised by all the talk about 'personality conflict' with Jayant Patel. And she was angry that Linda Mulligan believed the problems on the wards and in the Intensive Care Unit might be fixed by a book, *Coping With Difficult People*.

Dr Darren Keating had convinced himself and others that much of the criticism of Patel was the product of the surgeon's personality clash with Hoffman. On 18 October, Keating, Leck and Mulligan met to talk about the problems. They agreed that there needed to be mediation; the constant bickering was having an impact on the operations of the ICU. Keating was fed up with the stream of complaints against the star surgeon. He made time in his diary to meet Patel and Hoffman together. He doubted he could resolve their feud, but he might be able to placate them for a while. Keating had made no secret of his admiration for Patel. Hoffman believed that it verged on sycophancy. 'When you get to be as great as this man, you can do what you want,' Keating had told one of the ICU nurses in Patel's presence outside the hospital canteen.

When Mulligan again raised 'unresolved behaviour and communication issues' shortly before lunch on 20 October, Hoffman made her most forceful effort yet to bring about decisive action. 'Dr Patel's patients are dying because of his care!' she said.

Hoffman knew that her career would probably stall or even end, but to hell with it. In an angry outburst she spoke about Patel's dishonesty in describing the condition of patients; how Dr Peter Miach refused to let his patients undergo procedures by the Director of Surgery; how the number of post-operative complications was without precedent.

A few hours later in a hastily called meeting in Peter Leck's office, Hoffman repeated the serious allegations. She also told Leck about Patel's stubborn refusal to observe hygiene and how a probable consequence – wound dehiscence from infection – was not properly reported in the patients' notes because Patel knew it would give clues to his negligence. 'The death of Mr Bramich was the last straw,' Hoffman told Leck. 'They may come back and say he would have died anyway. But that isn't the point. It was about Dr Patel interfering in the process that would have got the patient to Brisbane in time for him to have the best chance.'

Hoffman reminded Leck of how she had gone to him eight months earlier with her concerns about Patel's behaviour; and how she and Dr Jon Joiner had warned Keating about the dangers of the oesophagectomies in mid 2003. She repeated other disturbing clues to Patel's incompetence, including evidence of the harm caused to patients in the Renal Unit because of his ineptitude with the placement of catheters. Hoffman gave the District Manager an ultimatum. Unless there was a rigorous and independent audit of the outcomes for Patel's patients, she would be forced to take further steps. 'I am quite happy to be proven wrong,' she told Leck.

In an email to Leck two days later, she documented the details of unnecessary suffering by a dozen of Patel's patients:

> I spoke with Dr Dieter Berens and informed him the nursing staff were going to report their concerns with Dr Patel to an official source.
>
> He stated he would support us, by telling the truth, but he was concerned he would lose his job and Dr Patel would be the one left behind.
>
> It is widely believed among the medical and nursing staff that Dr Patel was very powerful, that he was wholeheartedly supported by Peter Leck and Darren Keating and was untouchable.

Anyone who tried to alert the authorities about their concerns would lose their jobs. This perception was indeed perpetrated by Dr Patel on a daily basis.

Many of the [Principal House Officers] have expressed their concern, Dr Alex Davis and Dr David Risson, but were unsure of what to do because of the widespread belief Dr Patel was protected by executive.

On the day Leck received Hoffman's written report, Keating and Miach had an angry row over Patel's competence. But still nothing was done to restrict any of Patel's work. The surgical wards were full of patients. They were still being led into theatre like lambs to a slaughter.

Leck briefly considered suspending Patel on full pay. But Patel was much too valuable to the hospital and the campaign to reduce the waiting lists. Leck bought time. He decided to test Hoffman's serious allegations.

Leck and Keating interviewed Dr Dieter Berens, one of the anaesthetists, who questioned Patel's competence and judgement in undertaking some operations. Berens bluntly described Patel as dishonest about his mistakes and so rigid, he refused to consider alternative and safe clinical options for the patients.

Risson, a relatively junior doctor, revealed that he had concerns about the number of post-operative complications and infections. Patel's dismantling of one of the reporting mechanisms meant that the surgical audit process was a bad joke. When Risson had previously raised a wound dehiscence, Patel tried to change the definition of dehiscence. 'We should be careful what we call wound dehiscence and what we class wound dehiscence,' Patel had said. The Director of Surgery was trying to minimise the number of complications being recorded.

The next doctor to be interviewed, Martin Strahan, had nothing to lose for speaking his mind. He was a Visiting Medical Officer who helped out at the hospital when he had time away from his full-time job elsewhere. He described Patel's misdiagnosis of a woman upon whom the Director of Surgery was determined to perform an extremely complex Whipple's procedure. She died several days later. Strahan was concerned that Patel believed he was invincible – a 'Johnny come lately' with aggressive traits who was strongly supported by management to take a scalpel to the waiting lists. Strahan also emphasised the dangerous vacuum into which Patel had arrived – the Director of Surgery, who saw himself as a 'self declared expert from the First World to help the Third World of Bundaberg', had been permitted to operate without any form of peer review.

Keating and Leck did not bother asking Miach, the most qualified and experienced specialist in the district. But in early November 2004 Miach handed to Keating another scathing indictment of Patel. It was a letter written by Dr Jason Jenkins, a vascular surgeon at the Royal Brisbane Hospital who was held in high regard for his specialist skills and integrity. He sent it to Miach and to Patel. Only rarely would doctors lambast colleagues in writing over the care of patients, but Jenkins was enraged after he examined Marilyn Daisy on 1 November for her diabetes problems.

'When did you get that done?' Jenkins asked when he saw the bandage on her below-knee amputation.

'Six weeks ago,' Daisy replied.

'Do you mind if I have a look at it? Has it not healed yet?' asked Jenkins.

It was clear that not only had the wound not healed, the sutures were still in Daisy's amputation stump six weeks later. There was also an area of gangrene.

'So have you seen the surgeon since the operation? What's he going to do about this? Did he offer you a chance of saving your leg?' asked Jenkins.

'I haven't seen the surgeon since the procedure. No, they just said that I need my leg off.' Patel had not offered Daisy the option of trying to save her leg with a bypass operation.

In his letter Jenkins wrote:

These sutures were heavily buried within the tissue and very difficult and painful to remove. I find it mind boggling that someone could leave sutures in for this long.

It shows a complete lack of understanding of diabetic disease and how to perform an operation. I have suggested to her that when she comes to Brisbane that she will require a debridement of this stump and if it fails to heal then she may require an above knee amputation. I think if procedures can't be performed appropriate with the Bundaberg Hospital then they should not be performed at all...

In the months before Daisy sought help in Brisbane, Jenkins had noted a disturbing pattern in patients who underwent vascular surgery by Patel. Jenkins quickly determined that the Director of Surgery was doing more harm than good. He was astounded when Miach told him how he had tried to stop Patel to no avail. Patel would go and find patients in the wards and operate without Miach knowing.

Before writing the letter, Jenkins telephoned Patel and threatened to report him to the Medical Board if he kept doing vascular work. 'Look, you know if you keep doing this then there are going to be consequences,' Jenkins said.

Patel was unmoved. For as long as the hospital let him do such operations, he had no intention of stopping.

MIACH gave Keating the written complaint on the same day the Health Practitioners Tribunal in Brisbane was delivering its own verdict. The wheels of justice had turned slowly for Elise Neville, her parents and Dr Andrew Doneman, who was pleading guilty to unsatisfactory professional conduct to save himself and his family further trauma and crippling legal fees. District Court Judge Debbie Richards said:

The tragedy has had an enormous impact on the Neville family and, no doubt, others who knew and loved young Elise.

Dr Doneman must have been fatigued by the hours he was working. It seems extraordinary in this day and age that anyone, let alone someone in a position of such responsibility, should be asked to work such long hours.

One does not need medical evidence to know that anyone who is in the 20th hour of a continuous duty must have reduced capacity to assess the situation when it presents itself. If this tragedy leads to nothing else, it should lead to the abolition of such brutally long shift hours...

Richards concluded that Doneman's treatment of Elise 'was deficient in a number of respects'. She ruled:

> His interpretation of the history and physical findings based on limited examination and his lack of appreciation of the parent's concerns were wrong and errors of judgment which eventually denied Elise the chance of survival.
>
> Accordingly, the Tribunal concurs with the Board's submissions that stringent conditions should be placed on Dr Doneman's continuing right to practice.

The disciplinary orders compelled Doneman to work in a supervised position for 12 months, with ongoing assessment and reporting of his competence to assess patients.

After the delivery of the judgement I walked to a nearby cafe to talk to Gerard and Lorraine. They still had unfinished business, Gerard pledged. The system was yet to reform itself.

WHEN the pain in Trevor Halter's stomach had become too much, he went to see his GP, Dr Ken Hornsby. At 54, Halter regarded himself as being in reasonably good shape. 'As fit as a Mallee bull,' he half-jokingly boasted. But the pain was constant. Even Halter, a part-time race-caller who rolled beer kegs around the club where he did odd jobs, had to concede he needed help. Hornsby wrote a referral letter for him to attend the outpatients department at Bundaberg Hospital.

Halter had gallstones. Fortunately, he learned, the condition was easily remedied. 'You're probably better off having your gall bladder out because you don't really need it and so you may as well have it out,' Jayant Patel told him. ' I do four to five a week and there's nothing to it – it's keyhole surgery.'

The routine corrective procedure, laparoscopic cholecystectomy, was on a par with having your tonsils out. Halter learned he would need to stay just one night in the hospital.

He awoke after the operation in agony. Halter spent the next seven weeks in hospital. Two of those weeks were in the Intensive Care Unit as he fought for his life. His children were told his lungs had collapsed, his liver had failed and he contracted pneumonia and septicaemia. Then his heart went. He was finally transferred by helicopter to Brisbane on 4 December for lifesaving treatment. All from a routine gall bladder operation bungled by Patel. Months later, Halter was still in pain and undergoing corrective surgery.

The bloodletting

December 2004

WHEN Judy and Gerry Kemps looked back on their lives and the fruits of a close marriage of 50 years, they felt blessed. They were wed on 23 October 1954 in St Patrick's Cathedral in Melbourne. Judy had given birth to three healthy and happy children, Jacqui, John and Bernie. They had relaxed into the gentle pace and tranquillity of Bundaberg after a stint overseas. They set up a photographic studio and continued to raise their three children.

The couple remained active as they aged. They went bushwalking together and enjoyed regular tennis and golf. Kemps was one of those fortunate people who never had a sick day in his life, but by 2002 his health began to deteriorate. His blood pressure was erratic. He got gout. He suffered back pain. When he received a letter from Queensland Health offering a free check-up, an appointment was made for 24 November 2004 at the local Burrum Street Medical Practice. The tests on his urine sample pointed to a problem.

'You look yellow. You look anaemic to me,' Judy told her husband as they ate lunch ten days later.

By 6 December, further tests at Bundaberg Hospital showed Kemps was bleeding internally. The endoscope had identified a large, malignant tumour about 4 centimetres in size, in the lower oesophagus. The CT scans showed the cancer had spread beyond the oesophagus. There were shadows on both lungs. There were enlarged lymph nodes where the trachea splits into the left and right main branches.

Dr Dawid Smalberger was adamant that Kemps needed to go to Brisbane for keyhole surgery. Nothing too radical was proposed – the cancer was such that the patient might have just 12 months to live. Under the circumstances, Smalberger wanted to ensure Kemps received the best care and quality of life possible for the time he had left. He did not contemplate an oesophagectomy. Even for a highly competent surgeon, such a complex procedure was far too risky. But with the presence of secondary cancers, it was also pointless. Smalberger decided the best course of action was a stent to make it easier for Kemps to swallow his food.

The protocol for a transfer of a patient from Bundaberg to another hospital's surgical department required the decision to be signed off by a surgeon in Bundaberg. Unfortunately for Kemps, he was seen by Jayant Patel. The safe and conservative course was suddenly turned on its head by the Director of Surgery. Patel told the couple that the keyhole surgery recommended by Smalberger was 'patch-up work' – and that what he really needed was an oesophagectomy.

He explained how he would remove part of the stomach and part of the oesophagus and join what was left back together again. No problems. 'It is a big operation but it is nothing because I've done hundreds of them,' Patel said. His confidence was contagious. Neither Kemps nor his wife were given any reason to doubt Patel.

THEATRE nurse Damien Gaddes went to work early to start preparing for the operation on Gerry Kemps. But there was a problem: the Intensive Care Unit already had two patients on ventilators; they would be unable to cope with Gerry.

Gaddes called Dr Dieter Berens, who agreed the operation should be postponed. But when Gaddes reached Jayant Patel on his mobile telephone, the Director of Surgery was furious: 'That brain dead patient should have been switched off last night!' Patel said.

At 8 pm the day before, Patel had told a nurse to call Dr Jon Joiner and ask him to turn off the life support keeping a critically ill woman, Robyn Turton, 63, alive. Turton had slipped in the bath and hit her head on Saturday, suffering a cerebral bleed; her family was aware that her prospects were poor. Her death would free up an ICU bed. And Patel wanted it for Gerry Kemps.

But Joiner flatly refused. He was offended at the indecent haste to end the life of a woman who had not yet undergone formal brain death tests. Although it was probable from the CT scans that she was brain dead, Joiner prudently decided to wait.

Patel had little time for Joiner, the anaesthetist who, 18 months earlier, had expressed concern to management about the risks of performing oesophagectomies in a small hospital with a limited ICU. As Patel did his ward rounds on Monday morning, he badmouthed Joiner. 'I have a theatre case to do!' Patel told Martin Brennan, one of the nurses.

The theatre nurse was astonished at Patel's cavalier approach to ending Turton's life before the necessary brain death tests had been done. Brennan did not trust Patel. He had heard the surgeon intimidate and bully the nurses and threaten to harm their careers. Patel had created a climate of fear in the operating theatre and ICU. All the nurses doubted they would be backed by management in a showdown as Patel often boasted of his influence over Darren Keating. 'I can get what I want from Darren as I've just made this hospital $500 000,' Patel reiterated.

Patel stormed into Dr Martin Carter's office and denounced Joiner. He pressured Carter to end Turton's life and free up a bed for the oesophagectomy.

Nurse Vivian Tapiolas witnessed Patel's insistence on the withdrawal of life support for Turton, whose children were in the waiting room at the ICU as Patel pressed Carter to make a decision. After a review of the charts, Tapiolas and the two doctors spoke to the family about ending Turton's life.

Patel walked back into the ICU with a spring in his step. 'Now I can perform the oesophagectomy,' he said.

Carter switched off life support at 8.55 am on Monday. Despite the absence of the formal brain death tests, Carter decided there was sufficient clinical evidence to show Turton had suffered massive and irreparable brain damage. 'In view of the dreadful prognosis this lady has and following discussion with family, ventilator support is to be withdrawn,' Carter wrote.

Patel had his bed.

AT 9.52 am on Monday 20 December, less than an hour after the death of Robyn Turton, the operation on Gerry Kemps began. Patel was flanked in theatre by the anaesthetist, Dr Dieter Berens, two Principal House Officers – Dr Sanjeeva Kariyawasam and Dr Anthony Athanasiov – and the nurses. Kariyawasam had spent much of his time at the hospital as Patel's shadow. They got along well. Patel was only too happy to explain the complexities of surgery to his eager apprentice.

Together they used to undertake what Patel would call a 'blitz' – in one week there would be a swag of colonoscopy procedures; in another week there would be a run of gall bladder operations. It was part of Patel's ongoing assault on the waiting lists, and it kept him in management's good books. Kariyawasam often heard Patel boasting about how successful he had been in reducing the lists and establishing rapport with Keating.

The oesophagectomy went well at first. Kemps's abdomen needed to be opened to permit access to the oesophagus and the stomach. Suddenly, however, he became unstable, with plunging blood pressure and a rising pulse rate.

Kemps was turned onto his side for the thoracotomy part, the opening of the chest cavity. As Patel resected the tumour in the chest, the blood continued to pour freely into the drain. The heavy bleeding in the abdominal cavity was obvious to everyone. Berens was worried. Apart from the blood loss, he could see that the Director of Surgery lacked the skill to be attempting such an operation. Patel's roughness around the heart and the vessels was all too obvious. Nor did he appear interested in the monitoring being done by Berens of blood pressure and other vital signs. Berens was shocked. It was as if Patel could not acknowledge a major problem. Unless the blood stopped flowing, Kemps would surely die.

'Dr Patel, the Bellovac drain is over half full with no vacuum and is still draining freely,' said nurse Damien Gaddes.

'That's what drains are for, Damien,' Patel replied.

To the amazement of Berens and the theatre nurses who were alarmed by the obvious and heavy bleeding, Patel gave instructions for Kemps to go to the ICU. From that moment it was inevitable that he would not survive.

At 2 pm, Patel called Judy at her home: 'It was a great success – we have got it all. There's a little bit of bleeding there but that's nothing.'

When Judy went to the ICU soon afterwards, she saw a nurse frantically pumping blood into her husband's body. Kemps received more than 30 bags of blood altogether. His abdomen was distended as bright blood drained away. Three nurses were needed at his bedside for fluid management and one ran back and forth from the blood bank for products and to page the doctors. Berens was using large quantities of a drug to maintain blood pressure and support the heart.

Another nurse took Judy aside. 'Gerry is a very sick man and he is on life support,' the nurse said.

Judy, joined by her son John, went over to his bedside and gave him a kiss.

'I love you,' she said. He tried to sit up.

At 5 pm, Judy was told of the need for another operation. 'I have to take him back into theatre again. It can only be the spleen. I'll take it out because he doesn't need it anyway,' Patel said. But Patel had begun another operation on a different patient, which led to another complication. Kemps was not taken back into theatre until after 6.30 pm.

The situation was critical when Dr David Risson, who had not been involved in the oesophagectomy, came to theatre to help. Risson was surprised to see Dr Sanjeeva Kariyawasam, a junior doctor, identifying problems and tactfully pointing them out to Patel, who seemed out of his depth and at a loss to pinpoint the torrential bleeding.

Patel reopened the abdominal cavity and the chest cavity.

As scout nurse, Jenelle Law's tasks included finding sutures, sponges and anything else that might be needed for the operation. She lost track of the amount of blood spilling from Kemps on the operating table. But Law counted 75 large sponges and 15 gauze squares to absorb the blood. It was everywhere. As the nurses moved around theatre, they left footsteps of blood on the floor.

'This man's going to die! He's going to die on the table,' said Patel. 'I can't do anything. Get the family. Get the family!'

Law watched Patel becoming agitated, defending his surgery and saying the bleeding had nothing to do with him

'This isn't my fault. This has nothing to do with my surgery. This isn't my fault.'

But Patel also had a rare moment of insight. He was shaken by the demise of Kemps. 'Maybe they're right. Maybe we shouldn't be doing oesophagectomies. Maybe I should start thinking about not doing these types of procedures any more,' Patel said in the operating theatre.

Law opened the theatre door for Patel to go outside to talk to Judy and her two sons. Patel was covered in Kemps's blood.

'I have taken the spleen out but it was all right,' Patel told the worried family. 'I had a look at the lungs and they were all right so the bleeding must have come from the heart. I can't do anything about it but he will be lucky to last the night.' Patel repeatedly told the shocked Kemps family that his surgery was 'perfect'.

The longest night in Judy's life was spent with her dying husband in Toni Hoffman's Intensive Care Unit. His demise was inevitable; the equipment supporting him was gradually removed. Judy noticed something else – the nursing staff seemed strangely uncomfortable around her. Their body language was defensive. They avoided eye contact.

Gerry Kemps died at 9.20 am on 21 December. Patel had notched up another lucrative procedure for Bundaberg Base Hospital, which received its financial bonus irrespective of whether the patient survived the operation. And the ICU bed was vacant again already.

Dr Athanasiov, given the task of filling in the death certificate, was discouraged from referring the case to the Coroner by Patel. 'We know the cause of death, it was due to a bleed in the aorta,' Patel said.

The theatre staff were furious with Patel. Berens was alarmed. He could not understand why Patel would send a bleeding patient to the ICU. Nor could he understand Patel's inability hours later to discover the source of the bleeding.

Berens and Martin Carter agreed the death should be reported for formal autopsy – the Coroner's Act refers to 'a death being reportable where it was not reasonably expected to be the outcome of a health procedure'. But by the time the two anaesthetists had come to this view, it was too late. A notice in the NewsMail showed that Kemps was being buried in a few hours.

Berens was struck by the lack of interest Darren Keating showed in investigating, even when Carter explained his concerns about survival rates of Patel's patients.

Nurses Jenelle Law and Damien Gaddes decided to make a formal complaint. They believed Patel had killed Kemps.

In the afternoon after Kemps's death, Peter Leck saw a note blandly advising the outcome of the complex procedure performed by the Director of Surgery.

'The oesophagectomy concerns me somewhat. Have any of these patients survived?' Leck asked Keating.

26

Life and limb

Late December 2004 to January 2005

SHANNON Mobbs fell spectacularly from his friend's trail bike at 10 am on 23 December, the day Judy Kemps farewelled her husband at his funeral in Bundaberg. The teenager had struck a tree stump hidden by long grass on a winding track at Woodgate, south of Bundaberg.

Mobbs, 15, was flown by helicopter to Bundaberg Hospital after his friend sped 10 kilometres along the track to raise the alarm. By the time he was in the operating theatre for lifesaving surgery by Jayant Patel, the boy had lost a massive amount of blood from a deep slash in his groin and a lacerated femoral vein in his thigh. His condition was so perilous that the boy was initially transfused with blood that did not match his type: at least it kept him alive.

After the first operation, Patel emerged from theatre to reassure Mobbs's mother, Karen Orreal. The surgeon talked about himself for the first ten minutes, falsely claiming that he had been in charge of the trauma and emergency ward of a New York hospital for a decade. Orreal was relieved when the Director of Surgery told her he had stopped the bleeding. He assured her that her son was fine and would make a complete recovery – all thanks to his vascular surgery.

Over the next 12 hours Patel performed another two operations on Mobbs. Despite the initial lifesaving surgery, and then serious complications demanding more major surgery, Patel told the other doctors and Orreal that there was no need to transfer the boy to Brisbane. Patel left the hospital on Boxing Day to fly to the United States for annual leave, but not before instructing the medical staff to keep the boy in the surgical ward.

He had extracted something from Darren Keating on Christmas Eve – another 'Dear Jay' letter. It set out the terms of a four-year extension of his current contract. 'I would like to offer my congratulations on your ongoing appointment and hope that your work with the Bundaberg Health Service District will continue to be both beneficial and rewarding,' Keating wrote.

The many serious issues raised by Hoffman were yet to be formally investigated. She was at home, mourning the death of her grandmother at 98, preparing for the funeral in Sydney and worrying about the condition of Mobbs. Although Hoffman was supposed to be on annual leave and entertaining her parents, her sister Maree and husband Matthew, and their two kids, she could not let go of the problems with Patel. She stayed in touch with the hospital by telephone and repeatedly urged the nurses in the ICU to do what they could to influence the transfer of Mobbs: 'You've got to get that boy to Brisbane,' she said.

Her brother-in-law was also worried. He could see the high levels of stress Hoffman was under when she was supposed to be on holidays. Hoffman showed him the lengthy letter of complaint she had written and spoke to him about her pleas for a clinical audit. He said: 'At least you will be able to sleep at night.' But Hoffman was finding sleep difficult.

For most of the nine days Mobbs remained in the hospital, there was no pulse in his left foot. The foot was dying. Contrary to the claims Patel had made in the notes about repairing Mobbs's femoral vein, he had simply tied it off.

After Patel went on holidays, handing over to Dr Jim Gaffield, the boy was in excruciating pain with a fractured pelvis, huge muscle tears in his thigh, raging temperatures, sepsis and gangrene. It took until 1 January and a snap decision by an appalled Dr David Risson on his return from leave for Mobbs to be airlifted to the Royal Brisbane Hospital. There, Dr Mark Ray diagnosed him on New Year's Day as the sickest 15-year-old he had ever seen. Ray could smell the septic and grossly infected leg from the other side of the Emergency Department. He did not expect Mobbs to survive the night. If he did survive, he would need more surgery to amputate his leg through the knee.

The operation by Dr Jason Jenkins and Ray showed that both ends of the femoral vein had been suture-ligated instead of being reconstructed. Blood had been going to Mobbs's limb through the femoral artery, but it could not drain away through the femoral vein. This had led to gross swelling and a range of serious life-threatening implications. Dr Steve Rashford, who organised the emergency airlift, and the two Brisbane surgeons, Jenkins and Ray, were disgusted by the care Mobbs had received in Bundaberg. There was no excuse for the failure to send him to Brisbane after the initial surgery. They thought the athletic 2-metre tall boy, who wanted to be a professional basket-baller, might have kept his leg if he had been transferred immediately after the major operation.

On 4 January, Michelle Hunter, the nurse who had alerted the doctors to Mobbs's shocking condition on New Year's Eve, resolved to do something. She had come to the conclusion that Patel was a serial danger. She had never seen so many instances of wound dehiscence; and the Internet search she had done months earlier was still on her mind. Patel's treatment of Mobbs – the tying off of his femoral vein which effectively destroyed his leg – persuaded Hunter to act.

She went to see Hoffman, who was back from Christmas leave. But the nurse in charge of the ICU had still not heard anything from Peter Leck or Keating about an investigation, despite her increasingly detailed and grave complaints made during 2004.

Hunter decided to make her own complaint. She considered going directly to the Health Rights Commission. First, she sent a memo to Linda Mulligan setting out her concerns over the Mobbs case: 'My concerns are with the surgeon that performed his initial three opera-tions...I am concerned that if the patient had been transferred to Brisbane initially he may not have lost his leg or be in such a grave condition. I would like his treatment at the hospital investigated as I fear his health and well being has now been compromised by inade-quate, substandard treatment by the medical team,' Hunter wrote.

There was a similar expression of concern from Dr Rashford in Brisbane, who wrote to the most senior administrators in Queensland Health – and copied his memo to Leck and Keating. Pressure was mounting. But Keating, who wanted Patel to return from holidays to a new four-year contract, produced a report stating no external probe was necessary.

Mulligan was now starting to worry. From the beginning she had downplayed Hoffman's concerns. She believed the nurse and the top surgeon simply loathed each other and that Hoffman's complaints were motivated by emotional rather than clinical issues. But on 7 January, three distraught nurses from the operating theatre – Katrina Zwolak, Damien Gaddes and Jenelle Law – had decided to unite in an unprecedented complaint. They went to Mulligan and told her Patel was a shocking surgeon whose patients were dying unnecessarily. Weeping, Zwolak and Law told of the falsification of patients' records by Patel and of how staff had felt powerless because of his claims to have management in his pocket.

Mulligan immediately tipped Leck off about this dramatic new development. 'They displayed different degrees of emotion, to the point of one stating the whole issue is keeping them from sleeping,' Mulligan told him.

All of Hoffman's claims were being corroborated. And still, a clinical audit of Patel's work was not begun.

27

Executive decisions
13–14 January 2005

PETER Leck was showing the first signs of acute panic by the time Jayant Patel had returned to work in early January. Leck worried about his own failure to conduct any sort of review of Patel despite a trail of dead and maimed patients and a string of complaints. He had broken his promise to Hoffman to have the concerns properly checked. He had not even told her what he was doing. Leck had dithered. He had been indecisive, weak and interminably slow.

On 13 January, Leck raised the concerns for the first time with the acting Director-General of Health, Dr John Scott: 'I was just wanting to flag that I actually do have some concerns about the outcomes of some of Dr Patel's surgery,' Leck said. He told Scott about the nurses' fears over injuries and deaths, adding that Darren Keating believed the concerns were 'completely driven by the personality conflict'. 'However, he has now expressed some concern although he still believes most of the issues are personality-driven,' Leck said. He was mute about the backing of Hoffman's concerns by the three doctors, Dr Martin Carter, Dr David Risson and Dr Dieter Berens, who had been interviewed.

Keating was angry that it had come to this. He did not like confrontations with Patel, particularly as he had exceeded the surgery targets and made Keating and the hospital look good. But the ICU and theatre staff were close to rebellion. Something had to give. 'Look, we need to make sure that Dr Patel is aware of the investigation and give him as much information as possible,' Keating told Leck.

In a meeting in Leck's office on 13 January Patel was told for the first time about the complaints concerning his handling of Shannon Mobbs as well as other patients. He was told there would be an investigation and that, in the meantime, he could continue doing surgery – just not cases requiring admission to the ICU.

Patel scoffed at the very notion that his surgery was below standard. But for the third time in his career, he faced a thorough investigation with potentially grave findings. 'I will be considering my position,' he said indignantly.

The next day Patel told Keating he would not be taking up the four-year contract after 1 April. But he had no plans to leave Australia. Patel still believed he could remain as a surgeon on a special contract. Despite the trouble he would be in if the easily discovered details of his past came to light, he chose not to flee. At least not yet.

'I would like to thank you for your support over the past two years,' he told Keating. 'My stay at Bundaberg has been challenging at times, but mostly enjoyable and rewarding.'

Keating replied with a glowing appraisal of Patel's troubled time at the hospital, thanking him for his 'sustained commitment, ongoing enthusiasm and strong work ethic'. 'I have greatly valued your advice, insight and support over the last two years and I wish you well in the future in whatever endeavours you make [sic] take,' Keating wrote. Patel kept the note for his CV. It was the sort of adulation not dissimilar to the praise bestowed by his peers in New York State and Oregon when he had been in trouble.

Seeking further reassurance and comfort, Patel turned to the junior surgeons, Dr Anthony Athanasiov and Dr Sanjeeva Kariyawasam. They were upset at the story told by their mentor, the man who had bought their meals and passed on his surgical prowess. They immediately teamed up with three other junior doctors to lobby on Patel's behalf. In a note to Keating they wrote:

> Dr Patel is now in a position whereby he feels it is not in his best
> interest to stay at Bundaberg and we believe the hospital should
> consider this very carefully.

Dr Patel's approach to his work is nothing short of admirable. He is dedicated, hard working, efficient and knowledgeable. His efforts to ensure that his patients receive the best care go above and beyond the call of his duties.

He constantly goes out of his way to provide timely, expert management for a wide variety of surgical problems. In summary, we are concerned about the circumstances surrounding Dr Patel's departure and we believe his leaving would be a great loss for the hospital, and also for the Bundaberg community.

By the end of January, Keating had hatched a devious plan. He was annoyed that impertinent nursing staff had dashed his hopes of retaining Jayant Patel as the Director of Surgery until 2009. Keating decided to flex his management muscle, pander to Patel and put the nurses back in their place. All with one big decision. In early February, he offered Patel a senior surgical role with a daily rate of $1150 – a significant enhancement on his existing $200 000 a year package. Keating had also given the Medical Board another glowing appraisal of Patel's work: 'Dr Patel is a very committed and enthusiastic clinician who has continued to be a very effective member of staff and Director of Surgery. He has a very strong work ethic which is a model for others.' There were 'nil significant' areas for improvement in Patel's performance, according to Keating, who rated the surgeon's performance as 'excellent'.

Keating had paved the way for the four-year contract extension offered previously. He wrote to the Department of Immigration and affirmed that the hospital planned to employ Patel until 2009.

'They're going to pay me as much for three months as what I get in a year!' Patel boasted to nurse Jenelle Law in the operating theatre during an endoscopy procedure.

Law was appalled. She had been looking forward to seeing the back of Patel and all the problems he brought to the hospital. Now it seemed he was to be showered with money and kept on.

28

The investigation

February to March 2005

GERRY FitzGerald spread the email printouts, memos, reports and letters across his desk at Queensland Health headquarters in Charlotte Street. The Chief Health Officer had given himself an unenviable assignment: a clinical audit of Jayant Patel's surgical outcomes.

The documentary material was the first part of the puzzle. Dr FitzGerald had already been advised by Leck that there were personality differences between Patel and his principal accuser, Toni Hoffman. FitzGerald also knew how valuable Patel was to Bundaberg Hospital. His role in slicing through the waiting lists had been repeatedly stressed by Leck. Mindful of the sensitivities of the people involved, FitzGerald made plans to visit Bundaberg to interview Patel as well as the nursing and medical staff. He told Leck:

> At this point we will be simply collecting information and not seeking to validate or evaluate any particular concerns raised.
>
> Would you mind asking Dr Patel if he can spare some time to meet with me to discuss any concern he may have? Dr Patel is definitely entitled under the principles of natural justice to be confronted with the details of the complaints made against him.
>
> He may decline to meet with me until he has had the opportunity to respond to the complaints. I hope he does not do so. Our main intent is to find the facts and to seek a resolution ASAP.

Anyone else who risked being exposed as a clinical fraud would have skipped overseas on the eve of an investigation by the Chief Health Officer, but not Patel. His ego and self-belief refused to entertain the idea that he might be found out.

Patel also knew that the hospital still desperately needed him. On 8 February Keating had all but pleaded for Patel and other staff to work harder on those waiting lists – the hospital was 92 operations behind its target: 'Should the target not be achieved, Bundaberg Health Service District will not get another chance to upgrade the target and hence lose flexibility and significant dollars...therefore it is imperative that everyone continue to pull together and maximise elective surgery throughput until 30 June. All cancellations should be minimal with these cases pushed thru as much as possible,' Keating wrote in a memo to senior staff.

In the executive meeting room on 14 February, FitzGerald and a Brisbane colleague, Sue Jenkins, began working their way through a list of about 30 nurses and doctors. Some of the interviews lasted just 15 minutes. Others went for over an hour. Nurse Karen Jenner wondered how seriously it was being taken when told during her interview: 'This is not an investigation of Dr Patel. This is us gathering information to find out whether or not it is important to have an investigation into Dr Patel.'

When Patel strolled in he acted as if he did not have a care in the world. He had spared about 25 minutes for the Chief Health Officer, who immediately identified an arrogance bordering on megalomania. Patel's self-confidence was almost pathological. It was a personality that FitzGerald, a naturally shy and disarming man, could not easily understand.

Patel proceeded to boast about how much surgical experience he had in the United States. He repeatedly spoke of his expertise in complex procedures. He was clearly agitated at the scrutiny being applied to his work, but he brushed it off as the product of flaws in other people. 'Nurses have been complaining about doctors for centuries. Some of them are lazy. They don't want to work hard,' Patel told FitzGerald.

Patel offered an olive branch: 'Well, if you don't want to do these procedures anymore, we won't do them here.'

After hearing from Dr Peter Miach and several nurses about the catheter problems and the lack of hygiene, FitzGerald, too, was doubting the competence of the Director of Surgery. But was the hospital better off with Patel than with no senior surgeon at all? When FitzGerald asked Toni Hoffman this question, she was certain of the answer. She told him that the patients would be much better off if Patel were immediately suspended. 'We don't like this guy but that's not the issue,' Hoffman told FitzGerald. 'The issue is he's doing these things here and it's harming people.'

'Well, we can't do anything because nothing's been proved at this stage,' FitzGerald replied.

Hoffman was crestfallen. 'What on earth can we possibly do to stop this man?' she wondered.

'What do the patients feel?' FitzGerald asked Darren Keating. 'What's the level of patient satisfaction? Have there been any complaints against Dr Patel by patients?'

Keating had a folder of complaints, but he assured FitzGerald there were none.

Patel had given an undertaking to stop doing the oesophagectomies and other complex surgery needing ICU support, but he was still causing serious damage. Three days before FitzGerald's arrival, Jenny White was the scrub nurse for a procedure to remove part of the cancerous bowel of a patient, Jean Stuart-Sutherland. Patel cut the healthy part of her bowel. If he noticed his error, he did not acknowledge it until a junior doctor pointed it out. White shook her head in disbelief. How Patel could have overlooked the four centimetre cut was unfathomable.

When Stuart-Sutherland returned to theatre in late February because of the inevitable complications from the earlier incompetence, White saw the terrible state of the bowel. It was leaking – more than one litre of bile-stained fluid needed to be drained. There was also a gross infection.

THE blood from the carotid artery of Harry Petrohilos spurted in a fine but steady stream. It happened suddenly when one of the doctors in the coronary unit tried to put a central line into his neck, missing the vein but piercing the artery. Because arterial pressure is greater than venous pressure, Petrohilos began losing blood. Fast.

Petrohilos was already in poor shape. He had suffered a heart attack and was also battling severe kidney failure, which made him anaemic. He took blood thinning substances for a condition called atrial fibrillation, an irregularity of the heart. He had one more disadvantage: Petrohilos was a Jehovah's Witness, which meant he would not be a candidate for blood transfusion. His delicate condition and complications meant he had to be handled with extreme care. Any operation was a grave danger because of the potential for Petrohilos to bleed to death.

When Jayant Patel saw the commotion on 4 March and asked what was going on, a nurse explained that Petrohilos was one of Dr Peter Miach's patients. 'Okay, I won't touch him then,' Patel replied.

The rift between Miach and Patel had only widened in the year since the Director of Medicine banned the Director of Surgery from handling certain patients. Miach had made it clear in his interview with Dr Gerry FitzGerald in February that Patel was dangerous and incompetent. Miach had even taken the unusual step several months earlier of asking to see Patel's personnel file and CV. He flicked through it in a couple of minutes, expecting to find a red flag pointing to the incompetence of the man. But it seemed in order. Miach had walked back to the ward perplexed.

But Patel could not walk away. He told the theatre nurses to prepare for an operation. Patel wanted to operate on the punctured artery of Petrohilos.

The nursing and junior medical staff were immediately alarmed. Someone called Miach and asked him to come to the ICU urgently. He walked into a bizarre and tense situation. Patel, all scrubbed up in his surgical gear, was intent on taking Petrohilos into theatre. The nurses were pleading with their eyes and body language to prevent another death.

'Just put pressure on it,' Miach said to one of the doctors. Patel loudly insisted on an operation to put a couple of stitches in the carotid artery. It was a delicate procedure under ideal conditions, but in the hands of Patel it promised to be a disaster.

Miach refused to budge. He believed that there was absolutely no chance the man would survive the operation that Patel seemed determined to perform. 'Look, the carotid doesn't need fixing,' he told Patel. 'His priorities are his heart, his anaemia, everything else.' Miach knew that by maintaining pressure on the small hole in the carotid, the bleeding would eventually stop. He gave firm instructions to a junior doctor. But he still had to silence Patel, who was angry and embarrassed. 'Look, this man is not going to theatre and that's the end of it. He's going to Brisbane,' Miach told Patel.

Toni Hoffman watched the drama with mounting alarm. Why had it come to this? She had prayed that an investigation by the Chief Health Officer would result in decisive and immediate action, but instead Patel was still wreaking havoc, still boasting about the renewal of his contract and a massive salary boost.

'Whatever you do, don't you leave this patient's bedside,' Miach instructed Hoffman. 'And if Dr Patel goes near him, telephone me immediately.'

As Hoffman stayed by Petrohilos to await the Royal Flying Doctor for an emergency flight to Brisbane, a leader of the Jehovah's Witness church in Bundaberg came to the ICU.

Hoffman already knew from contacts close to the church that Patel had ingratiated himself with the church. She had been suspicious when first told of the charm offensive. Now, one of the men who knew Petrohilos as well as Patel was in the ICU. 'Is Dr Patel available?' he asked.

Hoffman was in a panic. If she put a call through to Patel, the patient's fate would be sealed. Hoffman knew how persuasive Patel could be. He would tell the church elder that an operation to repair Petrohilos's carotid artery was absolutely imperative. He would prevail upon the elder to demand that the operation by Patel should go ahead.

'Dr Patel isn't here at the moment but the patient is going to be fine,' she said.

Ten days later, Dr Martin Strahan decided to use an endoscope to examine the stomach of Joan Cameron, who had been admitted to the medical ward with vomiting and bleeding. Strahan discovered an obstruction in the second part of her duodenum. He strongly suspected it was a secondary tumour which would require further investigation and, possibly, surgery in Brisbane.

In the corridor outside the theatre, Patel asked Strahan about the finding.

'Oh, well, that will be a primary tumour in the duodenum. The patient needs an operation to remove it and I'll put the patient in the surgical ward and I'll do it early next week,' Patel said.

Strahan suspected that Patel was wrong, and would attempt more complex surgery after opening the patient up. He was determined to prevent Patel operating. But how?

When Cameron developed a chest infection a few days later, Strahan seized the opportunity to remove her from Patel's grasp. He spoke to Dr Miach, Dr Martin Carter and Hoffman about a plan to hide the patient in the ICU, a safe refuge since Patel no longer ventured there. From the ICU, Cameron could be quietly transferred to Brisbane. They were all in agreement.

At the time Strahan regarded it as outrageous behaviour to have to resort to a ruse to keep an ill patient away from the Director of Surgery. He was also worried about how Patel would retaliate when he found out.

But the bizarre episode had made a more profound impression on Hoffman. Her mind was made up now. She had to expose Patel and worry about the consequences later.

PART TWO

COVER IT UP

29

Make or break

18 March 2005

THE two-lane road from Bundaberg to seaside Bargara was one Toni Hoffman had travelled often. Its red-dirt shoulders give way to waving fields of sugarcane, strawberry plantations, acres of beans and roadside produce stalls with hand-lettered signs.

The nurse noticed none of these as she gripped the wheel of her burgundy red Nissan Pulsar and sped through a storm and fierce rain to Rob Messenger's office. Hoffman was going outside the secretive Queensland Health system by approaching a local parliamentarian. She didn't know if he could be trusted. She didn't know if he would believe her. Her anxiety mounted as the familiar scenery flew by. She felt sadness. Anger. Fear. Tension.

After Patel's boastful announcement that his contract at the hospital had been extended, Hoffman and the nurses who supported her felt helpless. Hoffman had made up her mind to ring Messenger to set up an appointment. Afterwards, reflecting on what she had briefly told him in that first tentative telephone conversation, she feared Messenger would think she was unhinged. She confided her plan to Karen Fox, telling her: 'You know, I'm ringing him up and saying "patients are dying at the hospital". And he's probably thinking: "this woman's crazy, this can't be happening". But it is happening.'

Messenger's staff had gone home by the time Hoffman arrived about 5.30 pm at shop 7, Bargara Plaza. Her make-up was streaked by tears. He sat her down with a mini-disc recorder, his preferred tool when receiving sensitive complaints from constituents or sources. You could never be too careful in the cut and thrust of Queensland politics.

'Can I get you to state your name please?' Messenger started like a copper conducting a record of interview with a criminal. Except his delivery was gentle and patient.

'Yeah, Toni Hoffman.'

'Toni, do you want to claim whistleblower status?' Messenger asked, hoping the nurse would seek the limited protection afforded to public servants making a serious disclosure to a local politician.

'Yes.'

'Have you come to me because you believe that Dr Patel is incompetent and is killing people?'

'Yes. Yes, I do.'

There. It was done. She would not turn back now. For the next 90 minutes, Hoffman let Messenger know the entire dreadful story.

Messenger asked Hoffman if she was fearful. She replied:

I guess I'm more distressed than scared because I've watched patients die. I feel that every time I see him walk in the unit, I feel sick because I just think who's he going to kill now? What's he going to do now? And we all feel like that, all the nurses feel like that.

They feel physically ill when he walks in because they just know that he's going to try and interfere with something, operate on someone and cause more of a problem and a complication, or stop a transfer which has been arranged.

He says he trained in the United States. We did a search on the Net because there's a site there that you can look up physicians' qualifications and it says that he trained in India in 1973 and that he has a general qualification.

He continually tells us all sorts of things like he's been a trauma surgeon for 25 years and that he has been a cardiothoracic surgeon for about 15 years. He seems to have a new qualification every time he talks about it but we've not seen any of that. He also stated he studied medicine when he was only 15 years old so, you know, like, we sort of don't believe very much of what he says because, you know, it's just impossible.

Messenger wanted to know about the culture of the hospital. He had his views about how a moribund or incompetent management might be impotent to act against a dangerous doctor. Those views were about to be strongly reinforced.

'I think of all the places I've worked in, I've never worked in a place like this. There's bullying, intimidation, you can't trust that anybody is going to tell the truth...the nurses hold the hospital together and there are some great doctors but these few people hold the hospital together and the district manager takes the credit for it,' Hoffman said.

'You say,' continued Messenger, his quietly effective interviewing style honed as a commentator behind the microphone in the local ABC radio studios, 'in some of that literature that I've read, Dr Patel insists on keeping patients longer than what the unit is equipped to keep. Can you explain that?' Hoffman responded:

Well, as I said, we only keep patients for 24 to 48 hours. We do try and keep them for longer and we often do keep them for longer. And we substitute our staffing with overtime.

But Dr Patel refused to transfer his patients to Brisbane. He said he wasn't going to practise medicine like that. And he would go up to Dr Keating and throw a tantrum and say he was leaving or resigning. Or just refused to transfer them out.

Sometimes we would have a bed in Brisbane for a patient, especially if they were quite sick, and Dr Patel would stop the transfer and then we would lose the bed because Brisbane would need the bed for someone else. So he consistently would interfere and stop the transfer to Brisbane which caused enormous problems for us as nurses.

I mean, we were continually putting people on overtime. It blew out our budget for the first time in four years, because we had patients, we kept patients for so long, and the thing is that the patients weren't getting the care that they needed anyway because he's not a good doctor. The complication rate was so high. All these patients had huge complications that weren't being addressed properly.

What we've tried to do through Queensland Health is go through the right channels and address this properly, but it doesn't seem to have worked.

I've come to you because, I guess, as a last resort. Because we didn't know what else to do. I mean, I'm here not only as a representative for my own concerns but I'm here representing the concerns of a lot of people who are too scared to come. We've been told that we're not allowed to come and see you.

We literally are at the point where we are just about throwing ourselves over the top of the patients to protect them from this man, you know. And this is just ridiculous. This is crazy stuff. This is 2005. This should not be happening.

You know we've got this Code of Conduct that exists in Queensland Health and we're supposed to have all these things that protect us and the patients in place. And nothing is working. And that's why I guess I'm here, I'm asking you, who has nothing to do with the hospital whatsoever, to try and do something to save these patients from this man.

We don't know what to do or where to go. Like, who else can we tell? You know, we joked about it the other day and said: 'What else can we do? Strip naked and hang from the tree outside the Red Rooster and scream out to Bundaberg that this is what's happening at the hospital?'

So this is what I hope – that he gets stood down while there's a proper investigation done.

It was dark outside. Still pouring with rain. Almost 7.30 pm. Messenger had everything he needed. It was sensational. More powerful than any of the information brought to him in the past by people wronged by the hospital where his mother had given birth to him. Where his mother died.

There was something else. Serendipity? Whatever, it was a year to the day since his maiden speech in State Parliament when he pledged to campaign on health. He had ended the speech with a comment about evil prospering while good men remained silent. Now he wanted to shout the Patel disaster from the rooftops.

He reassured Hoffman. The poor woman, a lifetime Labor loyalist who had not voted for Messenger and never supported his National Party, looked a wreck from worry and sleeplessness.

'Okay, we'll leave it there,' he said. 'I know what to do.'

Hoffman eyed the dark rain-streaked windows and sighed as she prepared to go back out into the storm.

30

Political football

19–22 March 2005

IN a booming electorate few expected him to hold after his surprise 2004 triumph, Rob Messenger was run off his feet. The needs and expectations of working-class families and sea-change retirees were constant. He and his constituents were fortunate. Messenger had great stamina, patience, a methodical personality and dedicated staff.

He had been shaken by the intensity of the secret meeting with Hoffman and her shocking revelations. The documentation she handed to him was extensive and worrying. It corroborated her emotive story. He had been told by too many staff and patients that Bundaberg Base Hospital was a house of horrors. He had witnessed his own mother's battle with cancer there. He intuitively knew Hoffman was right. But he had to play it safe. A bad call now could stall his political career. Within his own beleaguered National Party, one or two colleagues envied his increasing popularity. They would not mind seeing him trip up.

His speeches and press releases highlighting the problems at the hospital were routinely used against him by the Labor Party's Nita Cunningham, the elected representative for the adjoining seat. For hammering the local hospital and revealing its ills, he was regularly accused of demoralising the staff and worsening the problems by hammering the local hospital and revealing its ills. If he publicly took on the Director of Surgery, he would be picking his biggest fight yet. It was conceivable the man would resign, Messenger knew. Who would be around to repair the worn-out knees? Perform the colonoscopies? Cut away the cancer? And if Patel were not as bad as Hoffman claimed, the community would be up in arms. If Messenger forced an innocent surgeon out of the hospital, the politician's head would be on the chopping block and the voters would lop it off pronto.

After asking his staff to transcribe the record of interview, he went -to the country town of Calliope and then to Gladstone on the coast for National Party business. By Sunday evening when he checked for email, every word of his conversation with Hoffman two days prior was at his fingertips. He read it again on his computer screen, shaking his head at the seriousness of it all as he scrolled the text.

He spoke to Mike Horan, the reliable parliamentarian from Toowoomba, west of Brisbane. Horan had been a health minister in a former Coalition government. He listened intently to Messenger's version of the meeting with Hoffman. Horan gravely told the young understudy he had a duty to act with urgency.

Before meeting his political colleagues to explain the bombshell and work out a strategy on how best to drop it, Messenger called Dr Martin Strahan, a highly qualified physician in Bundaberg. Strahan was known to Messenger. In the confidential October 2004 memo Hoffman had written to Peter Leck setting out the concerns over Patel, she specifically related one of her conversations with Strahan. It followed the death of Des Bramich. Messenger read the passage in the memo again.

> The day after the patient's death, when I thought he had safely been transferred to Brisbane, Dr Strahan came to talk to me in the office and found me very distressed. He offered to talk to some of the other doctors and get back to me as the representative of the AMA in Bundaberg. He did this. He stated 'there is widespread concern, but at the moment no one is willing to stick their neck out'. He urged me to keep stats on my concerns.

Messenger dialled Strahan's number. It was a confidential query, Messenger explained to Strahan, before candidly revealing how he had received statements and information about Patel and the serious concerns over his competence. He asked Strahan, a dry-humoured Seventh Day Adventist who abhorred unhealthy habits like smoking and drinking, about the chain-smoking, wine-loving incompetent surgeon. Did other doctors at the hospital, or the Visiting Medical Officers who had contact with Patel and his patients, share the concerns about the Director of Surgery?

'Yes, I know about Dr Patel,' Strahan replied. 'We think he's going to resign in June and we'd like this matter to go away quietly. However, if this man was to stay on for another 12 months, we'd have serious concerns.'

The response floored Messenger. Knowing that the matters were under review by Queensland Health, Strahan, a former secretary and president of the Bundaberg and District Local Medical Association, urged Messenger not to go public with the issue. If Messenger outed Patel, Strahan added, every patient who had been operated on by the Director of Surgery would be anxious.

Messenger found this attitude hard to comprehend. Later, he would be furious. Strahan was effectively corroborating the story about Patel being dangerous. Messenger did not know what was worse: the confirmation, or the reluctance of the doctors to act. He decided to smash their protective nexus. If nobody said anything and Patel left quietly, he would wreak more damage at the next hospital he went to.

Messenger became excited and a little apprehensive as his opportunity to go public with the scandal loomed. He planned to rely on parliamentary privilege, the protection afforded elected politicians. It permitted him to speak without fear of legal retribution. It was a permanent immunity. He would get his chance soon. On 22 March, State Parliament would convene for the seventh sitting day of 2005. Messenger began rehearsing his questions.

The plan he had developed in the party room would be a double act. To reinforce the seriousness of the issue and lend support, the party's shadow health minister, Stuart Copeland, would join in. That way, it would be harder for the media or the minister to write it off as the baseless outpourings of an inexperienced politician suffering relevance deprivation syndrome.

The day began unpromisingly for Messenger. As he took his seat on the Opposition benches, waited for the moment of truth and mentally reworked his speech, he was jolted to attention. At 9.30 am, the Speaker of Parliament, Ray Hollis, went to his grand chair. The journalists in the gallery above milled around with notepads as media officers handed out press releases and briefing notes. But, already, one of the Beattie Government's more experienced head kickers was on his feet, accusing Messenger of lying. Robert Schwarten, the Minister for Public Works, Housing and Racing, put the boot in. The issue turned on claims of bungling over the installation of air conditioners in a Bundaberg public school. Messenger had raised it in Parliament a fortnight earlier. Now, Schwarten was questioning his honesty. 'It is important that honourable members in this Parliament reflect accurately the facts and not mislead the House,' Schwarten thundered. If it was a pre-emptive attack with the specific aim of undermining Messenger's credibility before he went public with Patel, it meant something had leaked. It could presage a plot or a set-up.

The parliamentary session that morning featured the usual verbal fisticuffs between members of the Opposition and those of the Beattie Government. Emergency Services Minister Chris Cummins was wounded. Cummins, one of the lightweights in Cabinet, was exposed by National Party leader Lawrence Springborg for trying to dodge payment of parking fines. Liddy Clark, the former ABC *Playschool* presenter who had been sacked after a brief stint as Indigenous Affairs Minister, resented Springborg for describing her as less than truthful. She called him an 'absolute grub'.

Beattie sang the praises of the Smart State and trumpeted that Queensland's public hospital waiting times for elective surgery were the best in Australia.

Health Minister Gordon Nuttall pledged improvements at the crisis-torn John Tonge Centre, where thousands of forensic samples needed urgently by police and the courts were awaiting scrutiny by too few overworked scientists. It was a story I had been writing after a helpful leak from the embattled staff there.

Messenger tensed as Copeland stood and spoke:

My question is to the Minister for Health. I refer to the fact finding process conducted by Dr FitzGerald, the Chief Health Officer, into serious allegations made about the clinical and surgical competence of Dr Patel, a surgeon operating at Bundaberg Base Hospital.

The allegations involve approximately 14 patients who have suffered serious post-operative complications, including death, following surgery performed by Dr Patel. As the findings of the process have not been released publicly to date and to ensure that first-class patient care is provided at Bundaberg Base Hospital, will the minister now release these findings?

Will the minister have the allegations independently investigated? Will Dr Patel be stood aside while he is under such investigation?

Nuttall, who had no idea what Copeland was talking about, tried a stalling tactic. 'In relation to the issues raised by the honourable member, they are matters for the Medical Board. I am not aware of the issues raised by the honourable member. I am more than happy as the minister responsible to investigate those matters,' Nuttall said. 'I will meet with the CEO of the Medical Board today and speak with him about those issues. I am more than happy to give the member the details of what I find out from the CEO of the Medical Board.'

Mike Horan, a parliamentary ally to Messenger, exploded. 'You should have known about this – there were deaths! A 100 per cent strike rate.'

By noon, Messenger was ready for his speaking part on Patel. He wanted to make sure nobody misunderstood the significance.

For the protection of patients at the Bundaberg Base Hospital Intensive Care Unit and the wellbeing of the medical staff, I make public and table a letter from the nurse unit manager of the Bundaberg Base Hospital ICU.

This letter alleges serious concerns relating to the behaviour and clinical competence of Dr Patel, an overseas trained surgeon working at the Bundaberg Base Hospital ICU.

The letter submitted to the management of the Bundaberg Base Hospital on or around 22 October 2004 lists the cases of approximately 14 former patients of the Bundaberg Base

Hospital ICU who the writer believed required formal investigations.

I am astounded that the Minister for Health, as witnessed by his reply this morning to a question without notice from the shadow health minister, was ignorant of the investigation.

Messenger began reading aloud paragraphs of Hoffman's October 2004 letter to Peter Leck. He emphasised how Dr Patel was feared by nursing and medical staff as very powerful and that 'anyone who tried to alert the authorities about their concerns would lose their jobs'. Messenger issued a plea to Nuttall to release the findings of FitzGerald's clinical audit report and start a thorough review of the entire hospital and its administration:

> I challenge the minister to guarantee that all staff members who choose to give evidence be afforded full whistleblower status and that they be protected from any vindictive administrative action.
>
> Pending the results of this investigation, the minister must immediately stand aside and suspend from work surgeon Dr Patel and senior administrative staff Peter Leck and Dr Darren Keating. The staff of the Bundaberg Base Hospital ICU are desperate.

After Messenger sat down, Liberal leader Bob Quinn lamented a 'government that does nothing to address emerging problems until those problems become full-blown crises'. Health, according to Quinn, was one of those crises.

Malcolm Cole, the *Courier-Mail*'s political correspondent, was on the telephone in the parliamentary press gallery. He half heard the attack launched by Messenger, whose credibility was yet to be proved to some of the journalists covering politics. 'We'll need to file on this,' Cole said to his colleague, Rosemary Odgers. She, too, had heard the attack. Odgers doubted the veracity of the story. Still, the *Courier-Mail* was the paper of record. She decided to write a few paragraphs.

Behind the scenes, the political machinery began to move.

BY the time Rob Messenger had finished his parliamentary spray, Gordon Nuttall was close to having a ministerial meltdown for being left out of the loop by his top departmental staff. He furiously ordered his staff to find the Chief Health Officer and demand answers. Fast. So much for the policy of 'no surprises', Nuttall seethed, as he relived the embarrassment of being ambushed by Stuart Copeland and Messenger. 'What is going on at Bundaberg Hospital?' Nuttall asked.

Paul Dall'Alba, the senior departmental liaison officer, telephoned Gerry FitzGerald and explained the questions in Parliament. At 10.53 am, Dall'Alba emailed FitzGerald:

> Mr Copeland stated that you are investigating post-operative complications and asked if the Minister would release the report and suspend Dr Patel.
> Can you please provide some dot points by return email to allow the D-G to verbally brief the Minister this afternoon.
> We may then need to organise a Parliamentary Question-time brief for tomorrow so the Minister can respond to the question in Parliament.

Dall'Alba was ordered to summon FitzGerald to a 6 pm meeting with Nuttall at Room A37 in Parliament House. 'Glenda Viner will meet you at Main entrance to Parliament House,' Dall'Alba told him.

Dall'Alba asked David Potter, the media manager for Nuttall, to transmit the parliamentary Hansard transcript and the statements tabled by Messenger to Queensland Health's two media managers, Leisa Schultz and Phil Nickerson. Peter Leck was also to receive the material. Paranoid about the probable media interest, Dall'Alba then briefed Schultz, Nickerson and another public relations flack, Paul Michaels:

> Due to the nature of the statements made, it is likely that media attention will result.
> D-G has advised that Q Health response should be along the following lines:
> – District Manager has sought assistance in evaluating the appropriateness of surgical services at Bundaberg.

– This review is underway and Queensland Health will consider recommendations when complete.

In his naturally disarming manner, Gerry FitzGerald explained to Steve Buckland the background to the Bundaberg audit and its preliminary indications of Patel's competence. 'He's not as good as some, but he's not as bad as others,' the Chief Health Officer told Buckland. FitzGerald, who was waiting on comparative figures for wound breakdowns, complications and organ injuries, confirmed that Patel had a high infection rate and attempted too many complex procedures. He hoped to finalise his report in the next 48 hours.

Already, however, FitzGerald should have been alarmed by some of the findings. One stood out. Too many patients had suffered bile duct injuries after routine surgery by Patel. The procedure, laparoscopic cholecystectomy, involves the removal of the gall bladder via tubes inserted through small incisions in the abdominal wall. It is a common and uncomplicated operation for people in pain from gall stones. Before Patel arrived at the hospital, the rate of bile duct injury was zero. Over the ensuing 18 months, Patel's patients appeared to have suffered bile duct injuries at an alarming rate – 28 times the national average. For someone supposedly as experienced and senior as a director of surgery, it was horrendous.

At his desk, FitzGerald produced a document for Nuttall to rely on if he were asked more questions by Messenger. The first part of the document was confidential, and not for public release. It told Nuttall:

> Procedures have been performed at Bundaberg which are beyond the capacity and facilities of the Bundaberg Hospital.
>
> The significant issue regarding the competency of Dr Patel appears to relate to his preparedness to take on cases which are beyond the capacity of the Bundaberg Hospital and possibly beyond his personal capacity.
>
> There is no evidence that his general surgical skills are inappropriate or incompetent.

FitzGerald prepared the second part of the document for public release. Under the heading 'Suggested Response', he helpfully provided a page of points, setting them out so they would sound like Nuttall's handiwork should he read the page in Parliament to fend off Messenger.

I have now been informed of concerns raised by staff at the Bundaberg Hospital in regard to some general surgical services provided at the hospital.

The Chief Health Officer, Dr Gerry FitzGerald, has undertaken a review of clinical outcomes at the hospital and is currently finalising his report.

Dr FitzGerald has identified a number of issues of concern at the hospital and will be making recommendations in regard to those concerns.

There is insufficient evidence at this time to take any particular action against any individual, and to suspend anyone would be unjust and inappropriate.

The Bundaberg Hospital has taken certain action to limit the scope of some general surgery performed at the hospital which should address the majority of issues raised by staff. The report will also make recommendations regarding the management of staff conflict at the hospital.

However, the report has also identified that there is a relatively high satisfaction amongst patients and that waiting times for elective surgery have been reduced considerably in recent times.

Junior staff have been very complimentary in regard to the teaching and guidance provided to them.

However, Dr FitzGerald has raised concerns about the clinical judgement exercised by one member of staff and will be referring these concerns to the Medical Board for consideration.

Later in the day, after his documents had been emailed to Dall'Alba, the Chief Health Officer briefed Nuttall personally.

Back in the office, I watched the 6 pm TV news which featured the silliness of Chris Cummins in his efforts to evade parking fines. Colleagues Des Houghton and Jamie Walker, watching with me in the office, made jokes at Cummins's expense. Rob Messenger's revelations went unnoticed.

Paul Dall'Alba knew the *Bundaberg NewsMail* would run the Patel story. Peter Leck told him the *NewsMail*'s reporter had a copy of the document Hoffman had compiled in October 2004 when she detailed the Patel concerns and the bad outcomes for patients.

31

Natural justice

23 March 2005

'TRUCK OFF BRIDGE', reported Bundaberg's *NewsMail* on its front page the next day. '"Very, very lucky" was how Emergency Services described a 56-year-old man who survived a 5m fall in his truck and endured two hours trapped in the cabin yesterday.'

Rob Messenger had tipped off the *NewsMail*'s Dan Nancarrow about the Jayant Patel allegations. The young journalist's two articles were relegated to page 5 under the heading 'Taking an in-depth look at issues of interest to people in our area'. Peter Leck had told Nancarrow: 'It is important Dr Patel receives natural justice and is given the opportunity to respond to any allegations that have been made.'

In the *Courier-Mail*, the story barely rated a mention – just a brief summary under the heading 'Fast News'. Blink and you would've missed it. I saw the item while scanning the newspaper at home. When I went to work and logged on to the parliamentary web site, I felt distinctly uneasy. I pointed the item out to the *Courier-Mail*'s news editor, Graham Lloyd. 'I think we've seriously underplayed the story,' I said. 'Look at the allegations – an incompetent surgeon whose patients are dying. It all came out in Parliament.'

I told Lloyd of my earlier contact with a concerned nurse. I explained how I had wanted to launch a proper investigation when the yellow A4 envelope arrived a few weeks earlier, but had been unable to see my way clear of other stories.

Lloyd knew what to do. He said he would ask Ryan Heffernan, a tenacious newsroom colleague, to follow the story in the meantime.

WHEN Gordon Nuttall spoke in State Parliament at 10.20 am, he went on the front foot, describing Rob Messenger as 'totally irresponsible' for airing the Patel matters while Gerry FitzGerald's clinical audit was incomplete. Messenger, according to Nuttall, had circumvented 'all natural justice processes' to vilify a health professional:

> I can tell the House that some of the allegations made by the Member for Burnett are not only inaccurate but could also be considered deliberately misleading.
>
> Should any issues be raised regarding the professional performance of an individual clinician as a result of the clinical audit into surgical services, these will be referred to the Medical Board to be investigated.
>
> I am advised that at the conclusion of the audit of surgical services, the director-general will refer any outstanding issues which are appropriate to the powers and function of the Medical Board to that board.

Nuttall's incomplete response omitted FitzGerald's own advice that he had formed concerns over Patel's clinical judgement.

Despite everything the nurses had told FitzGerald, despite the figures showing the remarkable complication rates, despite the failure of the Bundaberg Hospital administration to ensure Patel had been credentialled, the Director of Surgery was still safe. He was still operating. Still being given the benefit of the doubt.

When Toni Hoffman saw Dr Martin Strahan in the Intensive Care Unit he told her: 'You'll be lucky to keep your job after this.'

As the hospital seethed with rumours, Strahan also visited Leck. Divulging the telephone call he had received from Messenger, Strahan told Leck that no doctor would have stooped so low in leaking details about a fellow medical practitioner to a parliamentarian. The clear implication was that the culprit must be a nurse. Strahan, who suspected Hoffman, also tipped off Leck about something Messenger had indicated: the information was leaked to him by a nurse.

Patel, who had been briefed by Leck about the furore in distant Brisbane, passed Hoffman in the corridor and stared straight ahead. He was full of swagger and confidence as he walked to the theatre to wield the scalpel again. One of his patients that day would suffer an avoidable complication. Gail Aylmer considered Patel's rhinoceros-thick hide. She would have had a grudging respect for the man – so stoic in the face of adversity – had she not already decided he was a psychopathic narcissist.

With Linda Mulligan away on holidays, the acting Director of Nursing, Deanne Walls, was in the hot seat. She called a meeting of ICU staff. Hoffman had devoured the brief reports in the *NewsMail* and fretted over the lack of attention by the *Courier-Mail*. When she heard of the upcoming meeting, she felt her worries and fears easing. 'We're going to be supported now, everything will be fine,' Hoffman told the other nurses. She called in those nurses who were on days off. Hoffman wanted all who had joined her in raising concerns to come in to receive the support from management.

After Hoffman and nurses Karen Jenner, Jan Marks, Karen Fox and Vivian Tapiolas went to the tea room in ICU, Walls arrived with Leck. The District Manager was visibly furious as he waved around documentation and spoke of the severe consequences of leaks. The nurses believed the papers he held were sections of the Health Services Act and the Code of Conduct, setting out the penalty of two years imprisonment for staff who leaked information: 'In the course of their work, health service staff come in contact with information that must be kept confidential at all times. All employees are reminded that irresponsible discussion of any matters regarding the health service facilities, staff and, most importantly, the patients, is regarded as an offence.

'I'm appalled!' Leck said. He repeatedly condemned the handover of statements to Messenger, saying 'very high sources' had confirmed it came from an ICU staffer. 'I have good information as to who this person is,' he said, adding the leaker had brought shame to the hospital.

Hoffman was paralysed with shock and fear. She had only told one person, Karen Fox, about her meeting with Messenger. Leck's claim to know the source was almost as worrying as his failure to address the issues of patients dying unnecessarily. How did politicians operate, Hoffman wondered. Was it all a big game? Did they rat on sources?

When Leck claimed the airing of the Patel issues had 'caused a rift between the medical and nursing staff', Karen Jenner was astonished. In her two years as a nurse at the hospital, she had not met Leck until now. She could not recall him ever visiting the ICU. Shortly before the 1.30 pm meeting, she had been told by Jan Marks that the Patel story was on the radio.

Hoffman had warned several nurses that the media might try to contact those nurses whose names were on the document tabled in Parliament. Jenner, who hurriedly read the *NewsMail* before going to the tea room, figured that Leck had come to give advice on dealing with any journalists who might call for comment. She expected his backing, not a barrage of vitriol. There was no chance to ask him questions or put another side of the story. Immediately after his outburst, he got up and left. 'How dare he speak to us like that,' Jenner said.

Walls, who had no prior knowledge of the complaints and the depth of feeling in the ICU over Patel, told the nurses that management had spoken. 'Let it go now,' she said.

At 2.30 pm Leck fronted another meeting in the conference room outside the executive offices. He berated the more senior nurses this time. Robyn Pollock, the nurse in charge of the Renal Unit, learned by email that attendance was mandatory. She was a few minutes late. When she arrived Leck was admonishing her colleagues. Pollock wanted to say 'if management had handled this matter appropriately and dealt with the complaints about Patel back when they were made, you wouldn't be in this position now'. But Leck's anger was intimidating. He said the leaker was a nurse.

'Are you sure? How do you know that,' asked one of the nurses.

'I have it from a reliable source, but it is not just one source, I have two or three people that can verify it was a nurse,' Leck said.

Gail Aylmer bridled at the accusatory tone in Leck's furious diatribe. She resented being blamed over the leak and felt powerless to defend herself and her colleagues. She feared a nurse would be made a scapegoat for the leak when the bigger issue was the lethal incompetence of a surgeon. What sort of mixed-up management shot the messenger and ignored the message?

'Are you going to track this person down?' one of the nurses asked Leck.

Leck said something about it not being his immediate priority. At the end of the tirade he stormed out.

The afternoon was filled with tension. To the nurses, Patel appeared unmoved. But the surgeon seized the opportunity to confront Leck and demanded his complete backing. Leck could see that Patel was incensed at the questioning of his competence. 'Unless you send a letter of support to the *Bundaberg NewsMail* in relation to my work, I will resign,' Patel said. The Director of Surgery pledged to quit within 24 hours if he did not see signs of rock-solid backing from management. Patel spoke about launching legal action against everyone involved in what he saw as a plot to oust him.

When Leck could get a word in, he tried to placate Patel by apologising. Despite his grave concerns about the surgeon's incompetence, Leck was more worried about the need to continue churning through the waiting lists than the welfare of the patients being injured and killed.

'He acknowledges the support provided so far by myself, the Minister and others but wants some further backing,' Leck explained later to Dall'Alba. 'I'm advised that Dr Patel is the only general surgeon who will be in Bundaberg over the coming Easter weekend. His departure at this time would be critical to service delivery.' Leck told Dall'Alba he 'found only one patient letter of complaint relating to Dr Patel – from a family whose father was treated mainly by another surgeon'.

He sent to Dall'Alba a draft of the letter he would soon despatch to the *NewsMail*.

I refer to the article of March 23 concerning allegations made against Dr Jay Patel.

The fact that a number of allegations have been made public without completion of a review process designed to ensure the application of natural justice, is reprehensible.

At this time, I have received no advice indicating that the allegations have been substantiated.

A range of systems are in place to monitor patient safety and the community can be assured that we constantly work to improve our service delivery.

Dr Patel is an industrious surgeon who has spent many years working to improve the lives of ordinary people in both the United States and Australia.

He deserves a fair go.

PETER LECK
District Manager
Bundaberg Health Service District

A little while later, Leck went to the evening meeting of the District Health Council, which was part of a Queensland Health public relations exercise to pretend it was interested in the input of hand-picked community members. Its chairman, Viv Chase, who was cranky and in poor health with diabetes, received a nominal $500 a year to attend meetings.

Chase no longer wielded much influence – certainly nothing like when he was the local mayor – but this evening he was prepared to take a stand. Messenger was at it again, running down the local hospital. Chase knew little about what was really going on in the hospital; Leck simply didn't bother briefing him on the sensitive issues. In his ignorance of the situation, Chase had become sick and tired of the constant carping by Messenger.

As Joan Dooley, Leck's secretary, took the minutes of the meeting, Leck gave an overview of the Patel issues. One of the members, Dr Denise Powell, the president of the Local Medical Association, briefed everyone on the media interest, including TV follow-ups. Powell stressed that the local medical community was standing behind Patel. There was no mistaking the mood of the meeting. Whatever the significance of the allegations, the patients ran a poor second to the interests of Patel.

The meeting gave Powell the green light to speak to Messenger. Perhaps a chat could reassure the maverick parliamentarian or quieten him down. And everyone on the District Health Council was in favour of providing a letter of support to Patel.

32

Damage control

24 March 2005

BERYL Crosby is the type of down-to-earth person described by TV reporters and producers as 'great talent'. Although unknown in the media world, she had a story that might make or break a ratings night for the Nine Network's *A Current Affair* in its perennial war with Seven's *Today Tonight*. Her story and picture on the front page of the *NewsMail* and on an inside page in the *Courier-Mail* had excited Paul Ransley, Queensland chief of *A Current Affair*.

'Beryl Crosby was organising her own funeral when she found out being diagnosed with cancer had been a medical mistake. Mrs Crosby claims the doctor responsible was Jayant Patel – the man at the centre of malpractice allegations read out in State Parliament by Member for Burnett Rob Messenger this week,' the *NewsMail* had reported.

'I thought it was a one-off case,' Mrs Crosby said. 'I hope by not taking action back then I didn't add to anyone else's grief.'

Ransley, a former investigative journalist with the *Sunday* program, hoped the morbidly fascinating story would beat whatever *Today Tonight* might serve up. Its sharp new producer, Karin Cooper, was closing the gap in the ratings. He held an early-morning phone-conference with his counterparts in Sydney. They liked the angle. It was one of those back-from-the-dead stories with universal appeal. Ransley asked his veteran foot-in-the-door reporter David Margan and a crew to rush to Bundaberg to interview Crosby.

'Oh my God. It's like a frigging movie,' said Crosby as she did her first TV walk. The crew needed footage of her strolling. Smelling the roses. It was part of the package.

Crosby's transition from obscurity to public limelight had happened quickly. It started after her daughter saw the first day of local headlines about Patel. She called her mum and told her to buy the newspaper. Crosby sat transfixed as she read the brief stories. She wondered if her own brush with Patel was relevant. A sales representative between jobs, she plucked up the courage to call Messenger's office at Bargara and explained how Patel had treated her. She was told to expect a call from Messenger, who was still in Brisbane attending Parliament.

When Crosby explained how Patel had misdiagnosed cancer, Messenger cried. He still grieved for his mother. Just recalling her death at the hospital after a fight with cancer reduced him to tears. It was the moment Crosby decided Messenger was a good man. She felt she could trust him.

'When I come back up I would love to come and see you,' Messenger said. 'You should get a damn good lawyer and sue them for everything they've got.'

Messenger was a pragmatist. He knew that Crosby's story would help to validate some of the concerns about Patel. It might also ease the pressure he was under for naming Patel in Parliament. He asked Crosby if she would do some media. He wanted her to tell her story to the newspaper and TV reporters. He even offered to make the arrangements.

A short time later, the *NewsMail* arrived on Crosby's doorstep. My colleague Ryan Heffernan from the *Courier-Mail* had also telephoned her. And that was just the start of the media interest. The print articles were the bait for the follow-ups by *A Current Affair* and *Today Tonight*. The pressure on Patel, his bosses in Bundaberg and the bureaucracy in Brisbane mounted with each new headline.

Patel had it out with Peter Leck again, accusing the district manager of failing to rally robust support. Patel walked off in a rage.

'Dr Patel has just resigned effective immediately,' Leck wrote to Dan Bergin, the Queensland Health zonal manager, and Paul Michaels, one of their media advisers, just after lunch. 'He has indicated that he plans to take legal action against a variety of staff as well as Queensland Health for failing to stop the leak of confidential information and for not providing definitive support in relation to the allegations. There are no general surgeons in Bundaberg (privately or publicly) as from 8 am this morning (except Dr Patel).'

As the media scrambled to reach Bundaberg, Gerry FitzGerald, having received the data he needed to verify Patel's off-the-scale rate of complications, gave his final report to Steve Buckland. They met to talk about it. The clinical audit dealt with carnage on a grand scale, yet it was written in such a way that the reader might not be immediately alarmed. It began like this: 'Bundaberg is a progressive modern city with a population of 44,670, where residents are catered for with excellent shopping, medical services, education facilities and a diversity of recreational pursuits and experiences including the coral isles, coast and country.' On page 7, the report states:

> In general, staff have enjoyed their work at Bundaberg Hospital and only recently have issues arisen which have caused concern. However, as well as raising concerns, some staff made complimentary comments about the divisional director's commitment to teaching and mentoring of junior medical staff. In addition, there has been a significant improvement in efficiency, especially in the operating theatre, and in meeting elective surgery targets with significant reductions in waiting times for surgery.

FitzGerald compiled the report with regard to what was known as a 'no blame' protocol. Patel's name did not appear in the report. He was referred to by title with comments such as: 'The Director of Surgery has high standards and this has led to some degree of conflict with staff.' Only by reading between the lines and analysing the figures on complications at the back of the report would it have been possible to ascertain the seriousness of the matter. But as the report remained under a strict veil of secrecy, none of the patients or staff of the hospital would know.

Buckland, however, received an additional piece of advice. FitzGerald had attached a confidential memorandum to the report. The memorandum was alarming. For Buckland's eyes only, it stated:

> In February this year I was asked to undertake a clinical audit of general surgical services at Bundaberg Hospital.

As you are aware, the events which triggered this audit have now been the subject of questions in Parliament.

The report of the clinical audit is now complete and I have attached a copy to this memorandum. There are issues which I need to bring to your attention.

There is evidence that the Director of Surgery at Bundaberg Hospital has a significantly higher surgical complication rate than the peer group rate.

In addition, he appears to have undertaken types of surgery which, in my view, are beyond the capability of Bundaberg Hospital and possibly beyond his own skills and experience, although his surgical competence has not been examined in detail.

I believe his judgement, both in undertaking these procedures and also delaying the transfer of patients to a higher level facility, is below that which is expected by Queensland Health. I would recommend that these matters should be examined by the Medical Board and have written to the Executive Officer – Mr Jim O'Dempsey, bringing the matter to his attention.

The audit report also identifies that there has been a failure of systems at the hospital which has led to a delay in the resolution of these matters.

The credentials and clinical privileges committee has not appropriately considered or credentialed the doctor concerned. The executive management team at the hospital does not appear to have responded in a timely or effective manner to the concerns raised by staff, some of which were raised over 12 months ago.

While the report makes a number of recommendations for system improvements, I would recommend that some discussion should occur with the hospital management, reminding them of their responsibilities to put such systems in place and ensure they respond appropriately to reasonable clinical quality concerns.

Dr Gerry FitzGerald
Chief Health Officer
24/03/2005

FitzGerald wrote also to O'Dempsey: 'I wish to formally bring to your attention and seek assessment of the performance of Dr Jayant Patel who is the Director of Surgery at Bundaberg Hospital.' FitzGerald advised the Medical Board of evidence that the outcomes of complex operations performed by Patel 'were relatively poor, with at least two of the patients dying in the immediate post-operative period. In addition, data produced during the audit demonstrated a significantly higher rate of complications than the peer group average, however, we have not been able to exclude the impact of differential severity on this complication rate.'

But FitzGerald did not send his report to the Board. Nor did he send it to Peter Leck in Bundaberg. And despite the preliminary findings, neither Buckland nor FitzGerald considered suspending Patel. Based on what he knew at that time, Buckland, the man in overall charge of all the hospitals and staff in Queensland Health, would not have permitted Patel to come near him with a scalpel. But Buckland's priority was to keep Patel operating.

When Buckland spoke to Leck in the late afternoon, Patel was still threatening to sue everyone, including his employer. Patel also knew that without him, there would be no surgeon on duty over the Easter break, when thousands of families would be on the roads. There were always smashes. Broken and twisted limbs. Damaged organs. Hospital staff would be run off their feet and the nightly news could be counted on to grimly update the road toll each evening. It was the hospital's most critical time of need. By threatening to refuse to work unless certain conditions were met, Patel put Leck, who was not coping under the pressure, into a state of dread.

In his time of need, Patel was being flattered by fellow doctors who rushed to defend him. 'I would have no hesitation of having this highly qualified surgeon operate on any member of my family or myself,' Dr Kees Nydam wrote in a public declaration of support. Nydam regarded the primary role of newspapers to be the publisher of comics and his letters. Furious with the nurses, Nydam, who was in the chair as acting Director of Medical Services when Patel was first employed at the hospital, said he was 'vacillating between sadness and disgust' over the public shaming.

As president of the Local Medical Association, Dr Denise Powell was urged to show her support for Patel. She said the organisation felt he had made a 'positive contribution to the community'.

In Brisbane, the big guns lined up on Messenger. They had the politician in their sights. Dr David Molloy, president of the Australian Medical Association's Queensland branch, said Patel had spent many years training and practising in the United States. 'There is every probability that there was no negligence involved in the surgeon's practice and the issue before the Medical Board mostly relates to the scope of surgery being completed in a country centre,' Molloy said. 'The Opposition has acted irresponsibly by accusing a Bundaberg surgeon of professional incompetence in the interests of cheap political gain, and perverting the course of justice.'

At 5.25 pm, the relentless Rob Messenger launched another broadside in State Parliament against Nuttall, accusing the minister of instructing his department to run Queensland Health with the 'pretend I am a mushroom' approach:

> If we listen to the minister, everything is rosy and fine with the Bundaberg Hospital. There are no shonky surgeons, no access block, no shortage of beds and no mental health crisis, and nurses and hospital employees are not being bullied or vilified by the administration.
>
> But the facts of the matter are quite different. I repeat my call that not only should surgeon Dr Patel be suspended. Administrators Mr Peter Leck and Dr Darren Keating should also be suspended.
>
> They have lost the confidence of the staff and the patients of the Bundaberg Hospital. The minister can trust me not to hide the reality of what is happening in our wards and operating theatres.

In an angry aside not recorded by the Hansard reporters, Nuttall shouted at Messenger across the chamber: 'I hope you're satisfied that he's resigned. You are responsible for the lack of a surgeon in Bundaberg over the Easter break.'

Leck dashed off an email to Buckland to update him on Patel's latest demands. He had changed his mind about quitting – and was weighing an offer of a four-month contract from 1 April 2005. His current contract would finish in six days, on 31 March. In his email Leck said:

> I offered support by suggesting he take a few days' leave to consider his position and the future.
>
> Dr Patel indicated that he had been doing that and was prepared to return to work tomorrow if he was offered a contract of $1500 – $2000 a day (he wants something close to $2000) from 1 April through to July.
>
> He also wants the organisation to fully support him but was no longer explicit in his demand that we back him in relation to all the procedures he has undertaken in Bundaberg.

Buckland's day was worsening. The story on *A Current Affair* had given the Patel fiasco a national profile. It suggested the surgeon was about to quit. Messenger's latest attack had made Nuttall angrier. And the PR flacks were under pressure.

The loss of a patient's life was of far less concern to the organisation than damaging headlines. According to Queensland Health's little-known Risk Matrix, an official policy developed by a senior bureaucrat strictly for internal use, an adverse clinical incident is weighted as 'major' if someone dies. Publicity that significantly damages the organisation's reputation, however, has a heavier weighting of 'extreme'.

Apart from Bundaberg Hospital, Buckland had another problem. It was my story that day in the *Courier-Mail*, disclosing how Queensland Health staff at the John Tonge forensic laboratories were being threatened with imprisonment over the leak about serious testing problems and maladministration. Nuttall went on morning radio to attempt damage control. He expressed surprise at the suggestions that his organisation was secretive.

Although no patients' details were disclosed, the scientists had been warned by senior staff that an internal investigation would be followed by a police probe, which could lead to criminal charges. They were told to get independent legal advice and prepare for questioning. The crackdown terrified Toni Hoffman. Queensland Health issued a bland statement saying it was usual practice 'to investigate any unauthorised release of confidential documents as such actions are breaches of the Code of Conduct'.

Meanwhile, Buckland told Leck the surgical service had to be supported over the Easter break. They needed to keep Patel operating. 'I think he should work over Easter and we would look at his contract from 01 April during next week. The offer of $2000/day is unacceptable and would never be supported.'

Patel, larger than life, was out for dinner at a popular restaurant overlooking the ocean at Bargara. With its stylish timber fittings and furniture and a vast menu, Kacy's was a local favourite. Patel loudly talked up his surgical skills. His dinner companion, Dr Ayesha Curtis, a bright young intern on secondment from the Mater Misericordiae Hospital in Brisbane, wanted the ground to swallow her up.

Two months earlier, Patel's sexual advances almost caused her to quit her stint in Bundaberg. Curtis was sure she had not misinterpreted Patel's crude repertoire. The man had said he wanted to marry her and start a new life. Before the tolling of any wedding bells, he promised to write glowing reports about her surgical performance. There was a catch. He wanted sexual favours in the meantime.

When he had come on strongly in January, Curtis was worried about how to reject Patel without offending him and jeopardising her career. She quietly sought advice and support from Judy O'Connor, the Medical Education Officer, and Dr Kees Nydam. Curtis decided she would politely decline Patel's suggestions and tough it out.

After Rob Messenger slammed Patel in Parliament, Curtis heard rumours that he was going to quit and return to the US. She felt sorry for him and accepted his offer of dinner. Curtis soon regretted it. Patel was coming on stronger than ever. Over a couple of glasses of wine, he was offering further inducements.

The next morning, Curtis decided to terminate her contract early. She did not want to wait to find out if Patel was staying or leaving.

33

Nagging doubts

Good Friday, 25 March 2005

I SAT at my desk on Friday afternoon and contemplated the imminent start of a week's holiday – a visit to my parents-in-law in Mackay and a family camping expedition at Hook Island farther north. As the Friday afternoon wound down and my colleagues headed to the Jubilee Hotel for a few drinks in the Journalists' Bar I remained troubled by Rob Messenger's revelations in State Parliament three days earlier. A yellow A4-sized envelope from Toni Hoffman – who had followed through on my request of months earlier to send documentary evidence supporting her concerns – was still gathering dust on my desk. It contained copies of the statements Messenger had tabled on 22 and 23 March. On a partition erected at my desk to give colleague Craig Johnstone and myself some privacy as we cajoled and flattered our contacts, I had months earlier pinned a list of stories I wanted to write. My most recent scrawl was 'Overseas Trained Doctors – the ticking time-bomb'. I wanted to launch again into an issue that had alarmed me when I wrote about it in November 2003. At the time it went nowhere. But the time-bomb had been ticking for some time now. Had Messenger sped it up?

I was also troubled on Friday afternoon because I had not found time to investigate the statements in the yellow envelope sent by Hoffman in late February. The clues to Jayant Patel's negligence fell between the cracks. In my determination to prove myself after two costly legal actions brought separately in 2004 by men who believed they had been unfairly injured by my reporting, I aggressively pursued a couple of big stories in early 2005.

The major one explored the circumstances surrounding a Crime and Misconduct Commission investigation into an alleged bribery attempt by Peter Beattie of an impoverished Aboriginal community on Palm Island, near Townsville. Beattie, who faced a prison term if found guilty, was severely rattled by the scandal. He was livid with me for reporting that he had been tape-recorded while making the bribery pitch: the waiver of an $800000 debt in return for a public truce with the community's Indigenous leaders. Beattie had sought their smiles, handshakes and a cessation of all hostilities. If they agreed, he would gain political kudos in front of a media throng which had arrived on the island. The bait was the cash.

When the scandal broke it threatened not just his career but also his freedom. After the revelation about the tape-recorder was published with Beattie's comments, which a reliable source had provided to me, the Premier faced immense pressure in State Parliament. Under relentless questioning by the Opposition, he admitted that he had made the comments attributed to him.

Subsequent investigations by the CMC showed the tape was blank. The tape-recording machine had malfunctioned. The comments which had been provided to me were based on a detailed written file note made by the lawyers who heard Beattie. Beattie, who had adopted the potentially incriminating comments as entirely accurate on the basis that there was a tape-recording, was furious. He felt he had been tricked by my sources into admitting the truthfulness of a conversation which could amount to a bribe.

My contacts and personal loathing of the government's hideous addiction to secrecy delivered another scoop as the dust settled on Beattie's problem. It came in the form of Cathi Taylor, a bureaucrat from Beattie's inner circle who was appointed Freedom of Information Commissioner. Taylor lacked qualifications for the job and failed to even make the short-list until the intervention of Beattie's top public servant, Leo Keliher, on the selection panel. Happily for Taylor, one of her referees was Keliher.

One of Taylor's first decisions as Commissioner was to sack Greg Sorensen, the deputy and one of the most experienced FOI officers in Australia. Sorensen had angered the Beattie Government for being too open with public information. Taylor's elevation and Sorensen's ousting appalled even some of Beattie's backers. Beattie had sent a message that the secrecy would become worse. As I developed this story of ugly opportunism, the yellow envelope lay dormant.

In early March, before Messenger's outpouring, I had fired up my reporting colleague Michael McKenna to join me in investigating the contents of Hoffman's envelope. 'Mickey, are you up for a trip to Bundaberg?' I asked McKenna, who was back from leave after reporting on the death and destruction in Sri Lanka following the Asian tsunami.

McKenna, whose father was a prominent and respected patholo- gist before retiring, had also written about concerns over the screening of Overseas Trained Doctors. He understood the issues. But until Messenger stood up, the other big stories had devoured our attention.

Now, on the afternoon of Good Friday, my plan was to take Hoffman's Bundaberg Hospital material to Mackay to show my father- in-law, Dr Iain Mathewson, a retired GP. If Iain reckoned the state- ments indicated potential wrongdoing, I would return to work ready to take the story further.

My last task for the day involved emailing Hoffman. I wanted to buy some time by assuring her that I remained keenly interested.

Dear Toni, I've been following with interest the revelations in State Parliament through your local member, Mr Messenger. I've got your statements.

And I'm aware that the whole story is yet to be told. I'm hoping to be able to come up to investigate a lot of the issues and speak to you, confidentially, and some of the other nurses, doctors, patients and their families in April. Would you be able to assist? I'll be away next week.

Regards
Hedley Thomas

Hoffman, worried sick and feeling increasingly isolated at her home in Bundaberg, replied a few days later:

I would very much like to meet with you and tell you the whole story, which is huge. As you can imagine, I'm in heaps of trouble, although I have denied all. To this point I have not 'breached the code of conduct' by going to the media. I have been threatened with the CMC, I have read your excellent journalism with interest and the issue surrounding John Tonge scares me. In spite of this I will meet you, as long as I can remain anonymous.

I don't know if anyone will want to speak out now because of the threats. What can you get with FOI? Can you get access to the 'fact-finding mission' by Gerry FitzGerald? Qld Gov employees desperately need some sort of agency we can go to when we have real concerns. At the moment the issue has been taken off the real issue (the patients' deaths, etc) and is focused on who leaked the information.

We really tried to go through the right channels and nothing happened. I will wait to hear from you, I will help you with what I can,

Thanks, Toni

34

Renewed interest

26 March 2005

THE kitchen bench at Iain and Mary Mathewson's modest house in Slade Point is often strewn with paper. Magazines and torn-out articles about medicine, science, the environment, inventions and current affairs vie for precious space, occasionally prompting Mary, who prefers a less cluttered life, to take matters into her own hands and file them in the bin under the sink.

Most of the time, my mother-in-law tolerated the eccentricities of her gentle husband, Iain. Like many extraordinarily intelligent people, Iain, who went to medical school in Aberdeen north of his birthplace of Edinburgh, could make a hash of basic everyday tasks. It took Mary an eternity to teach him how to double-click with a mouse. He would leave the house for hours at a time with the oven turned on. Operating the microwave was a major challenge. Occasionally, there would be an explosion of food or cutlery. Once, he managed to set a baked potato alight. Yet when it came to issues like the impact of genetics on the brain, advanced hydraulics and the history of space, Iain understood the detail and often developed new theories.

As a GP and senior partner for many years in the Central Medical Group, a private practice in Mackay, he was loved by his patients and colleagues alike. There were many tears over his retirement due to ill health. His patients felt they had lost a doctor who cared passionately about their health. He was one of the few GPs left who regularly did house calls for elderly or ill patients. Even in retirement he gave up his time to check on former patients. Whenever our children were unwell,

Iain was consulted first for an opinion. He listened carefully before offering a prognosis. It always turned out correct.

Years after leaving the job, he remained intensely interested in his profession, its development and policies. As he knew all the senior medical practitioners in Mackay, he was aware of the culture of bullying and the fears Queensland Health staff had about speaking out about problems. He had been surprised at the reluctance of some of his friends to speak frankly to me, off the record, about serious mismanagement issues they had witnessed in the hospitals and emergency departments in which they worked. They had confided to Iain and initially wanted to talk but backed off, fearing retribution. Iain disdained the culture of concealment in the State Government. Peter Beattie's hypocrisy over Freedom of Information stuck in Iain's craw.

He was still cranky that the Medical Board of Queensland wanted to take away from retired practitioners the time-honoured right to call themselves doctors.

'Politicians like Beattie get honorary doctorates. We went to university for ours. Why do they think they can take ours away?' he asked in his Scottish brogue.

After a few single malt whiskies from a favourite Highlands distillery, we sometimes convened a meeting of our own peculiar political organisation, the two-member Don't Vote For Anyone Party, with its platform of reversing the law that made voting compulsory. Our motto was taken from George Bernard Shaw. 'Politics is too dangerous a subject to be left to politicians,' he said.

On Saturday 26 March, Iain sat at the cluttered kitchen bench, absorbed in the statements Toni Hoffman had sent to me. Mary prepared dinner, a particularly spicy Indian chicken curry.

Having grown up in a hospital environment in Kuching, on the island of Sarawak in Malaysia, Mary slipped easily into nursing after leaving school. Her father, Thantoney Marimuthu, whose family came from Madras in India, was a manager and operating theatre superintendent at the hospital where his daughter won her first job. She quickly fell in love with the tall, gangly, bagpipe-playing Scot who had left the bitter winters of Scotland to practise in the little hospital in exotic Kuching. Their courtship had the blessing of Mary's mother, Clare

Guan, a Chinese woman whose marriage to an Indian man had caused a scandal three decades earlier.

After eight years together in Malaysia and then Brunei, where Iain anaesthetised the world's richest man when the Sultan of Brunei fell from his polo pony, the family moved to Mackay. Mary was for years a formidable force in the Central Queensland town, running the Red Cross Blood Bank and surpassing plasma donation targets. Donors and friends nicknamed her Bloody Mary.

'This does not look good,' said Iain, stroking his chin as he leaned into the kitchen counter and read about the avoidable deaths and injuries. 'It is very serious. The nurse in charge of the intensive care unit has a very responsible position. Her opinions should be taken seriously. I really think you should examine the matters more thoroughly when you go back to work.'

Iain's obvious concern surprised me. A fierce critic of lawyers who made money running legal actions against doctors, he had always been conservative and protective of fellow medical practitioners. Mistakes were inevitable. Doctors were not infallible. Iain, I knew, would almost always give a doctor the benefit of the doubt. I suspected he adhered to an unwritten code that discouraged doctors from speaking out about other doctors. One explained it simply: 'There but for the grace of God go I.'

Iain set out in layperson's language the unusual circumstances surrounding several of the procedures and deaths listed in Hoffman's statements. 'Some of the things described do not make sense,' he said. 'I don't doubt the documentation. I think this doctor has some serious competence issues.'

As it was a Saturday, I telephoned a friend, David Murray, a journalist on the *Sunday Mail* who was dating my wife Ruth's sister, Catriona.

'Are you guys doing anything about this doctor who was named in Parliament?' I asked.

Murray, busy with something else and facing an early deadline, was not aware of any interest in the Patel story.

'Iain has read some statements about the operations. You know how conservative he is about doctors. He reckons there's a lot more to this and I think he's right. He was shocked at some of the things this doctor did. He wants me to follow it up when I go back to work, but that won't be for another week. What do you reckon?'

Murray considered my unsubtle suggestion that he start investigating it. But he was bogged down. 'Sorry, mate, I can't do it,' he said. 'I hope you can pick it up when you're in next.'

35

Time to go

26 March to 1 April 2005

JAYANT Patel began organising his escape. Although he had told Peter Leck that he might stay on in Bundaberg, Patel prepared a contingency plan. Leck could keep his health system. Patel just wanted out of Bundaberg. He wanted to put as much distance as possible between himself and the bad news.

He went to see Peter Cronin, the operator of the local Jetset Sunstate travel agency. Patel said he wanted a one-way ticket to Portland, Oregon. Business class. Cronin looked at the schedule. It was a handy commission. Walk-in purchasers of an international business class fare worth $3500 were rare in Bundaberg.

Patel had been a good customer, spending a small fortune in the past on international travel for himself and his wife and daughter who came to visit.

Most of the locals who travelled abroad spent weeks planning their itinerary and poring over various options. Often they wasted the travel agency's time before buying a cheaper fare on the Internet. But Patel made the arrangements on the spot and said he would pay with cash. Cronin booked a flight leaving Bundaberg for Brisbane on 2 April, with an overnight stay at the Comfort Inn and Suites at Northgate, close to the airport. The onward flight from Brisbane to the United States would depart on 3 April, a week before Patel's 55th birthday.

After two years at Bundaberg Base Hospital, Patel had seen more than 1450 patients and performed more than 1000 operations. The damage he had wreaked was incalculable.

Now he was going to flee, scot free.

ON April Fool's Day Jayant Patel was about to have the last laugh. He was booked to return to the United States but even at this late stage, Queensland Health management and the Medical Board of Queensland expected he might stay on as Director of Surgery.

Patel packed his bags. He would miss the apartment at Bargara with its views east over the beach and the water.

At 8.30am, one of the hospital's administrative staff called Duncan Hill, an officer at the Medical Board, to find out if Patel's registration had been renewed since lapsing on March 31. Hill asked to be transferred to Peter Leck, who said he still did not know whether the surgeon was staying or leaving.

For the next few hours, Patel went back and forth from Leck's office claiming to be unable to make up his mind on whether to accept the offer of a new four-month contract.

Leck massaged Patel's ego. He bent over backwards trying to accommodate him.

When Patel saw Kees Nydam, his original sponsor from 2003, in the corridor at the hospital three days before the departure date, Patel explained he had already paid $3500 for a flight back to the United States. 'Am I able to claim this?' he asked.

'Yes, absolutely,' said Nydam.

Emboldened, Patel told Leck he wanted full reimbursement for the business class airfare and the overnight accommodation in Brisbane. It was duly authorised.

In the previous three days, Patel had enjoyed 'stress-related sick leave'. He used it well, hosting a farewell party at the Indian Curry Bazaar Restaurant. All his Bundaberg friends came. There were the nurses whom he had favoured, the doctors and a handful of the administrative staff. They championed Patel and condemned those responsible for smearing his good name.

Rob Messenger, steaming over the AMA's latest attack on him for naming Patel in Parliament, was watching ducks on a pond in Hervey Bay during an Indigenous youth leadership forum. They appeared to move effortlessly yet he knew they were frantically kicking beneath the water. Messenger was feeling like a sitting duck himself. Maybe even a political dead duck. Nobody apart from the anonymous hospital staff and a handful of patients had backed him since he outed Patel.

Dr David Molloy, head of the AMA, had gone out of his way to lambast Messenger. 'It's an absolute disgrace that Dr Patel has been forced to leave his job, based on a gross misjudgement on the Opposition's part,' Molloy said. 'Mr Messenger should realise that having no one to care for his constituents when they are injured and there is no emergency care for Bundaberg is a terrible problem.'

Using his mobile phone outside the forum, Messenger called Molloy to ask whether the AMA Queensland president had even read the letters tabled in State Parliament.

Molloy was conciliatory. No, he replied.

'Isn't it about time that you got your facts straight before you start making public comments?' Messenger said.

He heard Molloy say he had it on good authority that Patel was an innocent victim who had merely been 'trying to whip some lazy nurses into shape'.

Once again, the medical community was sticking together. In Brisbane, Kerry Gallagher, chief executive of the AMA in Queensland, put the finishing touches to a counter-attack on Messenger.

Gallagher enjoyed writing for *Doctor Q*, the organisation's glossy magazine. And he particularly enjoyed writing the article, 'Plumbing New Depths', which began: 'In Queensland you would expect, certainly at my age, nothing that came from Queensland parliament, Queensland politics, and most definitely from Queensland politicians would surprise. This week, however, Queensland parliament and one politician in particular did surprise. Sadly! Indeed, it is more correct to say disappoint and disgust rather than surprise.'

Accusing Messenger of 'plumbing depths of politics that would normally be too low even for the average bathysphere to reach', Gallagher scoffed at the notion that the local parliamentarian's cause might have been noble. He borrowed a quote from a British priest who had been dead for half a century and applied it to Messenger: 'A loud noise at one end and no sense of responsibility at the other.'

'Finally, I note that the Member for Burnett is the shadow minister for education and the arts. Oh dear, oh dear, oh dear!' Gallagher concluded.

Toni Hoffman had heard the AMA's blasts and its smug repudiation of Messenger. Hoffman feared the worst. She and the other nurses trusted only one Queensland Health executive – the Chief Health Officer, Dr Gerry FitzGerald – but they were bitterly disappointed at the time he was taking to do something.

Toni had kept his card since the visit in February, and called him. FitzGerald listened carefully as the experienced nurse broke down.

'We feel we are being made the scapegoats in this,' Hoffman told him through her tears.

FitzGerald was surprised. 'My report is not going to say that,' he said. 'It's going to validate what you have said.'

36

Calm before the storm

Early April 2005

THE few nights camping on Hook Island after staying with the Mathewsons in Mackay made for our best family holiday. Framed pictures of the kids in their snorkelling gear would soon adorn a shelf in the office.

Back at my desk, I had a new project – this shadowy fellow, Jayant Patel, and the nurse, Toni Hoffman. She was going to extraordinary lengths to out him.

John Doyle walked over to talk about the status of a few of our Freedom of Information applications. In his last job, Doyle had been a senior officer in charge of the Queensland Police Service's Freedom of Information Unit at Roma Street headquarters. Until his retirement he was one of the umpires who made decisions on the release of thousands of documents. He had dealt previously with Paul Whittaker, a relentless reporter and an experienced user of Freedom of Information, who had suggested to Doyle that in his spare time he should work for the *Courier-Mail*.

In early 2004 after Whittaker, my brother-in-law, resigned to go to the *Australian* in Sydney, I followed up with Doyle and negotiated his contract.

He began coming in one day a week to develop applications and reply to FOI officers when they used spurious reasons to justify concealment. Doyle was kept busy battling a culture of secrecy, fostered at the top by Beattie and his ministers and their political advisers. As a public servant he had been a part of the system, but he was never a political hostage. Doyle released documents during his time as FOI chief if the applications were appropriately targeted and there were no legitimate reasons to prevent disclosure. Now, working for us, he witnessed his former counterparts in other departments clutching at straws and relying on nonsense arguments to stymie a request.

We were awaiting a response from Queensland Health to one of our targeted requests, unrelated to Patel.

A source had explained how all FOI applications to Queensland Health, and particularly those made by journalists and the State Opposition or by patients where the information sought was sensitive, were vetted at every stage in the department and the minister's office. This was highly inappropriate. It put further pressure on the officers tasked with deciding whether documentation could be released. Before the FOI officers could release a single page, the political hacks in the minister's office were consulted and afforded every opportunity to sabotage the exercise. Principles of transparency and openness had been discarded. The game, sanctioned at the leadership level of government, involved concealing as much as possible for purely political reasons. The cover-up had been perfected. Democracy could rot.

Doyle grinned mischievously. Our latest application to Queensland Health aimed to catch them out at their own game. It sought all documents – created by policy advisers, media advisers, the FOI officers themselves, the minister and any other bureaucrats – which related to the handling of previous FOI applications. It was a nightmare for a secretive department full of control freaks because it could, potentially, show up the brazen efforts to hide material.

After Doyle walked away, I renewed contact with the nurse from Bundaberg:

Hi Toni,

I'm back after Easter hols – thanks for replying last week. You can be assured of a couple of things – nobody will know about our contact; and if asked, I will refuse to disclose your identity or anything that could identify you.

When would be convenient to meet or talk? What is happening now? I saw the AMA Pres, David Molloy, went on the offensive in attacking your local MP, which I guess he had to do in defence of one of his members (Patel) but it seemed to deflect attention away from the doctor's conduct.

While on leave I showed the statements to my father-in-law, a very experienced doctor, who was appalled at the many botch-ups and decoded the medical language for me.

I gather the report by FitzGerald is close to completion – do you know about that and what it is likely to find?

Regards
Hedley

Her reply came just a couple of hours later.

Hi Hedley,

Thanks for your reply, I have never been in this situation before and I am appalled at what has happened to the nurses in this situation. Everyone has the right of reply but us. At least 8 ICU nurses had made the initial and related complaints, the Report is with the DG now, I do know a little of what is in it, but I am so scared about being whistle blown I don't want to say much.

Gerry Fitzgerald is a really nice man and I would rather someone else say what is in it. Our concerns were valid. Rob Messenger has really gone out on a limb with this, but I feel he is a loose cannon and even more naive than me in some ways.

There is so much going on here and so many lies, and so MUCH politics, that it really bothers me about the veracity of people who want to work in this field. I am sure your father-in-law would be really horrified at what was in the letter. Imagine living through it on a daily basis. I am coming to Brisbane on Thurs for a conference at RBH. It is finished at 1530. If you think we could meet at the airport or elsewhere, we are catching the last plane back to B'Berg. I think it leaves about 1840.

If this is not a good idea, and you want to come up here, I will make myself available. At the moment this is the only thing I haven't done to break the code of conduct (which is supposed to protect whistleblowers), so I am quite worried about it all.

This is not politically motivated, I have always voted labor, I say this because my only concern is for the patients and the staff. I am disgusted with the AMA and Exec though. They all called Patel 'dr Death' and dr E Coli etc. Incredibly two faced.

Hoffman ended it with her mobile and home phone numbers.

Hi Toni,
Tomorrow afternoon would be fine – I think the airport – being such a busy place with people whom you and I may know coming and going – would not be a good location. Would you be able to come by the *Courier-Mail*'s offices in Campbell St, Bowen Hills. It is near the city, en route to the airport. We can have a quiet and discreet chat in the staff restaurant where nobody will know you or your friend. Please bring all relevant docs with you.

Regards
Hedley

Hi Hedley,
Hopefully we will be there around 1600 depending on when the conference ends, I don't have much with me as I have only just got home now, but I can always send what you want after we discuss,

Toni

37

What the...!

4–6 April 2005

DARREN Keating returned from his Easter vacation to a shambles. He had missed all the action: the furore over Rob Messenger's disclosures to State Parliament on 22 and 23 March, the fallout at the hospital and the sudden resignation and departure of Jayant Patel to the United States.

Keating was angry. Everything had spiralled out of control as he took a fortnight's break with his family. He knew that the Queensland Health chiefs in Charlotte Street would be decidedly unimpressed with the negative feedback and media interest. Thankfully, it appeared to have died down after a burst of reporting by *A Current Affair, Today Tonight*, the *Bundaberg NewsMail* and the *Courier-Mail*.

The official line for public consumption was being scripted out of Queensland Health's headquarters in Brisbane. Keating would leave the PR to the flacks. He had his hands full in dealing with the ramifications of losing Jayant Patel. The elective surgery targets would be even harder, if not impossible, to meet. All the work, the throughput of hundreds of patients, had blown up in management's face. It was humiliating.

Keating had made an educated guess about the probable source of the information that had fallen into Messenger's hands. Toni Hoffman. He would deal with her and any other collaborators later. The paperwork came first. Keating wrote to the Department of Immigration on 5 April, formally withdrawing the hospital's sponsorship of Patel's visa.

Leck was also busy writing. He drafted a note to Patel. Leck wanted it signed by the hospital's community representative, Viv Chase, and sent to Patel in Oregon.

Dear Dr Patel,

I am writing on behalf of the District Health Council to offer our support and to advise that we are deeply saddened and appalled by the disclosure in State Parliament of confidential information, which has subsequently led to your decision to leave Bundaberg.

I would like to express my thanks for all your hard work while you were here and for the care you provided to the residents of our community.

All the best wishes for your future.

Yours sincerely,

Viv Chase

Chairperson

Bundaberg District Health Council

05/04/2005

After Leck's secretary, Joan Dooley, had typed the draft and told Chase it was ready, he came in to sign and post it. 'It is probably not exactly what I would have said, but that will do,' Chase commented as he perused the letter.

The next morning, Keating – after reflecting overnight on the damage caused by the disclosures and the embarrassment being suffered by Queensland Health and the Health Minister – prepared a memorandum for distribution to all medical and nursing staff. Nobody, least of all management in Charlotte Street, which took a dim view of uncontrolled leaks, would misunderstand Keating's position.

Dear All,

Since my return from leave, I have become very aware that all medical staff at BBH are unhappy with the recent events leading up to Dr Patel's resignation. The lack of natural justice afforded to Dr Patel so as to respond to the allegations, due to the leaking of an internal letter to a local MP who tabled this letter in parliament to his political advantage, is scurrilous. The potential damage to the working relationship between medical and nursing staff at BBH is very worrying.

Nevertheless patient care must continue and I ask you to continue to perform your jobs to your normal high standard while continuing to build upon the professional links that exist in all departments. Locums have been arranged from 11 April while interviews are occurring shortly for the Director of Surgery position and I hope it is filled as soon as possible.

This incident provides an opportunity to ensure that nothing similar occurs in the future. I would welcome your feedback (in whatever form) about what strategies should be used to prevent a similar occurrence.

The memo flattened the nurses. They were copping the blame. In the wards, Hoffman noticed that some of the staff were avoiding her. A few of the doctors who had been extremely concerned about Patel's surgery changed their tune, siding with management as it worked to shut the issue down. Dr Kees Nydam was still stroppy. Some of the doctors believed they had to stick together.

Who might be targeted next, they asked, if the nurses thought they could get away with scandalous public leaks such as this?

Keating realised that several of the senior medical staff worried they could be in the firing line in future. Some of the Overseas Trained Doctors told him so.

The culture of concealment kicked back in. Hoffman doubted she had any future at the hospital. A few of the nurses who were Patel supporters whispered behind her back as word went around that she was the one who went to Messenger.

After stating management's position in the memo, Keating left his office in the early evening with a nagging worry. Having received so many complaints from different people about the bombastic surgeon, Keating knew Patel was trouble. 'Where there is smoke, there is potentially fire,' Keating thought. 'Does he have any history in the United States?' For the first time, he decided to do some independent homework. Maybe Patel had baggage elsewhere.

On 6 April, Keating did an Internet search on his home computer. He went to the Google search engine and typed in 'Jayant Patel'. But there were too many hits. It would take forever to read them. Keating then remembered that Patel's middle initial was M, for Mukundray. He tried it and noticed a reference to a Jayant Patel in Oregon. Something twigged. Keating recalled Patel saying that was where he had come from. Patel had also boasted about his work in New York State.

Keating went first to the Oregon Board of Medical Examiners, the equivalent of the Medical Board of Queensland. The result immediately stunned him. Under the heading 'Board actions taken between April 1, 2000 and December 1, 2000', the following entry appeared: 'PATEL, Jayant M, MD15991, Portland, Or: A stipulated order was entered on September 12, 2000. The order restricted licensee from performing surgeries involving the pancreas, liver resections, and ileoanal pouch constructions.'

Keating found the definition of 'stipulated order': 'An agreement between the Board and a licensee which concludes a disciplinary investigation. The licensee admits to a violation of the Medical Practice Act, and the order imposes actions the Board and licensee agree are appropriate. Stipulated orders are disciplinary actions.'

It was more than a dilemma. Keating had stumbled on a potential catastrophe. Patel, the man Keating was publicly defending, had been severely censured in the US – and banned from performing the same complicated surgical procedures which had led to deaths, injuries and a litany of complaints.

Keating delved deeper. He double-clicked on the links to the Board for Professional Medical Conduct in New York State. The revelations there were worse. The Board on the other side of the US had ordered Patel be 'stricken from the roster of physicians in the State of New York' on 5 August 2001 for his 'gross negligence, and negligence on more than one occasion' in complicated surgical cases. There was more detail on the New York site, including a PDF file containing correspondence between Patel and the Board. It was all there: a public portrait of incompetence.

The ease with which Keating had discovered Patel's background and fraudulent conduct meant others would surely also discover it.

Keating's career, his family, the hospital's future and everything else he held dear could turn on this unexpected discovery of Patel's shocking past. Everything sped up. He knew that the next day, Minister Gordon

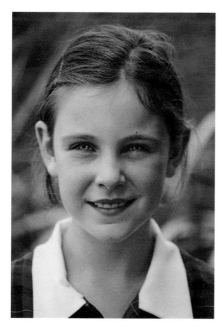

Elise Neville, whose avoidable death drew attention to the state of Queensland Health.

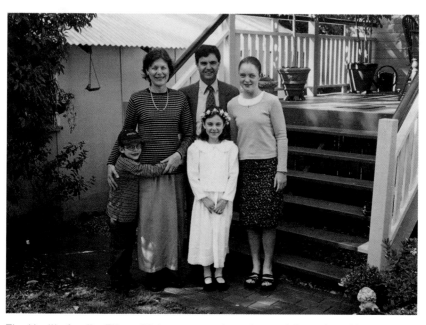

The Neville family: Elise with her parents Lorraine and Gerard, and her siblings Michael and Laura. (Private collection)

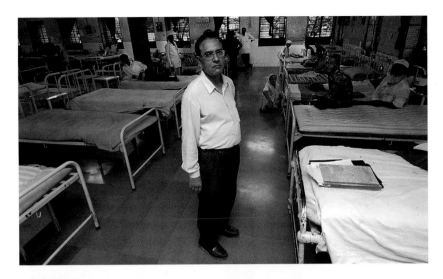

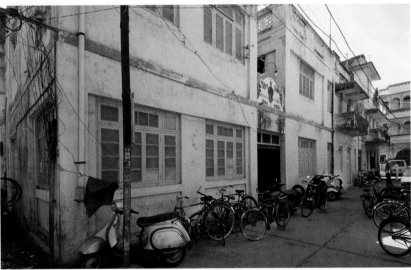

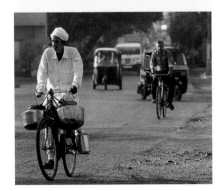

Jamnagar, June 2005:
(Top) Dr Mansurali Mamdani at the
Guru Govindsingh Hospital where
Patel was a resident.
(Above) the Patel house.
(Left) the Jamnagar streetscape.
(Courtesy of johnwilsonimages.com)

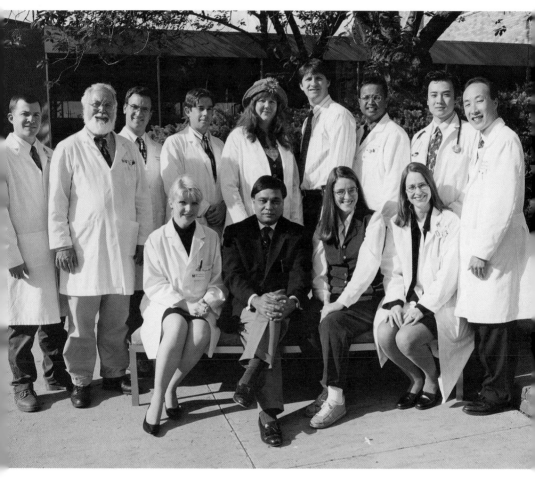

Portland, Oregon, circa 1996: Dr Patel, program director, with his students and colleagues. (Private collection)

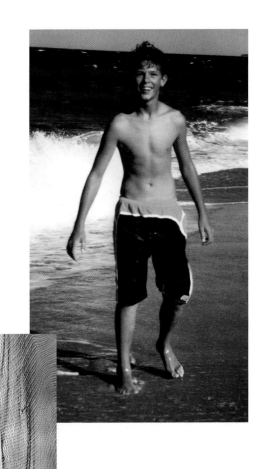

Shannon Mobbs as an active
young boy and after the accident
from which he might have made
a full recovery, had he received
appropriate medical treatment.
(Courtesy of johnwilsonimages.com)

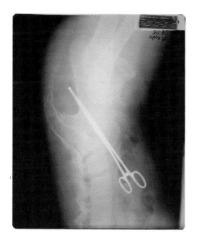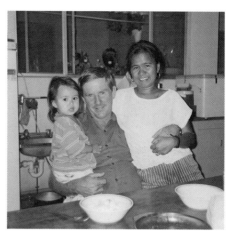

Left: This stainless steel clamp was left inside 27-year-old John Dulley after surgery by Patel. (Private collection) Right: Des and Tess Bramich with their daughter, Maria. (Private collection)

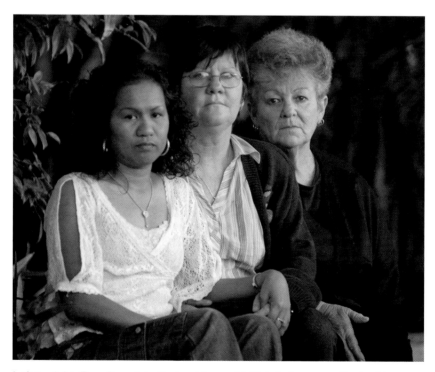

Left to right: Tess Bramich, Des's widow, with Patel's former patients, Lisa Hooper and Doris Hillier. (Courtesy of johnwilsonimages.com)

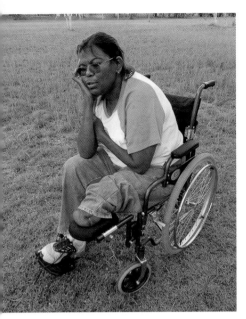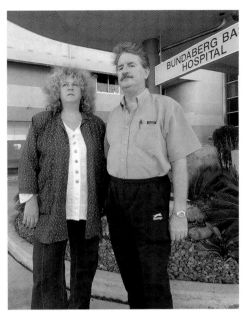

Left: Marilyn Daisy was not offered the option of a bypass operation that could have saved her leg. (Courtesy of johnwilsonimages.com)
Right: Survivors of Patel's treatment, Beryl Crosby and Ian Fleming, founding members of the Patients' Support Group. (Courtesy of johnwilsonimages.com)

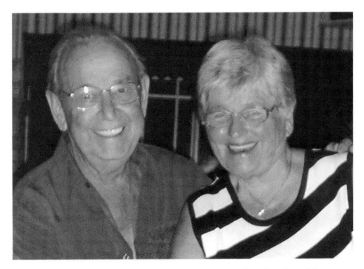

Gerry and Judy Kemps: Patel left Kemps to die after botching a complex operation. (Private collection)

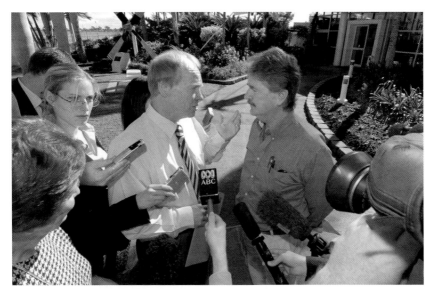

Queensland Premier Peter Beattie with Ian Fleming and the media at
Bundaberg Airport during the inquiry. (Courtesy of johnwilsonimages.com)

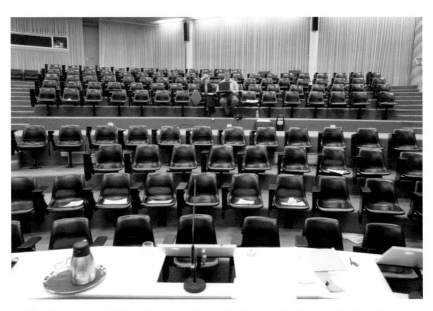

Hedley Thomas and his colleague, Amanda Watt, at the inquiry in Bundaberg.
(Courtesy of Philip Norrish)

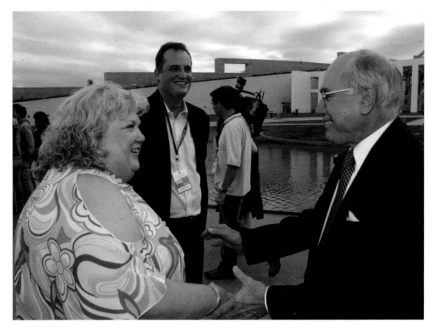

Australia Day 2006: Toni Hoffman, who received a Local Hero Award, with Prime Minister John Howard. Hedley Thomas is looking on.

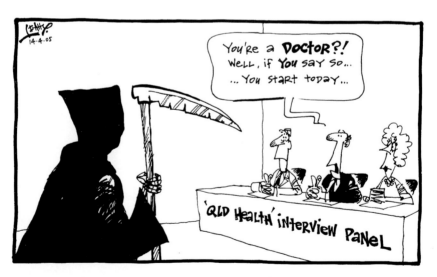

14 April 2005 (Reproduced courtesy of Sean Leahy)

Nuttall, Director-General Dr Steve Buckland and their entourage, usually a media adviser and a policy adviser, would be visiting the hospital.

Keating confided his discovery to his wife, Janine. He told one other person, a close friend whom he knew he could trust, Jennifer Kirby, who headed the District Quality and Decision Support Unit at the hospital. He talked it over with Kirby. She could scarcely believe the turn of events. Was it all true? Did the complaints she was supposed to take seriously really have substance after all?

Keating went to bed in a quandary. In the end he decided to share the pain. He decided to pass it to a manager with as much to lose as he did: Steve Buckland.

Keating, an administrator who routinely made file notes about innocuous conversations with staff or actions taken, printed nothing from his home computer. He made no physical record of the most remarkable discovery in his career. He withheld the information from Peter Leck. No paperwork would be handed to Buckland during his visit. It would be an oral briefing. Face to face. Less chance of it leaking.

38

Grind them down

3 pm, 7 April 2005

MARGARET Mears filed into the large staff dining room. The atmosphere was charged. Doctors, nurses, administrators, clerical staff – more than 100 people across every department of the hospital – had temporarily left their work stations for the visit of the Health Minister Gordon Nuttall and Director-General Dr Steve Buckland.

Mears, a highly experienced nurse whose job involved interviewing and preparing patients before their operations, booking the procedures and coordinating staff to deal with the admissions, was prepared to give Nuttall the benefit of the doubt as a politician. His previous two official visits to Bundaberg as Health Minister had been conciliatory and productive. She recalled him urging cooperation and trying to build a team spirit. On one of those visits, Nuttall had told Mears and her colleagues: 'We are sitting in a boat rowing and everyone should be rowing the same way. Those who don't want to row with us can get out of the boat now.' She liked his style. He was, she believed, working towards a better health system.

Mears, like most of those in the staff dining room, strongly suspected Nuttall's third visit was tied to the events two weeks earlier in State Parliament. Although she did not support the leaking to Rob Messenger of the documentation about patient outcomes, she was glad it meant the Patel debacle would finally be addressed.

Mears, too, had longstanding concerns about Patel's conduct. On two occasions after he had been aggressive and shouted at her, she talked to Carolyn Kennedy, the assistant Director of Nursing, but decided to take no further action. On many other occasions, the junior doctors with whom Mears regularly came in contact would confide examples of Patel's bullying and his reckless care of patients.

She had seen Patel speaking over the top of Dr Martin Carter and rudely interrupting other people in meetings involving issues of wound dehiscence, infection rates, mortality and morbidity registers, investigation registers and risk registers. The meetings became so heated, the animosity so obvious and the interjections from Patel so constant that little of substance was ever resolved. Since the Rob Messenger outpouring, Mears had also heard rumours that Dr Gerry FitzGerald's preliminary findings backed up the nurses.

Nuttall, shirt sleeves rolled up, strode to the front of the room. He could act tough, too, and in talks beforehand with Buckland they had decided to fight fire with fire. They were acutely embarrassed at being caught unawares by Messenger and Stuart Copeland. But the problem was now much worse. Patel had left. The rate of surgery was almost at a standstill. And some of those in the room were to blame.

Earlier that day, before the detour of the State Government King-Air to Bundaberg, Nuttall's visit to the nearby little town of Springsure had shown him what could happen when everyone in the same boat rowed together: Queensland Health went forward; nothing leaked; nobody was lost overboard.

'I have been to Springsure today, wonderful town, 900 people,' Nuttall told the staff at Bundaberg a little after 3 pm. 'And I have opened a community health centre which cost $250,000 and the town raised that money. What a wonderful town.'

Nuttall paused for dramatic effect before ploughing on: 'And now I am in Bundaberg.'

Mears heard Nuttall say that the only way to stop the nonsense involving Bundaberg Base Hospital was to vote Messenger out. The minister called on all patients affected by Patel's resignation 'to write to Mr Messenger personally'. 'Can we put an official report out relating to the allegations? The answer is no. There's no point in it continuing. There cannot be a report based on the lack of natural justice.'

When Nuttall stepped aside and Buckland took the floor, the Director-General went further, forcefully lecturing the staff about the damage they had done to the hospital and to the reputation of

Queensland Health and Patel. As a result of the leak, Buckland fulminated, the staff had completely screwed everything up. 'No decent doctor would want to come to Bundaberg to work in these circumstances,' he said.

The tone of the meeting was condescending and belittling. Instead of receiving feedback about Patel, the nursing staff were hit by recriminations for speaking out. Misleadingly, the doctors and nurses were told that not even the investigation by FitzGerald would be completed. As for any findings, Buckland said the staff could forget it. Nothing would be released because Patel had been denied 'natural justice'. He was now far away and unable to give his side.

Mears, by now infuriated, could not follow the logic. Surely just because a doctor goes missing does not mean an investigation cannot continue. If police reverted to such a policy, nothing would ever be solved. Did Buckland somehow imagine that had he stayed, a surgeon, particularly one with the arrogance and self-belief of Patel, would have confessed: 'Yes, it's all true, I am completely incompetent and those deaths and injuries are all down to my ineptitude'?

Mears asked Buckland what could be done about Patel.

'How are we going to get him back from America?' he replied. In other words, nothing would be done.

Karen Jenner listened in amazement. The Intensive Care Unit nurse walked into the staff dining room confident that Nuttall and Buckland were going to start a full inquiry into Patel's conduct. When she heard Nuttall and Buckland dismissing the deaths, the injuries, the incompetence and everything else she and the other nurses had strived to document after witnessing carnage on a dramatic scale, she became enraged. From the back of the dining room, she shouted out: 'Dr Patel can reply to the allegations from the United States.'

But Buckland responded with a rallying call, saying he supported his staff 100 per cent and would not tolerate anyone being tried by the media and denied natural justice. Jenner was disgusted.

'If you support your staff 100 per cent, then where is the support for the nurses who made the multiple formal complaints about Dr Patel?' Jenner replied. 'Just because one letter was leaked does not mean that the nurses are not entitled to your support.'

Buckland slapped the question and plea for support away. His patronising rejoinder stung Jenner. 'What part of "there's going to be no inquiry" don't you understand?' he said.

Even Dr Kees Nydam believed Buckland and Nuttall were overly harsh and severe.

Gail Aylmer, whose job as the nurse consultant in charge of infection control had put her in regular conflict with Patel, became angry. 'Are you trying to say that we're not going to find out the outcome of that report?' she called out.

'The report can't be released,' Buckland answered.

She wanted Buckland or Nuttall to publicly acknowledge the dire problems, not bury them with such a ludicrous justification. Even if they had said, 'Look, there are some issues with Dr Patel and we will investigate them, but we can't release them because Dr Patel has left,' Aylmer would have felt vindicated for the stand she and the other nurses had taken. Instead, she felt the nurses who had done the hard work were now being held up as the villains. At the very top, despite everything that had happened, the chiefs still weren't listening. Aylmer feared it had all been a massive waste of time. All the emotional energy and tears, the late nights preparing documentation and checking charts, the battle to produce the evidence were trashed. Their careers might be next.

Mears also feared the repercussions. As she left the meeting, still furious, a senior staff member said to her: 'Don't you like your job? Is that why you spoke up?'

Buckland was rattled.

Across town, Messenger was angry. 'The minister can't get away with covering this up,' he told the reporter from the *Bundaberg NewsMail*. 'This is an issue I will continue to pursue and keep fighting for staff.'

DARREN Keating could hold on to the explosive information no longer. But he was not going to tell Peter Leck.

After Gordon Nuttall and Steve Buckland finished their official duties, alienating most of the nurses and several doctors with stern lectures and a shutdown of the Patel issue, Keating approached the Director-General. Nuttall had left to visit a relative in a nearby private hospital in the hour before the party was due to return to Brisbane.

Buckland stepped away from the staff cafeteria.

'Can I talk to you?' said Keating. The Director of Medical Services related his stunning Internet finding of the previous evening, repeating the words 'negligence', 'gross negligence' and surgery bans in Oregon and New York State. Buckland sighed.

'This guy, he has got problems with his registration,' Keating said.

A truly awful day was turning into a disaster. And it was still early. Buckland had backed the wrong horse. Now it had bolted and he was the biggest loser.

Keating, nervous and uncertain about what would come next, studied the stocky bureaucrat's face for emotion. Buckland was a hard man to read. Keating continued with the hurried, harrowing briefing. He told Buckland that after doing the Internet search at home, he had checked Patel's personnel file, including the documentation related to his registration by the Medical Board of Queensland, and had made a further discovery. The surgeon had also lied about his past when he sought the job in Bundaberg. 'There was a copy of his application for registration as a medical practitioner and in that application, the individual...has to, yeah, declare whether they've got any restrictions, and he said no, he had no restrictions,' Keating said.

By the time Keating stopped talking, he could read Buckland like a book. The powerful bureaucrat's eyebrows were raised high on his forehead. The briefing over, Buckland headed for the airport, his head swimming. Damn. Could it get worse?

On the flight back to Brisbane, Buckland decided to hold back almost everything Keating had told him about Patel. He wanted to do his own research first. He covered his bases by telling Nuttall: 'There is more to this guy than we know. I will have a look at it. We need to continue to have a look at this guy. He's not what we think he is. I will go and have a look at him and I will come back to you.'

Above the drone of the engines powering the State Government's King-Air, Nuttall and his principal media adviser, David Potter, talked about the negative feedback from the staff meeting. In a town the size of Bundaberg, a high-powered ministerial visit to the local hospital to read the riot act to dissatisfied staff was news. Local news. They hoped it would not play out too badly in the local newspaper.

ROB Messenger was nothing if not persistent. After writing to the Medical Board of Queensland on 23 March about Patel, he wrote again on 7 April to urge action.

Michael Demy-Geroe, the Board's Deputy Registrar, reviewed the latest correspondence in the file. It was up to him to respond to the politician's muckraking. It would not do much good now that Patel had left. For Demy-Geroe, the surgeon's sudden departure was a blessing. It would save the Board the expense and trouble of investigating.

Demy-Geroe prepared his reply to Messenger, writing that it 'had been contemplated that conditions may be imposed upon Dr Patel's registration'. His resignation, however, meant 'issues of ongoing public protection and assurance of professional, safe and competent practise' were no longer relevant.

Messenger interpreted the letter as a brush-off. If you were a doctor, all you needed to do to avoid serious scrutiny was quit and try your luck elsewhere.

Strange meetings

3.50 pm, 7 April 2005

TONI Hoffman giggled nervously in the foyer of the old orange-brick Queensland Newspapers building near the top of Campbell Street, Bowen Hills.

She had come from a conference in, of all places, the Clinical Practice Improvement Centre at the nearby Royal Brisbane and Women's Hospital. I could see the massive complex from my desk. The fortunate timing of the conference in Brisbane meant she had an opportunity to meet me while many of her colleagues in Bundaberg were feeling severely bruised by Gordon Nuttall and Dr Steve Buckland.

'Karen is here to give me back-up,' Hoffman explained, introducing her friend and colleague, Karen Fox. 'She doesn't trust journalists. And she thinks I'm mad for meeting you.'

The blunt honesty moments after meeting at the front counter was a good start.

As a precaution Hoffman elected to sign the visitors' book as Jane English. Her friend signed in as Sue James. They liked their assumed names.

It was a relief to leave my desk. My previous meeting, with an elderly man who had been battling his local council for a decade over the use of an asbestos-linked product in road-base near his home, was heavy-going. His story had potential but I doubted it would get a run unless there were people who could say, 'I'm dying of mesothelioma now because my incompetent council put this lethal stuff near my home despite the obvious risks.' Stories warning of safety risks paled beside stories in which the result of unsafe practice was at once obvious.

I walked Hoffman around to the staff cafe, pointing out departments on the way. She seemed keen to talk. About anything, perhaps just to lower her anxiety levels. Her friend eyed me suspiciously and refused to utter a word.

'Can you tell me about the complaints involving the surgeon?' I asked.

Hoffman began talking in a rushing torrent of names, dates and medical terms. It was a struggle to keep up. And then she went faster. Her nervousness was driving her to try to spit out the entire two-year-debacle in a few frantic minutes as *Sky News* blared on the overhead TV and her friend stared daggers at me. Something had to give. I started to wonder about her state of mind. Clearly she was deeply agitated. Clumsily, I tried to calm her down but it sounded more like a rebuke.

'Toni, can we do this slowly, one fact at a time, please. I'm starting from a long way behind.'

She paused and began again:

There were so many botch-ups with patients and it continued on and on until this one big incident, the straw that broke the camel's back, and it took five months after that complaint.

The nurses from the Renal Unit complained. The infectious control nurses complained. In between all this we would be having the patients with complications coming into intensive care. And pretty much on a daily basis we would have a patient in ICU with some stuffup because of what he had done.

Since this all came out [in Parliament] the doctors have stood up and defended him and they were the ones who two days before had been trying to get us to defend and protect their patients. All we were trying to do was stop him from operating on patients and harming them.

He would tell us he was a cardiac, thoracic and trauma specialist. When we looked him up on the web, he just had a MBBS from a university in Pakistan. He thought that he could do everything. Even the acting Director of Medicine Dr Kees Nydam sent a letter saying he had full faith in him and would allow him to operate on his children.

Peter Leck has got up and said he was appalled that it had been leaked and that it was not due process. But where was the due process for the patients? The district manager stood up for the hospital. Nydam stood up for the doctors. But the nurses were gagged. Nobody stood up for the nurses.

Gerry FitzGerald when he interviewed me did not even have a copy of the complaint. He had not read it. His report is with the Director-General now.

A physician was hiding a patient in intensive care so that Patel would not get him. And this was just recently. We literally were throwing ourselves across the patients to stop him from getting to them.

After all that we were seeing, this guy got employee of the month. We were seeing this guy being rewarded while we lied to families and protected patients and felt sick about what was happening. We have been crying for months.

Patel had a 100 per cent complication rate with catheters. Every one of his patients got infections. He used to lie in the patients' notes. One was on 100 per cent oxygen and being kept alive with medication and Patel wrote that he was stable in his notes.

The nephrologist refused to let him operate on his patients; the hospital knew that this was going on because they had set up an alternative way for their fistulas and vas catheters to be put in.

Hoffman's account was shocking. We spoke about Patel's claim of earning the hospital an extra $500 000 a year. 'To meet the budget and surgical targets, hospitals have to do a certain amount of surgery,' she told me. 'Hospitals make money from surgical procedures. Because he was churning through the surgery, he was making them money.'

'Where is he now?' I asked.

'We have been told that Patel has left for good,' she said. 'Martin Carter, the director of IC and anaesthesia, he called him all the names under the sun; he called him Dr Death. But when the chips were down they supported him. The doctors called for the whistleblower to be identified and made an example of. I was told that they perceived the nurses have all the power and that they could be next.

'Some of the patients really liked him because he talked a lot. He was incompetent and he had a God complex. He was not malicious. He just did not realise how incompetent he was. The system has failed us. It does not allow us to be taken seriously.'

At that moment, Hoffman's mobile phone began to ring. She apologised and reached into her handbag. As she listened, her face lost colour and she balled her free hand into a fist. The caller was Gail Aylmer at the hospital.

'I can't believe it. They said what? No!' Hoffman ended the phone conversation. The composure she had worked hard to maintain in our interview was gone. She dabbed her eyes.

'The Director-General and Gordon Nuttall were just there,' she said. 'And they said that seeing as it was leaked, they are not going to release the report. They had nothing to say to vindicate the nurses.'

The chance call to Hoffman's mobile clinched it for me. The visit by Nuttall and Buckland to the hospital was unusual and, to the best of my knowledge, had not been foreshadowed in media releases. If the essence of the stern talk by Nuttall and Buckland had been conveyed accurately to Hoffman, it was, I suspected, a crude attempt to contain the Patel problem while waving a big stick at any staff who might have been involved in the allegations being aired. It felt like the start of a cover-up.

'The issue of Patel's competence might take ages to investigate, but the meeting today gives me an opportunity to put the story back on the agenda,' I told Hoffman. 'I'll call Nuttall's office and find out why they're trying to shut this down.'

We walked back to the foyer and resolved to stay in touch. Hoffman and Fox were booked on the last Qantas flight back to Bundaberg.

DAN Bergin, one of the managers for Queensland Health, remained angry about the leaking. He emailed Leck shortly after 5 pm as Buckland stewed over the Patel negligence revelations: 'Peter, Is there a process going on, involving Internal Audit, to investigate this?'

Leck, still in the dark on Patel's United States secret, was uncertain how to manage the problem.

I must admit that I'm not entirely sure where to go from here.

In the meeting with the staff today, the DG advised that we would not have a witch-hunt and that we needed to move on from this incident.

Bottom line is that regardless of whether an investigation is held or not, I don't believe the culprit who leaked this information will be found. While on one hand I would like to send a strong message to the person(s) concerned that they are on very dangerous ground – I am concerned that such an investigation could prove very destructive resulting in nurses and doctors going after one another.

Perhaps we have the Audit team come up and deliver some training sessions around the Code of Conduct and deliver some firm and scary messages? I would welcome your advice especially if the DG's office is expecting action in a particular way.

Peter

40

Fluke

6 pm, 7 April 2005

NEWS coming out of left field late in the day is always more difficult to place in any newspaper. As the story has not been the subject of a briefing in editorial conferences, it has to knock something else out to get in. Unless it is momentous and urgent – perhaps an aircraft crash or a political upheaval – its prospects of a good run are poor. Such stories are often held for the next day and that can kill them slowly. Stories held over can appear stale, despite not having been run. Something else invariably comes along to compete for the space.

Sometimes on a slow news day or when the best-laid plans go awry because the promised stories have failed to materialise, the late and unexpected ones are hailed as saviours. But most of the time they are a nuisance: the night editor has to change course and rebuild pages in the face of an unforgiving deadline.

I was keen to publish the story about Gordon Nuttall and Steve Buckland going to Bundaberg and telling staff nothing would be done about Jayant Patel. It was breaking news. It had been presented on a platter.

A few minutes after showing Toni Hoffman and Karen Fox out of the building, I saw Graham Lloyd, the news editor. Perfect. After I explained the story, Lloyd suggested postponing it: 'The paper is full. Do it as part of your bigger yarn for Saturday and it will get a much better run,' he said.

After working closely with Lloyd for six years, I had enormous respect for his judgement and advice. We had jointly delivered some powerful scoops from the newspaper's features section when he was in charge of it.

Although disappointed that Nuttall and Buckland would be off the hook for the moment, I figured it might make my scheduled lunch with the minister the next day less uncomfortable. One of Nuttall's closest friends, Brendan McKennariey, had called me earlier in the week to confirm the low-key meeting at the Hellenic Club in South Brisbane. When he first set it up, McKennariey, whom I knew through a mutual contact, explained that Nuttall wanted to develop a working relationship with a few senior journalists. Nuttall had big plans for Queensland Health. The private lunch at the Hellenic Club would give him an opportunity away from his minders and advisers to set out its future.

I went back to my desk for my keys as David Fagan, the editor, wandered over. He was unhappy. 'What a shocking day,' he said. 'We haven't got one story worthy of putting on the front page. You haven't got anything in your back pocket, have you?'

In the past six years at the *Courier-Mail*, neither Fagan nor his predecessor, Chris Mitchell, had come to me to ask for a story late in the day. They were too busy, for a start. They relied on their staff to talk about the big fish in a news editorial conference after the reporters had reeled them in. For Fagan to come into our section, sometimes known as Writer's Block or Poet's Corner, he must have been desperate. He was looking for a splash, the major story for the front page.

'I've got a great yarn,' I told him, relating the suspected cover-up in Bundaberg and the meeting I had just had in the cafe.

'All I need is confirmation from Nuttall's office. I've got heaps of background. The doctor has left Queensland. Do you want me to write it as the splash?'

Fagan was noncommittal. 'Possibly. Write it as soon as you can and we'll take a close look at it,' he said.

I called David Potter's mobile phone, but it was turned off. He was still in the air en route from Bundaberg to Brisbane. He would hear my message on landing. The next call was to Cameron Milner, Potter's PR sidekick in Nuttall's office.

'He's on the plane,' Milner said of Nuttall. 'He went to open the Springsure community centre and on the way back he dropped into the Bundaberg Hospital. He spoke with staff before doing a tour.'

The conversation became farcical when I asked about Gerry FitzGerald's clinical audit and report into Patel's surgery at the hospital.

'It's not a report into Dr Patel,' he said. 'It's a clinical audit to look at the range of services and surgery done at the hospital to determine whether appropriate surgery is being done there. The complaints about Patel were about particular types of surgery he was carrying out.'

Having heard at length from Hoffman about the surgeon's incompetence, the deaths attributed to him, the work of FitzGerald and the surprise visit that afternoon by Nuttall and Buckland, I responded aggressively to the spin from Milner. It was nonsense to suggest that Patel's competence was not under scrutiny. Why did these people always twist the truth? For a few minutes we went back and forth, arguing about the clinical review.

Milner stuck stubbornly to the script. When I questioned him about what had triggered the review, given that it was not a routine matter, he dropped his guard. 'It was prompted by the complaints arising from surgery being conducted by Dr Patel,' he said.

Finally, we were getting somewhere. I asked Milner to tell Nuttall and Potter to contact me urgently.

My next call was to the mobile telephone of Dr John Scott, the Deputy Director-General of Queensland Health. As I did not have a contact number for FitzGerald and it would be at least 30 minutes before I heard from either Potter or Nuttall, perhaps Scott could shed some light on what was unfolding. I wanted to see or hear about the report which, Hoffman had told me, FitzGerald had already completed. How did the report's completion square with what Buckland and Nuttall had apparently told the meeting earlier, that the denial of natural justice and Patel's departure meant it would not be finalised?

Scott knew little about the report by FitzGerald. 'Here we are looking at an individual and there's a range of things including natural justice that you have to consider when thinking about release,' he said. 'This is the Chief Health Officer doing a review of a particular person's conduct.'

Exasperated at being told nothing, I began hitting the keyboard to write the story Fagan wanted. I could write the bones of it and add flesh upon hearing from Nuttall's side. I called a medical source and explained the issues. He became angry at his employer's cover-up culture.

Potter returned my call at 6.30 pm. I told him I was preparing a story about the meeting a few hours earlier at the hospital and asked him to have Nuttall call me. Potter rang back and said Nuttall would not be available.

I didn't know if Potter had been told about the lunch planned with Nuttall for the next day – maybe there had been a deliberate decision by his boss not to brief him – but I decided against using the engagement as leverage. But it incensed me that the minister would not speak for himself about the meeting in Bundaberg.

'Why doesn't he have the ticker to talk about the meeting?' I asked Potter.

The likable and efficient media adviser, a former *Courier-Mail* colleague with whom I had worked on a number of stories, ignored the barbs. For the record, he told me Nuttall had not seen the report; the department had not seen the report; and the minister 'does not now expect to get a report because it can't be completed without going back to Dr Patel. Obviously, we can't go back to him because he has packed up and gone,' Potter said. 'Due process was not followed. We have said we are very disappointed about that.'

After goading Potter again about Nuttall's timidity, he agreed to double-check. He called back to advise me that Nuttall would definitely not be calling me.

When I wrote the story I led it with the news of the visit: how Nuttall and Buckland had admonished staff and told them there would be no report.

Kim Sweetman, the Chief of Staff, looked at the filed copy shortly after 7 pm and asked me about a single line which stated that the nurses were asked to hide patients from Patel. 'So the nurses were literally trying to hide patients from him in the wards?' Sweetman asked. She seized on the angle and elevated it to the top of the draft. The mental imagery was too powerful.

Fagan liked the story but in his walkabout he had found another, relating to the Beattie Government's failure to address the dangers of asbestos in hundreds of public schools. My report led page three, beneath the headline: 'Nurses hid patients in wards from Dr Death'. It contained an embarrassing error in the first paragraph – I had failed to check on Patel's background. He was from India, not Pakistan.

Nurses at Bundaberg Base Hospital were asked to 'hide' patients so they would not be treated by a Pakistan-trained doctor dubbed 'Dr Death' by colleagues.

The doctor, who has fled the country since the beginning of an investigation into his work at the public hospital, has been accused of gross incompetence linked to the deaths of at least 14 patients.

But Health Minister Gordon Nuttall will keep secret a report detailing evidence about the deaths and a trail of serious injuries suffered by patients at Bundaberg Base Hospital.

The report, by Chief Health Officer Gerry FitzGerald, includes evidence gained from interviews with doctors and nurses at the hospital.

Queensland Health sources described the doctor, hired more than two years ago under the controversial overseas-trained doctors scheme, as 'dangerous and incompetent'.

They said his actions had been extremely harmful, and in some cases lethal, to more than 14 patients and were an indictment of the health system for its failure to respond to complaints two years ago.

Patients who have been harmed, and the relatives of those who have died, are demanding an explanation from Queensland Health about the doctor's proficiency and conduct.

The Courier-Mail has been told of how at least one specialist at the hospital was so concerned he pleaded with nurses to 'hide' his patients in various wards to prevent them being seen by the doctor.

But Mr Nuttall and Director-General Dr Steve Buckland yesterday went to Bundaberg Base Hospital to tell a confidential staff meeting that the evidence gathered by Queensland Health in relation to the doctor's conduct would not be made available.

They admonished staff for leaking some of the evidence, which embarrassed Mr Nuttall because it was revealed in State Parliament last month before he was aware that an investigation by his own Chief Health Officer was under way.

The doctor, whose Queensland Medical Board registration lapsed last week, quit his job and left Australia at Easter, days after the concerns were made public.

Accompanied by a file photo of Nuttall, the story continued with a quote from my medical source about how it was 'an outrageous cop-out' that the doctor's departure had been used by Queensland Health to end its investigation and pull down the shutters. It included the accusations made in State Parliament and a reference to the Queensland Health report I had been leaked in late 2003 warning that a growing number of Overseas Trained Doctors rushed into the public hospitals lacked 'medical competence and capability' and put patients at risk.

The adrenaline was still flowing when I left the office. On the way home I dropped into a bar for a beer with my colleague Des Houghton, who had been writing about the Beattie Government's Secret State culture. He was fascinated by the Bundaberg Hospital story. He reckoned there had to be much more to it.

STEVE Buckland left the taxpayer-owned aircraft and headed home.

As Darren Keating had done the night before in Bundaberg, Buckland went to his home computer to search for details about Jayant Patel's United States registration. It took him some time. After he located the relevant sites in Oregon and New York State, then navigated the options until the truth about Patel's incompetence appeared, he made printouts.

Buckland called Gerry FitzGerald at home and told him of the stunning findings. They agreed that FitzGerald should tell the Medical Board as a matter of urgency. Buckland knew he had to deliver the political dynamite to Nuttall, too. He decided to wait a day. More time would help him develop a strategy which might, if they were fortunate, limit the damage. If Patel's secret past leaked before everyone was back in a position of control, the damage could be incalculable.

Put it in writing

8 April 2005

STEVE Austin, 612 ABC Brisbane's gung-ho morning radio journalist, introduced the story with gusto. The line about nurses hiding the patients had grabbed his attention.

His producer tracked Rob Messenger down in Sydney and quickly put him on the air. Austin, relating the *Courier-Mail*'s page three lead, asked Messenger if he felt vindicated now. The novice Bundaberg MP, whose bosses in Brisbane had instructed their media adviser, Darrin Davies, to begin priming other media outlets to have another crack at the story, said he had never doubted the concerns about Jayant Patel.

'I'm supposed to be having lunch with Nuttall today,' I told Ruth as the radio program played out at home.

'It'll be an interesting conversation after the yarn today. I bet he doesn't front.'

My mobile phone would not stop ringing. Darrin Davies reckoned Dr David Molloy, the president of the Australian Medical Association's Queensland branch, should be asked if he still stood by Patel.

I wanted to talk to Molloy about whether he would support the release of the report by Dr Gerry FitzGerald or the establishment of a more exacting audit. Molloy began to distance himself from Patel. He told me:

> I have not defended the doctor. Dr Patel is not a member of the AMA and I did not feel compelled to defend him. We have been constantly arguing for better transparency in the health system.

And part of the tension between Queensland Health and the medical organisations and the doctors they employ is over truth. It is in the public interest that the truth is told here. If there is a bad doctor in the system, we have to wear that. We strongly support the findings being made public. Covering up this stuff is not in the public interest. The fact that the doctor has left town already is not a reason to not have these issues addressed. This is a serious inquiry. It is a serious issue and in the public interest that the findings be made public. Twenty kilometres from Brisbane, the public health system runs on Overseas Trained Doctors.

Given the dreadful publicity that usually accompanies ham-fisted cover-up attempts, I was puzzled by Gordon Nuttall's strategy in the staff dining room at Bundaberg Hospital the day before. Surely he did not think all the staff would suddenly go quiet. What was his motive? I asked Molloy.

'He doesn't want to undermine public confidence in the system that supplies hundreds of doctors,' Molloy said. 'To try to bury this is just so wrong. I'm concerned about the public interest aspects of this for the people of Bundaberg, for Overseas Trained Doctors and the health system.'

Dennis Atkins was blessed with finely tuned political antennae, in part the result of his years working for a former Labor Government in Queensland before returning to journalism at the *Courier-Mail*. Atkins reckoned the story was a cracker. He urged me to pursue it.

Darrin Davies called again from the Opposition's office. 'The police are looking now at criminal negligence,' he said. He wanted me to interview Messenger.

When I reached him in Sydney he told me how Tess and Mark Bramich had been to the police to ask for a criminal investigation over the treatment received by Des:

She supplied death certificates and all the information she has. I heard first-hand the devastation in their lives. I'm still feeling angry. I have told my staff to write to the Medical Board and I'm asking them to investigate this matter and I referred them to the previous correspondence. I have also written to the Health Rights Commission.

We would like to see the report. And if there's nothing to hide and nothing has gone wrong, they shouldn't need to keep it secret.

Messenger said Tess and Mark Bramich were among some 50 locals wanting action. 'There will be a public meeting at the Brothers Club on Thursday,' he said.

My next contact was with Mark Bramich, to confirm his visit to the police. 'We just want all the help we can get,' he said. 'Dad did not die because of the accident. He died because of what happened in the hospital. We can't bring Dad back but other people in Bundaberg might benefit.'

Tess told me: 'Dr Patel needs to answer a lot of questions that we have.'

My next call was to one of my original contacts from late 2003, Dr Chris Blenkin, who had told me about the debacle over the Fiji-trained doctors being falsely passed off as orthopaedic surgeons at Hervey Bay Hospital. He had seen the paper that morning. 'It's terrible. They're trying to bury it,' he said. 'The only justification is that the findings are so bad, it could cause an extraordinary loss of confidence in the public system. If it's seen to be a cover-up, that will lead to a loss of confidence.' Blenkin understood the dynamics immediately:

They should have some form of public inquiry into how he came to be there in the first place and whether mistakes were made in the appointment process. They need to appoint investigators through the College of Surgeons to perform a full audit into his surgery, as has been done for the Overseas Trained Doctors at Hervey Bay Hospital.

The patient files, notes and statements will all be there. There is such a smell about this that it is terribly important to maintain public confidence. An open inquiry should be performed.

Before leaving the office to meet Nuttall, I wanted Dr Peter Woodruff on the record. A Vice-President of the Royal Australasian College of Surgeons, Woodruff worked for Queensland Health as a vascular surgeon at the Princess Alexandra Hospital. I quickly briefed him on the issue and the circumstances. What should happen?

'There is no question that it has to be fully investigated and the public made aware of the findings,' replied Woodruff. 'There is no justification for not releasing it. If there are complaints about surgical standards, as the body vested with responsibility and a track record for striving to maintain standards, the college would happily investigate any perceived deficiencies and surgical outcomes. We should be a party to anything that smacks of substandard surgery in this country so we can address and correct it.'

If Queensland Health came under enough public pressure over the report it was refusing to disclose, I believed that its leaders would crumble and relent.

By the time McKennariey had called to say he was coming to pick me up from the *Courier-Mail* for the lunch meeting with Nuttall, I had more than enough in my notepad to form the basis for a strong follow-up story in the Saturday paper.

MICHAEL Demy-Geroe reckoned he had seen it all. A career public servant, he began as a junior clerk in the Mines Department. For the past 17 years he had been Deputy Registrar of the Medical Board. Even if he were ambitious, the prospects of career advancement were limited.

Demy-Geroe knew the job backwards. He developed and perused much of the paperwork, briefed perfunctory committee meetings and gave many of the doctors streaming into Queensland from overseas a legal rubber stamp to permit them to practise. But on Friday, the Medical Board's Executive Officer Jim O'Dempsey, who had been tipped off by FitzGerald, asked Demy-Geroe to drop everything. Demy-Geroe was instructed to investigate Jayant Patel's registration history in the United States. In particular, O'Dempsey wanted to know anything about past disciplinary issues.

Demy-Geroe performed his own Internet search and retrieved the data from the Oregon Board of Medical Examiners website. It

SICK TO DEATH

stunned him. It was inexcusable. When he went to Patel's complete file, he realised the travesty immediately. He and his staff had overlooked a crucial notation: 'Standing: Public Order on File, See attached.' Demy-Geroe turned the file over. There was nothing attached. It had been omitted.

The clue to the existence of disciplinary action, and the document setting out what Patel had been disciplined for, had been overlooked by the Medical Board's staff. Had they followed up the clue or investigated Patel's background with a few clicks on the Internet, the surgeon's incompetence in the US would have been plain. They would have seen another notation: 'An amended stipulated order was entered on 12 September 2000. The order restricted licencee from performing surgeries involving the pancreas, liver resections, and ileoanal reconstructions.'

Demy-Geroe went to the website of the New York State Office of the Professions. Its information was more damning. More succinct.

Effective Date: 5.10.2001
Action: License surrender
Misconduct Description: The physician did not contest the charge having been disciplined by the Oregon State Board of Medical Examiners for negligence involving surgical patients.

A bureaucrat to his bootstraps, Demy-Geroe began producing a report. O'Dempsey wanted a complete written explanation for this debacle. Under the heading, 'Learnings', Demy-Geroe would write: 'An incident such as this provides an opportunity to reflect on the effectiveness of procedures in place and to consider any changes which might ensure the circumstances which arose in this case cannot reoccur.'

42

The backlash

8 April 2005

TONI Hoffman went to work three hours later than usual. After her long day at the conference in Brisbane, her secret visit with Karen Fox to the offices of the *Courier-Mail*, the flight back to Bundaberg and another night of sleepless worry, she was glad to be starting at 11 am. It was a small mercy. She remained fearful.

The article about the visit by Steve Buckland and Gordon Nuttall, and the provocative headline about the nurses hiding patients from Jayant Patel, was the subject of gossip and speculation among staff in the wards.

Darren Keating kept his head down. He had told only his wife, Buckland and Jennifer Kirby, a colleague and friend at the hospital, about the results of his Google search. They each had as much to lose as he did. Peter Leck remained ignorant of the discovery.

Deanne Walls, the acting Director of Nursing, called a meeting of about 15 senior nurses after Hoffman arrived. In the seminar room on the third floor, Walls, who had cut the article from the newspaper, vented her anger over the latest blaze of publicity. 'I'm appalled,' she said. Walls told the nurses that anonymous sources were clearly trying to create unnecessary mischief and mayhem. She suspected someone in the meeting. A few of the nurses there were also angry over the leak. They felt threatened.

Hoffman believed that Walls had fingered her as the prime suspect. In Hoffman's favour, however, was her absence from Bundaberg during the dressing-down delivered by Buckland and Nuttall.

'Why is it appalling? It's all true!' she said to Walls from the back of the room.

Gail Aylmer had made a point of moving off to one side of the room. She very deliberately made herself a highly visible study of concentration. Aylmer had a pretty good idea that Hoffman was behind the article in the *Courier-Mail*.

In past months when Hoffman confided some of the actions she was taking to stop Patel operating, Aylmer half-jokingly told her friend and colleague she needed to see a psychiatrist. 'You're certifiable,' she would say. But Walls had not been joking in her efforts to persuade Hoffman to have counselling for mental stress. 'We're all really worried about you, Toni,' she had said. 'Peter Leck is especially worried about you. Please seek some help.'

Hoffman was going mad. She was mad with management for its inertia and its blinkered approach to Patel.

'I don't know about this,' said Aylmer, holding the article.

The other nurses looked at her. She emanated authority and credibility. She was about to throw Hoffman a lifeline.

'I've read it closely and I reckon the information in it has come from a doctor. It reads like something from a doctor. Not a nurse.'

Everyone bought it. They agreed a doctor was behind the leak. Hoffman sighed with relief. The meeting ended.

43

Mind games

8 April 2005

THE Hellenic Club in a timeworn building on Russell Street in South Brisbane is a favourite meeting place for the Greek community's senior citizens and their sons.

Its old tables on the outdoor patio sit uneasily on cracked tiles overlooking a neglected garden and driveway.

The club has none of the refinement of the riverside restaurants favoured by politicians and business leaders. Despite its authentic and remarkable food, friendly staff and casual atmosphere, it is the last place you would expect to find a Cabinet Minister. For Nuttall, it was the perfect venue for a low-key chat with a journalist who had become one of his government's thorns.

Leo Keliher, the Premier's Director-General, still wanted my guts for garters for exposing the Freedom of Information fiasco and the remarkable appointment, two months earlier, of Cathi Taylor. By meeting with me, Nuttall was fraternising with the enemy.

At an outside table as the Greek regulars savoured souvlaki and ribbed each other over card games, Nuttall and I talked. My estimation of him rose because he had fronted after being stitched up in that day's newspaper. At least he was not precious.

After a tentative introduction he spoke about the challenges confronting Queensland Health. As he sipped a beer he stressed the brutal reality: a finite amount of money and an infinite number of costly medical procedures. He came across as a realist being as honest as he dared about a system under strain.

We exchanged ideas and anecdotes. He told me of his respect for some of my colleagues and his contempt for others. At one stage he asked why I was labouring at the *Courier-Mail*, and wanted to know why I had not moved elsewhere. Like into a more lucrative job in government.

He was ambitious. When I asked him about taking on arguably the toughest job in Cabinet, Nuttall laughed. Despite Health being a huge promotion from the industrial relations portfolio, none of his colleagues had wanted it. He decided they were wimps. If he made a good fist of Health, he would prove his credentials as a premiership contender. None of the logs around the Cabinet table could see the potential of Health and how a competent chief might soar in the portfolio.

For all his ambition, Nuttall was not an insider. Beattie was wary of him. The Deputy Premier and Treasurer, Terry Mackenroth, and Racing Minister, Robert Schwarten, had little time for him. He had succeeded in bringing in anti-smoking measures which infuriated the major clubs and threatened to dent the revenues from poker machines. Mackenroth had opposed the proposals; the bottom line for Treasury was a loss. The bean-counters did not factor in the future savings from improving the health of individuals.

Nuttall's alignment with the Left meant his natural allies were Education Minister Anna Bligh, who was struggling to limit fallout from the tardy handling of the issue of asbestos in schools, and Attorney-General Rod Welford, who had been damaged by legal bungles and speculation over his conduct at a Christmas party.

Nuttall was also close to a former deputy premier, Jim Elder, who had quit over a vote rorting scandal. I had the unfortunate assignment of confronting Elder at his home with the evidence of the rorts, precipitating his sudden resignation.

Nuttall relied on Elder's wife, Leisa Schultz, for advice on media management. She had been his ministerial media adviser until transferring to the most senior media management role in the department, answering to Steve Buckland. I suspected that both Schultz and Elder were not among my fans.

Nuttall's big-picture analysis of health was interesting for its honesty, but it did not advance the issue I wanted to drive. I broached the Bundaberg story. I told Nuttall that I believed it had legs. His response baffled and angered me.

'I have to be fair to the doctor. He has not received natural justice,' said Nuttall. He asked me what I thought about the predicament.

'You've got a doctor who has forfeited his right to natural justice by leaving. And now you've got a hospital with a lot of angry staff who think you're covering it up,' I said. 'How does Dr Patel leaving Australia somehow prevent a thorough investigation or the release of the report? Surely you owe more to the staff and the patients than you do to Patel? If Patel turns out to have been a major problem, you're going to have to carry the can for him. I'm going to Bundaberg first thing Monday morning to try to find out exactly what has been going on there.'

Nuttall kept returning to the natural justice issue, which seemed to me either a red herring or an idea someone else, perhaps Buckland, had pressed and exaggerated. Natural justice never worried politicians when it came to launching attacks in Parliament on perceived enemies. Why was it suddenly so concerning now?

My mobile phone rang. It was Messenger calling with more information. He was determined to remain integral to the story he had kicked off in Parliament on 22 March. I did not tell him why I couldn't chat.

Nuttall seemed to grasp the need for a strategy. The meeting with Bundaberg staff the day before had rattled him. Realising the issue was not going away and might become a serious problem, he groped for a remedy; a circuit-breaker. He seized it when I told him I had spoken to Dr Peter Woodruff minutes before coming to the lunch. I related Woodruff's comments about the need for the College of Surgeons to be involved in any audit of Patel's surgery.

Nuttall was oblivious to the 2003 report by one of his senior advisers, Dr Denis Lennox. Its warnings about the dangers inherent in the Medical Board of Queensland's abysmal screening of Overseas Trained Doctors, a number of whom lacked competence, had been front page news before Nuttall's appointment. He asked me to repeat the full name of the report and its author. He made a note of it.

I explained how the report had been published in the *Courier-Mail* in November 2003, a few months before he took on the portfolio, and how its warnings and recommendations were backed up by respected practitioners such as Dr Chris Blenkin of the Australian Orthopaedics

Association, and Dr Anne Kolbe, President of the Royal Australasian College of Surgeons. Nuttall told me he would ask his department for a copy.

When I began writing in a mini-notebook, Nuttall chose his words carefully:

> These are matters of great concern to me. I understand that patients and families have concerns as well as staff. We are trying to be open and accountable. There is nothing in [FitzGerald's report] that we want to hide.
>
> But we are in a dilemma. I have a person here not able to respond because he's left. We are obviously concerned about both the patients and the families and that's why we need to talk with the Chief Health Officer to address those concerns.

When I asked about Woodruff's offer, Nuttall replied:

> I'm happy to meet with the college and talk about the issue. I'm not opposed to it. If that's the offer, I will talk to the Chief Health Officer.
>
> What he indicated to me was that there were concerns enough for him to refer the doctor to the Queensland Medical Board. Now if it can be sustained that these allegations were made two years ago, we need to have a really good look at the operations of the Bundaberg Base Hospital because I'm not happy that it's taken that long to be brought to my attention.

The interview and the lunch over, McKennariey fixed up the bill and drove me back to the office. I had everything I needed for the following day's story. It was headlined: 'Police open file on Dr Death's alleged killing'.

> A police probe into the alleged unlawful killing of a Bundaberg Base Hospital patient began yesterday as the dead man's grieving widow and son demanded full disclosure from Health Minister Gordon Nuttall.

Des Bramich, 56, was one of at least 14 patients whose treatment by the overseas-trained Dr Jayant Patel alarmed hospital doctors and staff, prompting a top-level investigation by Queensland Health.

Health professionals and heads of the Australian Medical Association and the Royal Australasian College of Surgeons called on Queensland Health to openly deal with the preliminary findings of Chief Health Officer, Dr Gerry FitzGerald.

Their calls came as Mr Nuttall revealed he was told by Dr FitzGerald that the issues surrounding Dr Patel were serious and warranted referral and further inquiry by the Medical Board of Queensland, which prosecutes doctors.

The article included quotes from Mark Bramich, David Molloy, Nuttall and Woodruff. For the second time in as many days, Nuttall's photograph ran as a single column picture, this time with a prescient caption: 'Trying times...'

44

Strategy

9–10 April 2005

PETER Woodruff slept soundly in the master bedroom of his motor cruiser, *Annabelle*. The 23-metre white-hulled beauty was gently rising on the tide at its Manly mooring when the leading vascular surgeon's mobile phone began bleeping about 6 am.

His wife, Maria, roused him. The phone was upstairs on the counter near the kitchen. Calls so early usually meant bad news, thought Woodruff, as he walked up the polished teak steps. Was it a clinical crisis at the Princess Alexandra Hospital? Or an accident involving someone in the family?

He had purchased *Annabelle* shortly after the September 11 catastrophe at the World Trade Center. He and Maria tried to escape to the boat most weekends and often succeeded in luring their eldest daughter, Samantha, her husband Roger Traves, SC, and their little ones for day trips to the beach at Peel Island. Since the children had grown up and moved away, the family home at Chelmer overlooking the Brisbane River had lost some of its appeal. But *Annabelle* turned heads on Moreton Bay. She was the perfect sanctuary after battles with administrators at the Princess Alexandra Hospital.

The caller was Deb Podbury, a bane in Woodruff's professional life. He suspected he was about to be reprimanded. A tough Queensland Health district manager with a reputation for toeing the corporate line and taking the clinicians to task, Podbury had attempted to rein in Woodruff in the past – his well-intentioned contact with journalists had caused alarm.

During one memorable made-for-television visit by Peter Beattie to the Princess Alexandra Hospital, Woodruff beat the Premier at his own game. As the cameras rolled and the self-proclaimed media tart talked up the hospital's capabilities, Woodruff told him the reality. Too few beds. Severely limited funding. Patients not receiving timely treatment. From a public relations perspective, it was dreadful for Beattie. Damning. The evening news played it up. It was the sort of spectacle the bureaucrats, who probably regarded *Yes, Minister* as a serious documentary, never forgot.

Podbury's tone and the hour of the call put Woodruff on guard. When she sounded sorry for disturbing his sleep, he relaxed. 'Have you read this morning's paper?' she asked him.

Woodruff, yet to see Saturday's edition of the *Courier-Mail*, wondered what it said. 'No, I haven't,' he replied.

'There's a rogue doctor. And the minister is going to have an inquiry into it. Your name has been suggested as an investigator. You will possibly hear from him or his department in the near future.' She was friendly, asking if he would have any objection to receiving a call from Gordon Nuttall.

'Of course not,' he replied.

About 20 minutes later, Nuttall called. Woodruff found the early morning activity a little hard to follow.

'I would like you to join a team to review the issues at Bundaberg Base Hospital involving Dr Patel,' Nuttall told him.

'No problem at all, Minister,' Woodruff said. 'We have had rogue doctors before. This should be pretty straightforward.'

'No, this is serious. Very serious,' Nuttall said.

After the call, Woodruff went to a nearby shop to buy the paper. When he read the article he still couldn't understand why Nuttall and Podbury seemed so worried.

At the same time, my enthusiasm for the story was now tempered with concern. The College of Surgeons wanted to be involved, the minister had begun to take it seriously, and the AMA also now urged a thorough review. What if the investigations determined that things were not nearly as bad as Hoffman had claimed?

'If what you're saying is right, I reckon there's a good chance it will come out,' I told her that Saturday morning.

My qualified comment angered Hoffman. 'You still doubt me, don't you?' she said crossly. 'You're not convinced yet? I promise you, it's much worse than people think. It's shocking.'

I was on the mobile at the Rocklea Markets while Ruth and the kids shopped for fruit. A leaflet for the local Subway sandwich outlet became my notepaper as Hoffman vented her anger:

> Queensland Health spends a lot of money teaching us about risk management and putting us through courses on open disclosure. And then when we need to disclose, the system fails. People went in for simple operations and came out missing a spleen.
>
> Doctors and administrators don't know how bad it has been. It's the ICU nurses who have had to go in each day and look after his complications and who had to lie to patients about what had gone wrong.
>
> He was still performing surgery until the end. On the day it was raised in State Parliament, he was operating that night and didn't seem at all concerned.
>
> He would ingratiate himself by buying the alcohol at parties and gifts for the other staff.
>
> There are lies in the death certificates. We don't know the full extent of it.

Hoffman's impassioned account bolstered my confidence and I felt guilty for doubting her. My plan was to head into the office to pick up the files I would need for the two-night visit to Bundaberg.

The latest story had provoked some strong reaction. On my office computer, an email from Darrin Davies flagged a door-stop media conference: 'Nationals Shadow Minister for Health Stuart Copeland will be available at Parliament House for comment on the Bundaberg Hospital Issue and Mental Health escapees from 11.30 am, or whenever required today,' it said.

But it was the email that had popped in at 12.26 pm from David Potter, the media adviser for Nuttall, that piqued my interest. 'Hed, this is release from Min for yesterday,' he wrote. 'Min has asked gerry fitzgerald to call you so I have given gerry your number – cheers – potter.'

April 9, 2005
MINISTER ANNOUNCES BUNDABERG HOSPITAL SERVICES REVIEW

Health Minister Gordon Nuttall today announced a comprehensive review of safety and quality at the Bundaberg Base Hospital.

Mr Nuttall said he has also been informed by independent Chief Health Officer Dr Gerry FitzGerald that issues regarding a doctor from the Bundaberg Hospital had been referred to the Queensland Medical Board.

In light of allegations, a full and comprehensive investigation of all clinical services will be carried out by a panel, including Royal Australasian College of Surgeons vice-president, Professor Peter Woodruff,' Mr Nuttall said.

'All appointees will be given investigative powers under the Health Act by the Director-General.

'The panel will report their findings to Dr FitzGerald. The report will be made publicly available.

'Dr FitzGerald's recently conducted audit of clinical services at the hospital showed 'issues of concern about individual patient outcomes'.

'I would reiterate what I have said this week that the correct process of investigating concerns at the hospital was circumvented by the naming of the doctor in State Parliament by the Member for Burnett.

'When concerns were first raised with my department and with Queensland Health, immediate action was taken through the audit by Dr Fitzgerald, but clearly we must do more.

'My major priority as Health Minister must be the welfare of patients and staff. The Medical Board investigation will ensure that any issues relating to the doctor concerned are thoroughly examined.

'I need an absolute guarantee of quality and safety at the Bundaberg Hospital to maintain not only my confidence but most importantly that of the public. Patients and staff who have aired their concerns deserve answers and, if needed, action.'

My only regret was the timing of its release: it fell right into the lap of the *Sunday Mail*. I emailed Hoffman and forwarded to her the media release about the clinical review. 'Toni, I came into work today to get some files – and this was on my email. The truth is coming out. You will be fine.'

When I rang Potter he said Nuttall and FitzGerald had just done a media conference to talk about the review. FitzGerald had been mowing the lawn at home when he received the call to come in and lend support to Nuttall.

45

Now they're talking

10 April 2005

THE 17th hole at Indooroopilly Golf Course is a long, dog-legged Par 4 with an elevated green. Making it onto the putting surface in two shots is a rare feat. My mobile phone was ringing and vibrating in my trouser pocket. The swing disintegrated along with a deep divot, which advanced farther than the ball. It was a dreadful misfire.

'Hello, it's Gerry FitzGerald, the Chief Health Officer. I'm sorry for interrupting your Sunday.'

As Potter had promised, the Chief Health Officer was calling about the review. He and Nuttall had announced it the day before. The *Sunday Mail*'s Darryl Giles went to the media conference along with the TV journalists. It made a brief story. FitzGerald, one of a few senior Queensland Health people who already knew about Patel's US background, explained he was happy to respond to questions about his audit at Bundaberg Base Hospital.

When I returned home and called him for a formal interview, he was friendly and open. He did not volunteer any clues to the highly sensitive revelation of the Oregon and New York disciplinary action. Patiently and methodically, FitzGerald told me about his clinical audit:

What we found came in two broad categories. Firstly, issues relating to the scope of practice. He would tend to do complex procedures that were outside the scope of a hospital the size of Bundaberg. Very complex operations that should have been done somewhere else. And as a result of that, in these complex cases, even in the best of hands there's a high complication rate, but certainly doing them at Bundaberg without the support, the complication rate appears to be higher than anyone would be happy with.

Secondly, there's the complication rate in general. We've got comparative data. It's evident that he has a higher complication rate in certain aspects. We measure infection rates, rate of wound breakdown and damage to another organ during an operation. Certainly, there were some higher complication rates.

The hospital, being a small country hospital, did not have the systems and structures in place to detect this earlier.

FitzGerald's answers did not tally with what I understood Toni Hoffman and the other nurses had detected. I asked about their disclosures and complaints. I believed that if FitzGerald backed Hoffman in print, she would be less likely to suffer retribution. FitzGerald responded:

I am aware that there was some informal raising of the issues. I'm not sure if that was raised in a written way. Certainly, the people who raised them were concerned that they raised them and concerned that not too much had happened.

I have to pay tribute to the staff up there. They were brave and persistent in their complaints and in raising their concerns.

The information they have brought to us is factual in what it says. They were honest about it. I do not have any reason to doubt them.

FitzGerald said he had about six cardboard boxes filled with files relating to the 14 patients pinpointed by Hoffman:

We did not have enough information to confront Dr Patel on all of those cases. We interviewed Dr Patel and asked him what was going on. He did speak about a higher level of wound breakdown and he suggested these were not really his fault.

He thought that it was largely a conflict with the people in Intensive Care. They did not understand him or support him and there was a personality conflict.

Even talking to him, it's probable that he does not see himself as a bad man and he believed what he was doing was possibly in the interests of those patients.

I asked about Patel's background and credentials. The Chief Health Officer, who had known since the previous Thursday of the serious concern over Patel's restrictions, did not miss a beat: 'I have a copy of his CV. All CVs are very broad in their description. I have not read one yet that says "I'm no good",' he told me.

46

Sugar town

11 April 2005

IT is known as a D.E. A Distant Engagement. Depending on how well you are perceived by the editor to have been working, the D.E can be a reward: perhaps, a junket to an exotic island where the most onerous task is to appear attentive as the guide provides helpful facts for a travel story.

Another kind of D.E is stressful work: dropping in on a community, usually after a tragedy. There might be a rough car trip over rutted roads after a wobbly flight in a light aircraft. A scramble to interview the locals, the injured and the relatives and friends of the dead. Sometimes they want to talk. But the intrusion on their grief is awful.

The trip to Bundaberg shaped as something in between. Patricia Holloway, the *Courier-Mail*'s travel organiser, had set up the Monday morning Qantas flight, the hire car and the motel accommodation for two nights. There would be interviews with the injured and bereaved, but I expected they wanted to talk.

I read the *Courier-Mail* on the flight. The story I had filed from home after the interview with Gerry FitzGerald ran as a page 4 lead. Page 4 was an ordinary space in a Monday paper, but I was glad to keep the issue alive. It had to maintain momentum. Hoffman, who I called after the conversation with FitzGerald to tell her about his praise for the nurses, was beginning to feel positive.

My father had been following the story with increasing interest. He emailed me shortly before the flight to Bundaberg. 'Good to see you have started an inquiry into the activities of our man from Pakistan,' he wrote. I winced, again, at being reminded of my earlier mistake about Patel's ethnicity.

Dad read the newspapers closely. He was always poised to pounce on the print media or the ABC for anything that could be seen as left-wing bias. A twice decorated former Royal Australian Air Force pilot, he had flown dangerous missions into jungles in Vietnam. He led squadrons in Australia and the Middle East before resigning to go into commercial aviation. He was my hero as a boy and he remained a steadying influence. Our political views were poles apart, but we agreed on the vital importance of a free media. We also agreed on the threats posed by the dishonesty and secrecy pervading the Beattie Government.

Dad was cranky with one of my colleagues who had written a weekend article on a military helicopter accident. Dad reckoned it was 'rubbish with a pile of codswallop thrown in for balance'. 'It was an irresponsible piece and ought not to have been published,' he said. 'On the other hand it was a fine example of how misreporting can mould opinion. Which leads me to my point: the truth, Pal, always the truth.'

The last time I had been to Bundaberg was in late June 2000, after fire destroyed a backpackers' hostel in the nearby town of Childers. Robert Long, an itinerant fruit-picker who bore a grudge against the hostel operators and some of its occupants, had lit a match in a bin in the downstairs lounge fronting the main road one chilly night.

When the volunteer firefighters combed the ruins of the historic building after the flames were finally extinguished, they counted 15 bodies. The victims were young, exuberant and hopeful travellers. Some died in their sleep. Others who realised their peril were unable to escape the smoke and heat because of bars on the windows. Unforgivably, the fire alarm system had been turned off.

Within minutes of landing and shutting the engines down, we wandered around a community in shock. The tragedy and the trespassing on the grief of the 69 survivors and the families of victims had a profound impact on me and my colleagues.

The *Courier-Mail*'s reporting team of Justine Nolan, Paula Doneman, Amanda Watt and myself filed dozens of stories in the first few days. Despite his sensitivity with a camera, photographer Anthony

Wheate was abused and physically assaulted by one traumatised survivor. It was a sobering reminder of the fine line we walked between the public's need for news and an individual's right to privacy.

Some of Bundaberg's retailers had asked the survivors to come to town for free clothing, backpacks and other kit. A bus was put on to ensure everyone arrived in Bundaberg safely. After a shopping expedition in which no money changed hands, the survivors and the journalists returned to Childers.

Our closest contact with the local community – our source for factual material about the rescuers, the police investigation, the suspect and even the shopping trip – came via a woman called Cathy Heidrich and her husband, Wayne. They owned and put together the *Isis Town and Country*, a weekly newspaper dedicated to local news. Everyone trusted Cathy and Wayne. They were generous with their news tips.

After arriving in Bundaberg on 11 April 2005, I called Cathy. She would know about the surgeon, Patel, and the problems at Bundaberg Base Hospital. We agreed to meet for lunch the next day.

My plan was to meet Hoffman after nightfall. It left me six hours to make calls, visit the hospital in Bundaberg and drive to the seaside at Bargara to drop in on the bold politician, Rob Messenger, for whom my respect was growing. Although I had told Gordon Nuttall and Gerry FitzGerald of my Bundaberg plan, it was my intention to keep a low profile while in town. There would be no dramatic attempts to door-stop hospital managers such as Darren Keating or Peter Leck to pose questions they would, I suspected, be under strict instructions to ignore.

After parking outside a private clinic on Bourbong Street, I was struck by the provincial feel and dilapidated condition of the hospital and its grounds. There were dying weeds ringing a faded concrete helipad a short walk from a dejected main entrance. I left my notepad in the hire car.

For all the staff and patients knew as I confidently pressed the elevator button, stopped to read the notices on the board and checked out the older wing of the hospital – with its suite of executive offices far removed in every sense from where the doctors and nurses improved or saved countless lives – I was one of them. Nobody challenged me.

Outside the Intensive Care Unit, I peered around corridors and into wards. After about 20 minutes I left for the drive to Bargara.

With the renewal of its seafront esplanade, a swathe of holiday accommodation, more buildings still coming out of the ground and restaurants promising all-day breakfasts and bottomless cups of coffee, Bargara, on the Coral Coast, had become one of Queensland's newest magnets for tourists. It was also where Patel had chosen to live.

I introduced myself to Rob Messenger's media adviser, Melinda Bradford, who told me the boss was still out of town. Bradford, 20, had her hands full: a middle-aged man, perhaps a constituent, sat transfixed as she offered advice. He seemed infinitely more interested in her than in the obscure problem he had brought to the office.

In a newsagency, I bought the *Bundaberg NewsMail* to check whether their reporters were still on the case. They had a story about Nuttall's backflip in establishing the review. I mentioned the controversy to the newsagent while passing over 90 cents. I was fishing. If she knew Patel as a customer, she might say so. Perhaps he spent $100 a day on instant lottery tickets. Maybe he subscribed to *Home Beautiful Magazine*. It was all grist for the mill.

'I don't know him,' she said sharply.

Bradford agreed to photocopy a handful of articles and a few written complaints from some of the people who had been to Messenger since his stand in State Parliament. She gave me names and phone numbers. Ian Fleming, Beryl Crosby and Nelson Cox had all been patients of Patel, she explained, and Ian Brown was their Brisbane-based solicitor, a personal injury expert from Carter Capner Lawyers. I knew the firm, having worked closely with one of their solicitors, Judy Teitzel, while reporting in 2001 on property marketeering and rip-offs. Teitzel had been targeting some of the people I was investigating and writing about. She launched legal actions to claim damages for their misleading and deceptive conduct.

By swapping intelligence, we both came out in front. I did not know Brown, but I figured he would welcome the *Courier-Mail*'s interest. Publicity was free advertising for Carter Capner to Patel clients who had suffered or who thought they might win some money. The usually symbiotic relationship between lawyers and journalists thrived on these understandings. We relied on the victims for their story. The lawyers relied on the victims for the money they could bring into the firm. The victims relied on the journalists and the lawyers to promote their case.

I was in the car reading the local newspaper and scanning the material copied by Bradford when Hoffman called my mobile phone. The onus was on her to set the evening meeting up. She offered her home and told me the address.

'I think a few other nurses will be coming to talk to you,' said Hoffman. 'I told them you were bringing the food.'

Earlier I had offered to buy dinner, a range of curries. Hoffman said the best ones came from the Indian Curry Bazaar, Patel's favourite restaurant and the venue for his farewell party. She giggled at the delicious irony and agreed to ring in the order.

Returning to the motel, I put in a call to the Bundaberg Base Hospital and asked to speak to Keating. Although certain he would not come to the phone or call me back, I needed to ensure he had been given the opportunity.

I contacted the local Channel 7 news reporter who had covered the visit of the Bramich family to the local police. She was too busy to meet for a chat about the story and she doubted anyone from the hospital would talk to me on the record.

My next call was to Mark Bramich, a quietly spoken bloke who missed his dad. 'Before this, everyone including myself bagged politicians,' he said. 'But if it was not for Rob Messenger, none of this would have come about. I really think he's trying to help us.'

Bramich had witnessed the accident which pinned his father, Des, beneath the caravan one day in July 2004, in the town of Agnes Water. 'A lot of people in the town knew him. He gave more than he took. He won respect. He was in good health,' he told me.

Des had appeared to be doing well when Mark visited him in the hospital. 'We went in there and he was stabilised, sitting up in bed and having a sip of coffee and talking. No worries at all. And that was the next day. He was just normal. He was thanking God that he had got out of the situation.

'I went home and started doing some work and the missus said "you had better come back, he's taken a turn for the worse". I got there at night-time. He was not conscious. We were up there until he died.' Bramich recalled Patel saying 'you had better pray because he has only a 10 per cent chance of surviving'.

'I did not know what to think. In a way, it was sad but in a way it was also upfront. It was arrogant in the way he said it.

'The nurses were crying. I will never forget that. They could see something was not right.'

After thanking Bramich for his time, I called the solicitor Ian Brown in Brisbane to clear the path for a meeting with his clients in Bundaberg. Brown and I talked about Queensland Health's decision to announce the clinical review. A few days earlier, Gordon Nuttall and Steve Buckland had firmly told the staff of the hospital that there would be no completed report and no finalised investigation. Now, a major inquiry was underway. Privately, I suspected that Nuttall had heeded at least some of my advice at our lunch. But I did not know how much he really knew about Patel.

'It all seems very rushed,' Brown told me.

'It could be a response to the Thursday public meeting that Beryl Crosby is driving. She's one of the patients. In the space of two days we have fielded a dozen people interested in making claims. The hospital staff are concerned about going to the meeting because they fear the hospital will send spies. We are still worried that Queensland Health is going to do a whitewash on this.'

Brown told me that Crosby was keen to set up a patients' support group. 'There's nothing better than shared experiences,' he said.

Cynically, I thought it was also a clever strategy adopted by personal injury law firms. It meant as many potential claimants as possible were brought together with a minimum of fuss and expense.

PETER Leck was feeling foolish. His earlier backing of Jayant Patel was backfiring. Now, after all the fuss, it seemed to Leck that the hierarchy was less concerned about the natural justice line. He was confused.

The report Dr Gerry FitzGerald had sent to Leck on 7 April was far from a clean bill of health for the former Director of Surgery. And Steve Buckland had to have known it when he visited the hospital that day. So why, Leck wondered, the angry condemnation of the staff at the time? And then the weekend backflip? Leck still had no idea how incompetent Patel had been. Nor did he know anything about Patel's lethal negligence in the US. FitzGerald, Buckland, Darren Keating and the Medical Board were holding that information back. It was too damning for them all.

FitzGerald had been asked to go to Bundaberg to meet the staff on 13 April and brief them on his findings. But he had not been asked to tell the staff about the discovery of Patel's United States history. Those findings were still a secret.

Leck thought it best for FitzGerald to meet first with the staff from the ICU prior to a general staff meeting at either lunchtime or afternoon tea time. Leck wrote to FitzGerald:

> This will allow for those staff who expressed the concerns to feel a little special in talking to you prior to a wider audience.
>
> Would be grateful if you confirm that you are happy to meet with the families of some patients before we make the offer.
>
> The ones getting most publicity are the Brammichs [sic] (crushed by caravan – case currently subject to coronial inquiry) and [Beryl Crosby]. You did not review this case but she has complained that she was wrongly diagnosed with cancer – and has had lots of media attention.

FitzGerald replied that he was happy to meet the families if that would be helpful. 'We should also meet with local press and the Minister asked that I try and give Nita Cunningham a briefing on the situation as well. That would need to be done discretly [sic],' FitzGerald said.

If any politician deserved a briefing from the Chief Health Officer, it was Rob Messenger. His outspokenness in Parliament had lifted the lid. But Messenger was from the wrong political party. Cunningham, who had done nothing but spout propaganda, was the first political cab off the rank. She was the Labor Party's representative.

Leck asked Joan Dooley to arrange a 'very discrete' [sic] meeting between FitzGerald and Cunningham. 'Would be grateful if you could make confidential arrangements,' Leck said.

The penny drops

Evening, 11 April 2005

BEHIND the counter at the Indian Curry Bazaar, the restaurant's owner, Pam Samra, her fingers and wrists dazzling with gold rings and bracelets, smiled and motioned me to a seat to wait for the takeaway meals. 'It won't be long,' she said.

At a table strewn with magazines and newspapers, the *Bundaberg NewsMail* from the previous Saturday stood out. The local paper had done its biggest story yet on Jayant Patel. Its front page screamed: 'Families to sue over "Dr Death"'.

The letters page, a potpourri of opinions, included a curt missive from Nita Cunningham, the Labor Member for Bundaberg, who was still criticising Rob Messenger for revealing the complaints against Patel.

> It is not proper for a Member of Parliament to rush in and defame a doctor before he has had the benefit of natural justice.
>
> But to do it in Parliament – to defame someone so badly under the cowardly protection of Parliamentary Privilege – has disgusted us all.
>
> Since then, as a direct result of the Member for Burnett's prolonged and vicious attacks, this surgeon has left our hospital.
>
> Many sick people will now face having their surgery postponed or being sent to another hospital in Brisbane or Hervey Bay to have this work done, and of course the waiting times in Bundaberg will blow out.

Meanwhile, the hospital has to find a replacement. It is encouraging to see that 'my disgust' at his lack of responsibility is being shared by so many health professionals throughout our district.

Knowing Patel had been one of the restaurant's best customers, I held up the newspaper's front page to use as a pretext for a seemingly innocent query: 'The story about this surgeon at the hospital has stirred up a lot of trouble – it's all over the papers,' I said.

'He's a lovely man,' Pam Samra told me. 'He used to come here all the time. He made a few enemies because he was very talented. Some of the people he worked with at the hospital became jealous. I don't believe the things they have said about him. I've heard from others there that it's all wrong. It's terrible he had to leave.'

Hoffman's directions were precise, but somewhere, it went bad. Late, hopelessly lost, speeding crazily and throwing the hire car into violent turns as the plastic containers of curry bumped and leaked on the front passenger seat, I almost crashed near the railway line. Even with a map and directions, I couldn't find her street just a few minutes from town. When I used the mobile phone to ask for help, she sounded exasperated. I wondered if she shared my thoughts – what sort of investigative journalist can't find a clearly marked street?

Her small weatherboard home, aglow with candles, ornate frames around pictures of loved ones, exotic trinkets, antique furniture, hangings and ornaments from the Middle East and Asia, had an immediate calming effect. As nurses Karen Jenner, Jody Girder (not her real name), Rita Black (not her real name) and Karen Fox introduced themselves, Hoffman set plates and cutlery around the kitchen table and opened a bottle of wine.

'I don't think I was followed here,' I said feebly.

After telling her what Pam Samra had said about Patel, I suddenly felt sick. Samra knew that Hoffman had telephoned the order for the curries, which I had picked up and paid for with a credit card bearing my full name. If Samra read the *Courier-Mail* and noticed by-lines, she would realise the connection. If the restaurateur spoke about it to one of Patel's friends, I feared hospital management would have the evidence it needed to go after Hoffman. I confessed and apologised for my carelessness. I should have paid cash for the meal. Hoffman and her colleagues had taken a big risk in meeting me under a veil of secrecy. I hoped it would not bring them more grief.

Between mouthfuls of roghan josh, garlic naan and chicken tandoori, we spoke of cardiac arrest, perforations of the bowel and pus-oozing infections. Hoffman had been through the charts during her shift that day to see the number of Patel's patients who had suffered serious complications – infections, wound breakdowns and death – since September. The exercise had made her more depressed. She told me:

> There's fourteen more.
>
> Dr Martin Carter is the one who should have stopped Patel earlier. I said to him that he should be ashamed of himself; that he had left it all to the nurses. And he said he realised that now and should have done more.
>
> The doctors cling together. They would not stand up and be counted. The doctors are commenting now 'well, none of us are safe anymore'.
>
> In ICU, you build up a special rapport with the families. You become surrogate families. They trust you. You see the patients at their sickest.

Black seemed naturally more reserved than the other nurses. Because of her quiet demeanour, her descriptions of some of Patel's procedures carried a lot of force. It was very difficult for nursing staff to complain about the doctors, she explained, adding Patel's antics were 'like something out of a movie'.

Jenner was more direct. Still furious about the attempt by Nuttall and Buckland to shut down the inquiry, she seethed over management's mishandling of a surgeon she regarded as a dangerous menace. 'Patel blew his trumpet so hard for himself and the hospital that he made it seem he was untouchable,' Jenner said.

Girder was blunt and brutally direct about Patel's incompetence. She had also tried to figure out what made him tick. Hours after

Messenger spoke about Patel in State Parliament, Girder had watched the surgeon going around the ward 'as if it was any other day'. His blind self-belief was abnormal.

Fox, who had been with Hoffman when we first met at the *Courier-Mail*'s Brisbane office, became upset talking about the death of Des Bramich. She had been there for his final minutes and heard Patel's heartless comments to Tess and the rest of the family. Fox had seen people die before, but never as violently as Bramich, with a surgeon standing over him stabbing his chest repeatedly with a long needle.

The stories of negligence, death and cover-up tumbled out. A man who died after Patel persuaded him to let him perform an oesophagec-tomy instead of going to Brisbane to have it done. A man whose bowel was perforated in surgery on the evening of Messenger's revelations in Parliament. They told how Patel's 100 per cent complication rate with the insertion of catheters for renal dialysis prompted the hospital to bypass him and have the procedures done privately.

They described Patel's obsession with performing surgery, even when the patients were not in his care. They spoke about the lopping of gangrenous toes with no pain relief. The delusional perception of his abilities. How he opened his wallet to shower gifts on the staff he regarded as supporters. How he would keep his patients in Bundaberg even when their deteriorating conditions were life-threatening.

'Why did he keep his patients?' I asked naively.

'Because if they went to Brisbane, the complications would be obvious,' said Black.

'In the public coffee shop he held court, comparing us to the Third World and referring to our substandard equipment,' said Girder. Hoffman continued:

> He worked long hours. I don't think he had a life outside. On weekends when he was not on call, he would turn up and in that time he would cause more mischief, telling the ICU staff that I did not support him and asking them whose team they were on.
>
> He wanted to be on every committee and every panel. And people thought that because he talked a lot, he was good. We

worried about what monsters he was creating from the younger doctors.

There were a lot of people who knew a lot and did nothing. And I think that's part of the culture of medicine that has to change as well. The doctors protecting doctors.

Away from the tragic accounts of those patients who died or were severely injured, the four nurses found humour. They laughed about the night his $200 Gucci shoes were stolen from theatre. They recalled his aftershave – so pungent the nurses knew where he was and how to avoid him. And his relentless flirting.

At the end of a five-way conversation which filled a dozen pages of notes, we stood in Hoffman's lounge room and began to say goodbye. It was after 10.30 pm. Ming, her pint-sized Lhasa Apso dog, and Sami, the Maltese terrier, were barking crazily.

'You know, he didn't become a bad surgeon overnight,' Jenner said matter-of-factly.

'What do you mean?' I asked.

'Well, he's in his mid-50s. He's worked as a surgeon for about 30 years. You don't suddenly go bad as a surgeon. He must have always been a bad surgeon. So there has to be a trail of wreckage everywhere he's worked.'

Jenner's words jolted me like a sharp elbow to the face. What she had said was so fundamentally sensible and logical. It meant an examination of Patel's US background was at least as important as his legacy in Bundaberg.

On the drive back to the motel on Bourbong Street, I decided to leave Bundaberg as soon as possible. There was a new priority. I wanted to return to Brisbane to run checks on Patel's employment in the US. Jenner's comment and the appalling horror stories kept me up most of the night thinking about the possibilities.

48

Close and personal

12 April 2005

AS the earliest available flight back to Brisbane would not leave until 2 pm, I still had time to meet some patients at the home of Beryl Crosby's parents on the rural outskirts of Bundaberg. For the second time in as many days, I became hopelessly lost and arrived late.

Crosby radiated genuine warmth and friendliness. She led me around the house to a backyard sitting area where Nelson Cox, an elderly man who had once been a handy boxer, sat with his doting wife, Harriet, and Ian Fleming, a former police officer. Of everyone there, Crosby's father, who had never laid eyes on Patel, looked the most unwell. He had a thick cough and difficulty speaking. Crosby's mother made sure everyone had a drink and a biscuit.

'I just went in for a gall bladder removal. I was as fit as a fiddle,' said Cox, keen to get the ball rolling. 'That was on 25 October 2004. The outcome? There was a mess-up in the operation and I had to go back into surgery again that night.'

Mrs Cox piped up: 'The surgical nurse said what happened in there should not have happened.' Cox continued:

That night I underwent another surgical procedure to fix the damage and then I was moved to the ICU for a day and a half. It was black and rotten. They were taking four or five litres twice a day out of me. I was that sick. Nil by mouth. For 16 days. Dr Patel did the first and the second procedure. Something was done or cut that shouldn't have been done or cut. All Patel said to me after five or six days was 'you were very lucky that you were fit and a good sportsman'.

He did the third procedure as well. That was a cut to put a drain in and get it all out of my gut. My stomach had swollen up so much. I was up there for more than three weeks. I thought I would only be there overnight.

Cox lifted his shirt. He carried hardly any fat on his wiry frame, but his abdomen was horribly distended. A bulge the size of one of the local mangoes jutted out. There was angry scarring.

'I reckoned there was something wrong from the start,' he said. But he was the doctor and he was that nice to me. He can't even put a staple in. The nurses would say to me "by gee, you had a hard time in surgery – you went through a lot". After the third operation he did not want to see me again. I had to go back for check-ups. I asked a couple of times for him. He was still seeing patients, but not me.'

I asked about Patel's personality. From interviews at Toni Hoffman's house the night before, and now with the patients in the backyard, Patel sounded like a man who believed he was flawless. Crosby said:

He had a lovely manner. We really believed in him because he was so positive – until something went wrong and he didn't want to know you. I told him 'I love you', when I was going under anaesthetic. He was so nice to me. He made you feel you could have faith in him. He told me that no matter what, he was going to buy me some time. He was a lovely man.

After things went wrong, he never saw any of us. He screamed at me. He passed the buck. Everyone knows someone who had a problem. A lot took the attitude that there's no point.

It was never the case that the doctors and nurses were not doing their jobs properly. They were wonderful. But they were gagged and forced to stand by while people were being hurt. Leck and Dr Keating should be held accountable along with the hospital board. They listened to reports and did not stop him. Messenger was the lynchpin.

'He deserves a medal,' chimed in Cox.

Fleming, who had been listening patiently as Crosby and Cox described their experiences, now spoke:

He made you feel that you and he would go through it together. Once it was apparent there was a complication, he became abrupt, rude and arrogant and he wiped his hands of you.

Complications in surgery are a fact of life. But the high complication rate he had goes back to when he started at the hospital and it was covered up. He was of an age where you expected he had 20 to 30 years of experience and qualifications and ability and competency. I didn't know his experience and I didn't know anyone else was suffering. He's delusional because he would convey a sense of absolute mastery of the subject.

He was very fluent and well spoken and I think he hoodwinked and befuddled the executives and administration at the hospital. I think the culture in the hospital maintains an atmosphere of suppression and repression. I have nothing but the highest praise for the nurses and staff there except for Patel.

Crosby took some telephone calls. She was torn. Ian Brown, her solicitor, had advised her not to meet the Queensland Health staff or Dr Gerry FitzGerald, due to arrive in Bundaberg the next day. Brown, unable to go to the meeting, was playing it safe. We spoke about the pros and cons.

Crosby feared she was out of her depth in her role as an advocate for the patients, dealing with journalists, lawyers and, soon, the Chief Health Officer. She had never been a political player. In her uncompli-cated life in Bundaberg, the single mother did not know or care which side of politics Peter Beattie represented. The slings and arrows of polit-ical theatre held no interest for her. She had a heart of gold and a capacity to keep giving to everyone around her. When she learned of Patel's errors and complications, Crosby's first concern was for those who might have escaped his attentions had she pressed her complaint.

I told her I thought there was nothing to lose in going to meetings with senior Queensland Health staff who would hopefully shed light on Patel and his legacy. Nuttall's backflip and FitzGerald's apparent openness were encouraging signs. Information was almost always power.

After leaving I sped back to Bourbong Street to meet Cathy Heidrich for a chat over lunch. She too knew one of Patel's patients, a woman from Childers who had died after surgery by Patel. She had been one of the town's stalwarts in the immediate aftermath of the blaze at the hostel. She had made herself available at all hours to give the survivors a shoulder to cry on, food, drink and clothing. Over a cappuccino and a toasted sandwich, Heidrich told me that the popular woman's demise was a great loss.

49

The bombshell

12 April 2005

FOR a few moments at the arrivals terminal at Brisbane Airport I considered going straight home in a taxi to Ruth and the kids. It was already after 4 pm. I was tired. I had barely slept. It seemed unlikely I would get much work done at my desk at the office in the late afternoon. But the doubts over Patel's background kept niggling at me. I had a sense there was something more. It was stronger than a hunch. So much of the double-speak of the politicians, bureaucrats and spin doctors did not add up. And there was Karen Jenner's haunting comment about the trail of human wreckage elsewhere. I went directly to the office.

There were 14 messages on my voicemail: one from an irate Pakistani doctor, furious that I had misreported Patel's ethnicity; one from someone in Mt Isa seeking someone to investigate his feud with the bank. There were several hang-ups. A couple of friends calling for a chat. My doubles partner for Tuesday night tennis asking if I would be available in an hour. And an overseas trained medical practitioner, Dr Jean Singh (not her real name), who had left three increasingly anxious messages.

There were too many emails to read. The last one was from Dr Singh:

My tears are for the 14 patients and their families.

My tears are also for the poor doctor whose life and reputation are now in shreds.

Certainly, lives could have been saved by more appropriately actionable systems.

And maybe a doctor could have been helped to modify his practice to the high standards of care, integrity and compassion the medical profession stands for.

The other email of interest came from Stuart Copeland, the Opposition's health spokesman, who declared Nuttall unfit to be Health Minister. 'Why did the Minister's office initially try and bury the findings of an investigation, claiming Dr Patel had fled the country and there was no point in pursuing the matter?' Copeland asked. 'What else is he trying to hide in relation to this sad and shameful cover-up that has clearly cost patients' lives?'

I returned to the online quest for clues to Patel's past. Were there other victims? Was there anything to hide? A decade ago, such a quest would have meant waiting up half the night to telephone a faceless stranger in an office on the other side of the world in the forlorn hope that the information would be made available to a journalist. The Internet changed everything. When organisations, including the registration bodies for medical practitioners, realised they could save time and money by making the data freely available to visitors in cyberspace, there were fewer boundaries. A couple of double-clicks could transport a journalist from Brisbane, or a patient from Bundaberg, into an online drawer of files setting out the disciplinary history, if indeed there was any, of a surgeon in the United States.

After unsuccessfully trying a few variations of Jayant Patel in search engines used by doctors, I went to Google and typed his name. I had done an identical search a few days earlier and nothing of interest came up. This time, a little after 5 pm, when Google presented me with dozens of pages of hits, I saw a reference to a Dr Jayant Patel halfway down the first screen. The word 'disciplinary' stood out. Double-clicking on the link brought a New York State Office of the Professions website to the screen. There was the distinctive logo for a PDF file next to the words Jayant M. Patel.

When I opened the PDF file, I felt the hair on the back of my neck stand up. The documentation was damning. Perhaps too damning to be true.

There were copies of correspondence between the Board's lawyers in New York City and Patel at his home in Oregon. His home address was published. His signature was there at the foot of several of the letters. The text detailed his negligence. There was a ruling that he be struck off for gross and repeated acts of negligence in surgery. The detail unfolding on the screen mesmerised me. Surely, I thought, this can't be the same Patel. I began to doubt the information. I doubted myself. I had to be mistaken – surely he would not have been registered by the Medical Board of Queensland without a background check.

But then I recalled the Board's track record of incompetence. Its naivety and complete lack of rigour in verifying the credentials of Overseas Trained Doctors when I wrote about the problems and the warnings in late 2003 had caused me and health professionals to be gravely concerned. With the Medical Board, anything was possible. The Board conducted fewer checks for doctors wanting to come from overseas than veterinarians applying to treat animals.

Stunned at the potential enormity of the discovery, I printed the pages and went to the equivalent site for the Oregon Board of Medical Examiners. Its built-in search engine allows visitors to type the surname of a medical practitioner to check for disciplinary or competence issues. When I clicked the mouse, it returned more information on Patel. More pages to print. The printer seemed to take forever to disgorge the documents. They were queued up behind page proofs of horse racing guides, court lists and other essential elements of the newspaper. They seemed so banal as I paced back and forth.

When the paper finally crawled out of the printer I walked over to Graham Lloyd who was leaning against a bench covered with bound files of month-old newspapers. He was planning the placement of stories for the following day's edition.

'Mate, you're not going to believe what a Google search on Dr Patel has turned up,' I said.

'What have you got?' he asked.

'It looks like he's been struck off in the United States for dodgy surgery. I mean, it all looks right. But I can't believe it. There must be some mistake.'

'What? Those stupid fucking idiots,' he said.

In six years I had never seen Lloyd, one of the most intelligent journalists in the industry, lose his cool. He might have looked like a well-dressed hippie, but he rarely believed conspiracy theories. He blamed incompetence first and foremost.

I showed him the documents fresh from the printer. 'What do you reckon?' I asked.

We looked faintly ridiculous. Two grown men jabbing at pieces of paper. One swearing and wildly waving his arms.

Stephen Sealey, the deputy editor, stopped to see what was going on. I told him hurriedly about the discovery. 'It looks right,' I said. 'I haven't been able to confirm yet that it's the same Patel. But what are the chances of another negligent surgeon called Jayant Patel coming from Oregon?'

Sealey shook his head. 'Well, you'd better start making the calls,' he said.

He urged me to get cracking on the confirmation. He turned to the back bench to explain to the night editor, Rory Gibson, and his deputy, Neale Maynard, the contingency plan to remake the front page in the event of the story being true.

Soon, there would be a newsroom clamour for images of Patel's patients in Bundaberg. Patients I had visited earlier that day without a photographer.

Over at my desk Lloyd restored calm. He methodically analysed the documents from the two medical registration boards. They were clearly dealing with the same surgeon. But was he our surgeon? Lloyd correctly synthesised the details.

'He was disciplined first in Oregon in 2000,' he said. 'So they banned him from doing surgery there. Then he's tried to obtain registration in New York State and he hasn't told them about his Oregon problems. When they found out they've struck him off altogether. He's agreed to go along with that as a kind of plea-bargain to avoid a greater punishment.'

We were still no closer to determining whether he was Bundaberg's Jayant Patel when I telephoned Gerry FitzGerald. It was shortly before 6 pm. Time was against me. The strategy I had decided to follow involved a few simple queries. I planned to ask FitzGerald to confirm

Patel's home address or his US physician licence number. Figuring that FitzGerald had access to Patel's file during the clinical audit, I hoped the details would be readily available to the Chief Health Officer. I would not volunteer what I had found.

The cryptic approach fell apart. I had delivered it clumsily. FitzGerald told me he did not have the basic information I sought. 'We have his CV showing his address care of the Bundaberg Base Hospital,' he said. 'It says he was staff surgeon at Kaiser Permanente. In Portland, Oregon. October '89 to September '02. And clinical associate professor, Department of Surgery, Oregon Health Science University.'

I changed tack. 'Gerry, I probably should have explained this at the start. I'm ringing because I've just done a Google search on Jayant Patel. It's come back showing him being struck off in New York State. He was also banned from doing surgery in Oregon. But there could be many doctors in the US with that name. I need to check if it's the same Patel.' Naively, I believed FitzGerald had no knowledge of what I was talking about.

'Oh really,' he said. 'I wonder if it's the same bloke. Probably is. There would not be too many in Portland, Oregon. He got a certificate of good standing from Portland, Oregon before he came here. They have to produce a certificate of good standing when they come.'

FitzGerald let on nothing as I asked about these certificates and how they were verified.

'We rely on the Medical Board from where they have come from,' he said. 'If they can't produce the certificate, then we make further enquiries.'

I read to FitzGerald extracts from the correspondence. When I asked him if he was hearing about this for the first time, he said he was. But although I did not know it at the time, I was preaching to the converted. FitzGerald had known about Patel since the previous Thursday.

I asked again if he had anything I could use to match Bundaberg's now-infamous surgeon with the Patel thrown up by the Google search.

'We don't have his date of birth,' FitzGerald said. 'It sounds like it's him. But he still appears to be registered in Oregon. What I'm intrigued about is the relationship over what has happened in New York and Oregon. It sounds like the New York Board has done a deal with him.'

At the time I was struck by FitzGerald's immediate acceptance that it was the same Patel. It was out of character. Senior public servants are always overly cautious. Doctors are the last to assume the worst about their colleagues. Or at least the last to share their views with those outside the club. At the time I did not comprehend FitzGerald's apparent confidence that it was the same Patel.

He suggested I contact Jim O'Dempsey at the Medical Board and ask him for the information about Patel's home address and US licence number. In previous exchanges with O'Dempsey, I had put down the phone infuriated by his lack of candour. We had invariably exchanged strong words. I doubted tonight would play out any differently.

'As Chief Health Officer, you'll have more luck than me,' I said. 'Could you please ring him, explain the situation and ask him to contact me urgently?'

Toni Hoffman was at home when I called her in the meantime. 'Do you have any documents signed by Dr Patel?' I asked. 'I've found something and I need to compare his signature with it as soon as possible.'

'I'll have a look,' she said.

Within 30 minutes, she had sent me a handful of emails. The attachments were documents bearing his signature. It was a lucky break. Hoffman had feared that the administration would deliberately lose the medical file for Des Bramich. So she had copied it and taken it home. Amongst the paperwork were documents bearing Patel's signature. She scanned and emailed the messy swirl as Jpeg files.

It looked very much like the signature on the letters. It was close but not conclusive. I asked if she knew anything definite of a New York connection or the medical college he had attended in India.

'He talked about his time in New York and Portland, Oregon,' she said.

Hoffman went on the Internet herself and called back later to say he had graduated from the University of Saurashtra in 1973.

'Peter Leck lost the plot at the hospital today,' she added. 'He had to be escorted from the premises. Someone said "he's behaving like an orang-utan". Everybody in Executive now is really very afraid.'

The editor David Fagan wanted an urgent briefing on everything we had. Lloyd and I sat in his office and showed him the material. The Oregon and New York documents. The signatures. And I read to him my notes of the interview with FitzGerald.

'I think we've got enough to publish,' Fagan said. 'It looks good to me. If it were not for the signatures, we'd fall short. They are pretty close.'

Fagan was more confident than me. What if we were wrong? I cringed at the thought of the consequences. The ABC's *Media Watch* would have a field day. As we talked in Fagan's office my mobile phone rang. It was O'Dempsey. He had stepped out of a scheduled monthly meeting of the Medical Board at Forestry House.

I figured he would have been well briefed by FitzGerald, a fellow Board member who was at the meeting, but he asked me what I was calling about. The question surprised me. Surely he knew. I told O'Dempsey what I had told FitzGerald and that I needed details to confirm whether Patel from Bundaberg was the same person uncovered in the Google search.

He said he had been in a meeting and would need to go away again to check Patel's personnel file.

'I think it's likely given he came from Oregon,' O'Dempsey said.

Like FitzGerald, the executive officer of the Medical Board was being casually optimistic about something gravely serious. It was out of character.

After ending the brief exchange with me, O'Dempsey made an urgent call in a desperate bid to minimise the probable damage. He knew the game was almost up when he telephoned one of Dr Steve Buckland's advisers, Jill Pfingst, on her mobile phone. Pfingst was on a road trip in Atherton in North Queensland with Buckland, Nuttall and one of the other advisers, Cameron Milner. They had been to Atherton Hospital after a visit to the Indigenous community of Yarrabah.

O'Dempsey, by now severely rattled, tipped off Pfingst, explaining that I had done an Internet search and discovered what they already knew about Patel and his disciplinary history. Nuttall winced. The worst secret was about to get out.

When O'Dempsey called back fewer than 30 minutes later, he asked me what address I had for Patel. I repeated the house number of the mansion in Northwest Bluegrass Place, Oregon. We also compared the date of birth.

'It matches,' he said. 'We have that date of birth in 1950 and that address.'

It was now conclusive. I told him the licence number of the Patel on the Google search. He confirmed it was the same number in the personnel file of the former Director of Surgery. I was incredulous.

'Jim, this is unbelievable. It means that he should never have been registered here in Queensland.'

O'Dempsey was ready with an explanation. He delivered it smoothly:

He provided the Board with a false statutory declaration and he removed part of his Certificate of Good Standing prior to providing it to the Board. On my review, that appears to be what has happened. I have asked my staff to undertake a full review. There was a reference to an attachment on the Certificate of Good Standing. We did not receive it.

If we had received it, it's still likely that we would not have had a sustainable case to refuse his registration totally. We may have had to put conditions on his licence.

They would not have addressed the issues in Bundaberg. The issues in Bundaberg were around the types of operations he was doing.

The justifications did not make sense to me. But there was no time to argue. A deadline loomed and there was much to write.

It dawned on me that O'Dempsey's explanation meant he already knew about Patel. O'Dempsey's routine of asking what I was calling about, going back for the file, asking me what I needed to confirm – it was a charade. I asked him when he discovered the fraud. He responded:

I got a review of the file over the weekend. We have been aware of the issues from Oregon and I was awaiting confirmation from Oregon. I'm not aware that the Chief Health Officer was aware of it.

I'm awaiting a brief from my staff member which is in draft form. He's looking at what went wrong. Can I stress that there have been no findings against Dr Patel. There has been a surgical audit that raised issues with Dr Patel.

The Medical Board is extremely concerned about this one-off incident. We are so concerned that I have instructed my staff tomorrow to commence a full review of every current Overseas Trained Doctor registrant to ensure that their certificates of good standing are accurate.

I questioned O'Dempsey closely on the timing of his knowledge. The answers to who knew what, and when, were essential.

'I looked at the Dr Patel file on Friday,' O'Dempsey told me. 'I saw the note regarding the attachment. I instructed a senior Medical Board officer to find out what it was and get the details from Oregon. We advised the Minister's office today on the basis of getting formal information back. I merely briefed the Director-General's liaison person.'

I asked him repeatedly when, precisely, he spoke to the Minister's office. I said that the findings about Patel's previous incompetence were startling and that surely he could remember at what time that same day he had advised the Minister's office, but he insisted he could not recall. He rejected my suggestion that there had been a shockingly negligent lapse by the Medical Board, with tragic consequences.

'Absolutely not,' he said. 'We have one incident of what would appear to be fraudulent activity by a doctor and an error in processing here. We rely on the certificate of good standing from the jurisdiction. We rely on the certificate rather than searches of the web. If we have a certificate of good standing that says they are okay, they are okay.'

It was immediately clear that the warnings of late 2003 about the lax screening of Overseas Trained Doctors had not been heeded by the Medical Board, which was little more than a rubber stamp. If doctors or complete impostors were capable of fraud or handy at desktop publishing, they might get away with the unlawful killing of patients. And maybe Patel had.

Hoffman must have been sitting next to the phone. She was on tenterhooks when she answered it on the first ring.

'We've got him,' I said. I explained the events of the previous two hours.

She cried. Hoffman felt immense and indescribable relief. She had been completely vindicated. But she was also disgusted and furious. How, she asked me, could her bosses and the board be so reckless? And, at what terrible cost for the patients and the nurses?

David Fagan wanted a maximum display. The rush for pictures became frantic. The *Bundaberg NewsMail* refused when we asked if we could buy one of their pictures of Des Bramich, Mark or Tess. The *NewsMail* had no idea of the story about to explode in their backyard.

Our photographer in Hervey Bay, John Wilson, rushed to the Bramich home to shoot a few frames and email them back before deadline. It was imperative to publish such extraordinary news as quickly and as prominently as possible. A little after 7 pm, I began writing the main splash under the banner heading, 'Why Didn't They Check?' The story began like this:

> The surgeon dubbed Dr Death by colleagues at Bundaberg Base Hospital had been found guilty of 'gross negligence' in the US and forced to hand in his practising certificate less than two years before coming to Australia. A Google search of public registers by the *Courier-Mail* revealed yesterday that Dr Jayant Patel, an Indian-trained practitioner, had been cited over serious problems with his surgery in New York State and Oregon.

Stephen Sealey made an astute decision to throw out the feature slated for page 13 and replace it with a lengthy read on the Patel case. As well as the splash, he needed a 1500-word inside story by 9 pm.

Before leaving the office I needed to respond to my source from late 2003. Dr Marsh Godsall, who had first explained to me the concerns over the proficiency and vetting of Overseas Trained Doctors, was following the Patel stories. He had emailed me the previous day, pointing out: 'The Bundaberg saga is an extension of what we discussed in 2003 – situation has not changed.' My reply a few minutes before 10 pm must have seemed somewhat cryptic: 'I've been thinking of you these past few days and recalling what we tried to achieve in late 2003. The news – in Wednesday's *Courier-Mail* – will blow your mind (or maybe it won't given your warnings) but it could also, finally, produce the sort of positive reforms you've been seeking.'

When I finally made it home and recounted the saga to Ruth, it was 11 pm. The *Courier-Mail*'s first editions were being printed. There was a window of about six hours before they would hit the streets and unleash waves of shock and anger. The story was still missing something. Its most important character. Patel.

From home I called our correspondent in Los Angeles, Nick Papps, who was waking up in another time zone. I explained the story, telling Papps he could take an early flight and be on Patel's doorstep in Portland, Oregon before the *Courier-Mail*'s revelations were read or understood by anyone else. Papps and his partner, a photographer, fought the rush hour to the airport.

PART THREE

EXPOSED

Shock

13 April 2005

THE scandalous revelations were irrefutable. As hard evidence poured in from Bundaberg, Oregon and New York, the authorities in Queensland had nowhere to hide. They had no excuses. How could even the most brazen spin doctors have attempted to justify employing Jayant Patel for two years, and maintaining his status as Director of Surgery, amid serious complaints, when all the time a simple Google or Internet search could have proved him to be a dangerous fraud? They didn't try.

Stephen Sealey's decision to emphasise on our front page the simplicity of the Google search had a devastating result. Ordinary Queenslanders directed outrage at those in charge of the health system. Everyone who had been on a waiting list for treatment, or who blamed a hospital for a procedure which had not been a complete success, was given good reason to vent spleen. The politicians, bureaucrats, Patel and the Medical Board were lined up for an unforgiving pasting.

In Charlotte Street, where the Queensland Health edifice stood, Gordon Nuttall saw his ministerial career disappearing down a drain. Dr Steve Buckland, trying desperately to run ahead of the crisis, had few answers pending feedback from the newly appointed investigative team.

Calls for sackings flooded radio talkback and the letters pages of newspapers. 'You can add my wife and I to the list of disgusted citizens of Queensland,' Troy Daniel, a reader, wrote to me. 'I feel sick in the guts for some of those poor people around the Bundaberg district. At least the deceased have no more pain to endure.' It was the start of an unprecedented crisis in confidence not just in the health system, but in the political structure as well. As one of the Labor Government's top advisers told me, 'Sometimes there are acts of incompetence that make even the hard men of politics shake their heads in disbelief.' A match had been struck and the fuse was well alight. It hissed angrily and headed steadily to the powder keg: the Beattie Government.

Peter Beattie's staff, in regular contact with their leader during his overseas trade mission, briefed him on the developing fury. Beattie was appalled. Even several thousand kilometres away in Japan, he realised the seriousness of this stuff-up. He valued, above just about everyone else's, the counsel of his wife, Heather, a highly qualified nurse with impeccable academic credentials and a sensitive political barometer. She told him it was bad. Very, very bad.

The acting Premier, Terry Mackenroth, gruffly rejected the predictable calls by the Opposition for an inquiry. Mackenroth, who as Treasurer had kept spending on Queensland Health to the bare minimum, reckoned Beattie needed a public inquiry like he needed a hole in the head. The money would be better spent on doctors and nurses, Mackenroth grumbled.

Nick Papps called me on the mobile phone as Dr Gerry FitzGerald tried to explain to ABC Radio 612's Brisbane morning radio host Steve Austin why the system had failed so badly.

'We've got him,' Papps told me. A seasoned news-hound from Melbourne, he had been to Patel's home, confirmed his identity and asked for comment as the photographer fired a dozen frames. They were transmitted to Brisbane in minutes. It was a paparazzi-style coup. David Fagan could barely contain his enthusiasm when he was told.

FitzGerald, who had flown to Bundaberg to meet the patients and hospital staff, was having a tough time. First with the rigorous Austin and, later, in a media conference, FitzGerald sounded well and truly beaten. 'I apologise unreservedly,' he said. 'The system has let these people down and we have to do better. Obviously, what worries us mostly is there will be a lack of confidence in the community towards Bundaberg Hospital, and the people I've met here, with the obvious exception of Dr Patel, are wonderful and dedicated caring people...'

In Brisbane, Gordon Nuttall demanded explanations from the Medical Board. 'This is an awful situation,' he told me. 'I'm very angry.

I'm as frustrated as everyone else that this was not addressed back in 2003 when it was first raised. I rely on the Medical Board of Queensland to say to me: "these are good [overseas trained] doctors who are well qualified to practise".'

Fagan raised the ante. At this early stage, it seemed possible that a story so shocking might have a fairytale ending. Reforms. Proper funding. A change in the culture of cover-up and shoot-the-messenger of which I had become all too aware. Fagan directed a team of reporters and photographers to go to Bundaberg to interview traumatised patients. Anyone who knew Patel was fair game.

Reporters from a dozen other news outlets flocked to the sugar town, including *A Current Affair*.

Karin Cooper, Queensland chief of *Today Tonight*, sent a crew to the *Courier-Mail* to film me doing a Google search. Just to rub it in.

Fagan wanted to know where Patel ate, drank, slept and partied. He wanted details on how his patients had suffered or benefited from his care. He wanted to know where loved ones of those who had died looked now for comfort and answers.

News editor Graham Lloyd urged me to continue working my contacts from Brisbane. The newest angle related to claims that the bodies of several patients who had died post-operatively were fast-tracked for burial to avoid autopsies.

Gay Hawksworth, for the Queensland Nurses' Union, raised the prospect of exhumations to ensure that death certificates accurately reflected the real cause of death. She wanted Peter Leck and Dr Darren Keating to stand aside pending investigations into their conduct. 'It is totally inappropriate for managers or other senior officials to downplay allegations such as those raised by the nurses at the Bundaberg Base,' she said. 'It is also totally inappropriate to personally attack and intimidate them and we believe this may have occurred on a number of occasions...'

It was not exactly business as usual at the Intensive Care Unit as the enormity of Patel's deception rippled through the wards. Almost all the nurses cheered Toni Hoffman.

51

Split personality

14 April 2005

'THE case of the elusive Dr Jayant Patel has medical boards across Australia reviewing the way they hire overseas-trained doctors.' After Tony Eastley, host of ABC Radio's *AM* current affairs program, had introduced the story, reporter Alison Caldwell revealed her scoop: an exclusive interview with a man purporting to be Dr Patel's brother in Oregon.

'Speaking from his home in Oregon on the West Coast of the United States, Ashish Patel says his brother Dr Jayant Patel has no intention of returning to Australia,' Caldwell reported. Patel responded:

And he doesn't give a damn about Australia, probably. I mean, this guy is, you know, he has a lot of money and he just wants to travel around the world, and he doesn't need to work, so I don't know why he was there.

I just picked him up from the airport one day, and that's all I know. He didn't tell me anything.

You know, I mean, essentially he was there for one year, and then he extended his contract, and his contract expired and he came back here. He's going to go back to New York and work, that's what I was told.

In the United States he was at a wonderful position, he was a program director of the training programs and he had a full professorship at the university, and he ran the whole residency teaching program here. He wrote several articles and his curriculum vitae is 30 pages long. He was at the top level in the position, to the point that he could retire already.

At 9.30 am in Brisbane, one of Queensland's leading TV reporters, Jane Hodgkinson, began a second and more comprehensive interview. Although he sounded agitated during the trans-Pacific call, he kept talking as Hodgkinson, tape-recorder running, peppered him with questions. Only a tiny portion went to air on the 6 pm news.

'Where is Bundaberg?' Patel asked. 'What's the town you say? Queensland? I have no idea what's going on over there. Would you please not call me at this number, please. You know, if you have a problem with my brother, you get hold of him. But you know there's no point of you talking to me.'

When Hodgkinson mentioned the widening investigations, Patel sounded interested: 'So what are the investigations? I don't know anything about this. But just for the curiosity, what does the investigation show? So who is investigating?'

Hodgkinson explained that separate investigations were being conducted by the Coroner, police and Queensland Health. Hundreds of patients, she told Patel, were being contacted.

'I think we are breaking off,' Patel said.

'No, I think you can hear me clearly,' Hodgkinson replied.

'I was away when he came back and then he went to New York,' Patel said. 'We didn't talk much about Australia because he was talking about going to India and seeing my mum, ah, his mum, our mum. And I don't know what's happened there.'

'Well, he's running away from a lot of trouble. There are many injured and dead people here that he operated on,' said Hodgkinson.

Patel became cranky and started to admonish his interviewer. 'Hey, listen. Listen. Listen. Calm down here, dear. I have nothing to do with you or my brother's practice in Australia. You don't have to be rough at me. I'm just trying to have a conversation with you. You know, I don't live in Australia. I've never been to Australia in my life and you are calling me out of nowhere and telling me all these things and you are kind of getting upset at me for no reason.'

He offered to take Hodgkinson's telephone number in Brisbane and pass it to his 'brother'. He continued:

> I live here with my family. That's why I don't want to get calls over here because I don't need my family members to get upset if he has done something wrong.
>
> I know he had a brilliant career over here. I know how well he did over here. I couldn't even figure out at the time why he wants to travel overseas. Because he says he was going to go and do some voluntary work in the Third World and everything. And apparently he has done well financially so he's travelling around.

Hodgkinson explained that apart from the poor surgical outcomes for patients, Patel was also in trouble for failing to disclose to the Medical Board the actions that had been taken against him in the US.

'Well, how did he get a licence in Australia?' Patel asked. 'Don't they check on people?'

It was the most insightful question asked all day.

Toni Hoffman, hearing the interview on the radio in Bundaberg, screamed.

After the report had aired she contacted me from home. 'He's lost the plot!' she said. 'It's him.' Hoffman knew the voice and the nuances of the Indian–American accent too well to be mistaken. She knew she was hearing Dr Jayant Patel, bizarrely pretending to be his own brother. 'Believe me, we have listened to that voice for two years,' she said. 'You guys got sucked in about the brother thing. God, it is amazing, isn't it? Never in my wildest imagination. I think I'm dreaming.'

Patel opened up more to our Los Angeles correspondent, Nick Papps, who reached him by telephone hours after appearing on his front lawn. Continuing the charade of pretending to be a brother, Patel described himself as a perfectionist. For days afterwards, Papps still believed he had spoken to a brother. Patel told Papps:

> He takes bad outcomes really seriously. If I told him this was happening, he would be really pissed. He had a brilliant career in the United States.

He told me the story about the train derailment. All the media were there but he stayed away from the media because he didn't like to take the credit from the staff. He did all the work and they took all the credit – that's what he was telling me. He doesn't brag much.

Having misrepresented himself to the Medical Board and Queensland Health, he must have decided it would be easy to hoodwink the media. Patel was one of several hospital doctors who treated passengers for cuts and bruises after the derailment of a Queensland Rail Tilt train near Bundaberg in November 2004. Now, he was pretending to be his brother to pat himself on the back.

Rob Messenger was being run off his feet as Bundaberg crawled with reporters, all of them seeking interviews with patients. Messenger, the conduit, raised the political stakes and targeted Nuttall. 'I doubt Mr Nuttall has the guts to look into the eyes of the victims and listen to their stories,' Messenger said. An emotional man, he found himself shedding tears while hearing about the pain and trauma. The revelations about Patel's history in the United States stunned Messenger, whose staff had also checked but come up with nothing.

'One of the first things Gordon Nuttall did when I exposed Dr Patel was to travel to Bundaberg and abuse staff for speaking out,' Messenger said. 'Make no mistake, had those courageous staff not gone public with their concerns, Dr Patel would still be operating at Bundaberg Base Hospital.'

Peter Leck was a spent force. The revelations had hit him hard. Unlike Darren Keating and Gerry FitzGerald, Leck knew nothing until it came out in the *Courier-Mail*. He was in no fit state for interviews. He wanted to step aside and leave the district manager's hot seat to someone else. Nobody could tell where this would end.

Through Phil Nickerson, tasked with managing the media for Queensland Health while Leisa Schultz remained on honeymoon, Leck issued a statement. He was unapologetic. He had been 'deeply saddened and hurt by political and personal attacks on my ability and character, which I believe have been unfair, unreasonable and unjust'. 'I firmly believe I have acted appropriately, based on information provided to me as manager, and responded swiftly to allegations raised,' Leck said. The stress and feelings of guilt and hopelessness weighed heavily on him. He needed to see a psychiatrist, Dr Jeremy Butler, but their meeting was a month away.

Butler's colleague in the Wickham Terrace practice, psychiatrist Dr Warwick Middleton, offered me an opinion on the mental state of Jayant Patel. 'Even now it does not seem that he can bring himself to acknowledge these terrible outcomes,' Middleton told me. 'I don't get any sense that there is any remorse, responsibility or reflection. At the same time he has an amazing sense of entitlement to be centre stage. Everything that has happened will be because of the mistakes and attitudes of others.'

Another psychiatrist whose opinion I sought, Dr Ian Curtis, said he suspected that for much of Patel's professional life, he had elevated his narcissistic needs and fantasies about a medical career above the welfare of other human beings. 'This man has had plenty of warnings to stop doing surgery. But he's continued to do it. It's almost as if he's a different species. He pre-empts rights over anyone else and he does not have the capacity to develop empathy for the people that he made an oath to care for,' Curtis told me.

Over at Forestry House in Brisbane, the Medical Board's management team had issued a plea to external public relations and media advisers for help. Jim O'Dempsey, the Board's executive officer, and Mary Cohn, its chairperson, questioned their own future there. Cohn signed off on a raft of stringent new rules and systems, which should have been introduced years earlier, or at least by late 2003 when clinicians expressed grave concerns in the *Courier-Mail*. 'From today, Queensland will have the most stringent registration process for Overseas Trained Doctors compared to anywhere in Australia,' Cohn said. 'The new system will ensure that doctors can no longer provide false and misleading applications to the Board without fear of being detected and penalised.'

As an audit of the credentials and background of almost 1700 Overseas Trained Doctors resorted to Google searches, with hits being returned for innocuous things like the membership of equestrian clubs, O'Dempsey gave Nuttall a report written by Michael Demy-Geroe, one of the Board's senior officers. It conceded that while Patel had been deceptive in his documentation, a thorough check by the Board should have identified his past. 'It is my view,' wrote Demy-Geroe, 'that a combination of circumstances coincided in this case with unfortunate consequences.'

In the early evening, scenes of utter despair were played out at Bundaberg's Brothers Leagues Club. When the meeting of patients was first planned by Ian Brown of Carter Capner Lawyers, nobody outside Queensland Health's top echelons knew of Patel's wrongdoing in the US. When the news broke it drew more than 140 patients and relatives of those who died to the club on the main road into town. As Rob Messenger walked around with a microphone to hand to anyone who wanted to speak, the TV cameras filmed outpourings of grief and anger.

Cheryl Johnson spoke about her husband Barry, 57, who had pancreatic cancer before his death in October 2003. His widow correctly feared he had died as a result of Patel's negligence. 'We thought we should get a second opinion and Dr Patel said he would perform a Whipple's procedure and that he had done hundreds of them before,' she said. 'He said before the operation that if he came out within an hour, that it was not a good sign. On 1 October, Dr Patel came out and told us there was nothing he could do and an hour and a half later Barry died.'

The raw emotion was affecting everyone. 'By that stage almost everyone in the audience was crying,' said the *Courier-Mail's* reporter, Jason Gregory, who found himself choking up. Dr David Molloy, the AMA Queensland president, tried to put on a brave face while comforting people who feared they had been butchered or left to die. He issued a heartfelt apology 'on behalf of the entire medical community'. He had come to share the pain and make amends for attacking Messenger just days earlier. It was a brave gesture by Molloy to turn up. He won plaudits and respect.

There was no forgiveness in the crowd for Nita Cunningham, Labor's parliamentarian for Bundaberg. 'Nita Cunningham, was it you a week ago who said we had lost a good doctor?' asked a furious Beryl

Crosby. Before being asked to leave, the politician was jeered and booed. She never fully recovered.

It was, according to National Party MP Jeff Seeney, seated in the second row, 'the most distressing and disturbing evening I have spent for a long time. Patients of Dr Patel who had been irreparably damaged from what should have been minor operations and families who had lost loved ones were there to desperately seek answers and explanations,' he said.

Gordon Nuttall, who was not invited, channel-surfed the TV news in his office at Charlotte Street. He found it almost unbearable. Although this burgeoning scandal was not directly his fault, it had happened on his watch – and, as the media kept reminding him, the buck stopped with the minister. The calls for his sacking would be shrill.

The political pendulum was not swinging, but it had certainly shifted a few degrees. The National Party leader, Lawrence Springborg, slammed the Beattie Government at every conceivable opportunity. In the *Bundaberg NewsMail* the next day, Messenger was hailed a hero on the letters page.

One patient, Doris Caville, stood out from the baying crowd. Dr Patel had operated on her in 2004 to remove a large growth. 'It was a very difficult and rare operation involving several organs, and normally would not be done in Bundaberg,' she said. 'He was a marvellous and very caring doctor. He was due to go on holidays to visit his mother in India, but did not leave until he was sure that I was going to be okay. If it was not for him, I would not be alive today.'

52

Bloody mess

15–17 April 2005

EVEN after Jayant Patel had been revealed as a charlatan, the nurse who had done more than anyone to blow the whistle was fearful of retribution. Toni Hoffman doubted Patel would attempt to harm her. His ego was so vast, he probably regarded her, a mere nurse, as a nobody. Hoffman felt sure he would want to return to Australia to tell his critics they were hopelessly wrong. She feared retribution from another source – the bureaucrats who had been severely embarrassed by the revelations.

We spoke at length on the telephone several times a day as an extraordinary news story widened into a major crisis. In all my reports, Hoffman remained an anonymous source. Astute readers and Queensland Health insiders no doubt speculated about her involvement, but there was nothing they could use as concrete evidence that she had breached the draconian Code of Conduct.

For the weekend I wanted to write a lengthy feature about Hoffman's struggle to be heard by her colleagues. I wanted to personalise the woman. Who was she? How had she coped? What did she look like? Everyone already knew Patel's history. They had seen his image. But the heroine remained a mystery.

When I explained this to Hoffman I suggested a way forward. I would interview her mother, Marie, and ask her for a photograph of her eldest daughter. As a public servant, Hoffman could be disciplined for speaking to journalists, but the Beattie Government had no such leverage over her mother.

'That's a cunning plan,' Toni said. 'I just don't know if I can trust my Mum to talk about me!'

Marie and her husband Warwick, both retired, were among a few people outside Bundaberg Hospital who knew what had been causing Toni's sleepless nights. They believed emphatically in her cause.

Since the story broke, Marie had left the home in Mooloolah on the Sunshine Coast each morning to buy every newspaper. Her friends and relatives were inundated with email as Marie copied and pasted the text from news updates on the Internet.

When it came time to do the interview, Marie spoke with the confidence of a seasoned professional:

> Toni is usually so funny and bright. But for two years she lost her vitality. I thought she was physically sick or depressed. The light in her had dimmed. She was under dreadful stress. She wanted to see something done about this doctor and now we can see why. If she had been taken seriously two years ago, none of this would have happened.
>
> If it had been anyone other than Toni, this doctor would still be operating on the patients. She is not one to stand back when she sees things that are not right. She is stubborn. She will not tolerate incompetence or stupidity. I can only imagine how awful it was for her as she saw what was happening to the patients. She felt helpless. Thank goodness she didn't give up.

Afterwards, Marie fretted. 'I hope I have not said too much. I take after my daughter,' she said. Toni laughed when I asked if this was true.

By lunchtime on Friday as I wrote the Hoffman story, headlined 'How One Woman Exposed Queensland's Deadliest Medical Fraud', the Opposition was demanding a public Commission of Inquiry. Stuart Copeland said:

> The Beattie Government has proved time and again to be the most dishonest, sneaky and closed government in the State's history.

We don't need Mr Beattie to get off his plane from Japan and promise again to get to the bottom of the problem while doing everything he can to shift the blame for this disaster onto everyone but his government.

A Royal Commission is needed to compulsorily demand all documents, summon witnesses and demand answers.

This whole issue is simply far too important to be covered up and glossed over by Mr Nuttall and his advisers.

David Fagan and the *Courier-Mail* were also demanding a public inquiry. The newspaper's editorial thundered:

The usual options of obfuscation and blunt denial do not wash with Queenslanders any more, if ever they did.

Quite apart from the ordeals suffered at the hands of one rogue doctor, this scandal has helped expose certain practices by health administrators which would appal even the most jaded observer of government misadventure.

Mr Beattie rejects the need for an independent judicial inquiry, citing the cost involved. He has instead indicated that the Crime and Misconduct Commission may want to examine the issue. But how is it that the Government considers it proper to hold an independent inquiry into the administration of horse racing, yet resists the clear need for a thorough and independent investigation of the health system.

The copy coming in from our reporting team in Bundaberg was powerful. The anger, shock and sadness of the community and Patel's patients were conveyed in thousands of words and dozens of images. Jason Gregory and Renee Viellaris, two dogged reporters, and their more experienced colleague, Glenis Green, had combed the town and surrounding districts.

At 6 pm Fagan began sketching a rough front page. He wanted it to make an impact like no other Saturday edition. He wanted it to hit our readers right between the eyes. He wanted to make the State of

Queensland, its institutions and Beattie appreciate the human cost of this disaster. Fagan doubted a conventional front page with picture and headline would suffice. He went for broke. There would be ten patients on the front page, three of whom were deceased. Ten photographs. Ten accounts of their pain and suffering. The main picture would be Patel.

Fagan agonised over the headline. If it struck the wrong chord we would undo a lot of the hard work and set ourselves up for blame. Shortly before deadline, the front page was finished. In white type against a black background it declared: 'Trail of Despair – The lives ruined because Queensland Health let this doctor practise'.

Beattie flew back into a storm of protest and recrimination. The coverage in the *Courier-Mail* that day confirmed everything his wife Heather had warned. He went into crisis meetings with his senior staff. But Beattie still wanted a Crime and Misconduct Commission inquiry. For any government, health was too dangerous to be left to a retired judge or an ambitious senior lawyer with wide powers and public hearings.

On Saturday evening, Fagan called me at home. He wanted to keep running hard. 'This is the only story people are talking about. We cannot let it slip now,' he said.

I told him that Hoffman had received a message from Beattie. The Saturday feature article on her had triggered a string of calls from TV stations and other media outlets. Hoffman told them all she was gagged. 'I can't say anything unless I receive an official clearance,' she explained to Channel 7's Peter Doherty. He subsequently pressured Queensland Health and the Premier's office. Beattie relented. He sent a message through one of his media managers, Fiona Kennedy, to Hoffman. She had his blessing to say as much or as little as she liked.

Michael McKenna, my friend and colleague who was feeling sick for not helping me pursue the unknown story in the beginning, had a saying: 'Feed the beast or the beast will feed on you.' The beast was the media. In a feeding frenzy a voracious beast might devour anything. If not fed, it became hostile. I wondered if Beattie was feeding Hoffman to the media to divert it from himself. Having witnessed too many examples of secrecy and cover-up, I doubted Beattie had suddenly embraced openness and transparency.

Under normal circumstances I would have remained silent about the top-level permission and Channel 7's potential scoop, but knowing how Fagan wanted the issue to maintain momentum, I tipped off Jane Hodgkinson at Channel 9. She told the network bosses at Mount Coot-tha to prepare the helicopter.

As word spread that Hoffman was no longer gagged, the networks dispatched crews and helicopters back to Bundaberg. Her little home looked like a film set as TV crews queued for the interviews. Her lawyers, barrister John Allen and solicitor Gavin Rebetzke, urged Queensland Nurses' Union officer Vicki Smyth to ensure things did not get out of hand.

The telephone in Hoffman's house rang just before the first of the interviews. It was Janine Keating, the wife of Dr Darren Keating. 'I am outside my house. Darren doesn't know I'm making this call. My husband is a ruined man,' she said.

Hoffman was taken aback. 'Janine, I have nothing against Darren. It is not about Darren, I'm actually fond of him.'

Keating's wife asked Hoffman to write a letter of support; a note that might help him get through the ordeal.

Hoffman doubted that under the circumstances she would be able to help.

'You have ruined my life. You have ruined my daughter's life. You have had your 15 minutes of fame. Now get back in your box,' Janine Keating said.

'It wasn't about me, Janine. What about the patients and their families? Darren should have listened to what people were telling him. This is out of my hands now,' Hoffman said.

The *Courier-Mail*'s reporter, Jason Gregory, agreed to talk to Hoffman after the TV reporters, all of whom had earlier deadlines. In all the interviews, however, there was no mention of the probable number of deaths which could be attributed to Patel's negligence.

I called Hoffman just before deadline. 'How many? Can you estimate the number?' I asked.

She was reluctant at first. 'It's more than you think,' she said cryptically.

Hoffman knew about cases involving the Intensive Care Unit. She believed that Patel was responsible for a number of other fatalities involving patients who had not gone to the ICU. In the end she was prepared to say, on the record, that she suspected he contributed to 20 deaths. But privately, she told me that the figure was probably higher.

53

Legal games

18 April 2005

'I THOUGHT this might interest you,' said Tony Morris, QC, at lunchtime.

A tall, strongly built lawyer reputed to have a brain the size of a planet and an ambition to be Chief Justice and Prime Minister (although not necessarily in that order), Anthony John Hunter Morris was an invaluable professional contact. In the past he had provided me with a free written legal opinion on the implications of the Brisbane City Council foolishly covering up research warning that the next big flood would be more damaging than the official projections had led ratepayers to believe. Morris had given up his time, which he could charge out at more than $5000 a day, to explain complicated judgements or points of law in stories I chased.

He had been the lawyer for the late Christopher Skase, Australia's fugitive corporate giant who remained in Spain out of reach of the authorities after the collapse of his business empire. He had worked with Federal Cabinet Minister Tony Abbott and the Liberal Party in their quest to demolish Pauline Hanson over the suspicious registration of the One Nation political party.

On this day, he briefly outlined a case involving a fellow who had purported to run a Swiss bank from his home at Reedy Creek on the Gold Coast. The case raised by Morris involved an elaborate but ridiculous scam with millions of missing dollars and a conman, referred to as His Royal Highness. Funds had been frozen amid scrutiny of the scam in the Federal Court.

A mercurial and enigmatic character, Morris was the youngest silk in Australian history when appointed Queen's Counsel at the age of thirty-two. Behind his back he was known by his peers as Lord Eldon – after Sir John Scott, a British lawyer who had enjoyed a remarkable career in the law, achieving silk at the age of 31 and going on to enter Parliament and high political office, aged 42, as Tory attorney-general.

In one of many articles on his vast website, a must-have legal resource for Queensland lawyers, Morris once described his mind as 'a down-market antique shop, crammed from the floorboards to the ceiling with useless bits of old junk', some of it valuable, but all of it hard to be rid of. Elsewhere on the website he expressed his admiration for Sir Samuel Griffith, another lawyer who became a Queensland premier in 1883, then promoted himself to Chief Justice. It was the sort of career path Morris might have envisaged for himself. Presciently, Morris wrote that 'of all human vanities, there is none greater than to contemplate one's place in history. Posterity reserves its bitterest mockery for those who presume to foresee how they will be judged in retrospect.'

Our connection became stronger after he acted in court for clients whom I had exposed as charlatans. His father-in-law, Cedric Hampson, QC, had chastised me in early 2003 for refusing to reveal a source during cross-examination in Southport Magistrates Court, almost resulting in a contempt finding and imprisonment.

Morris was friendly with a handful of journalists. I had called him in 2004 when Teresa Mullan, a Beattie Government media adviser, needed urgent legal advice after being sacked and threatened with prosecution for taking a bottle of red wine on the government jet to the Lockhart River Aboriginal community where alcohol was strictly banned. Within 90 minutes of agreeing to help her, Morris was meeting Premier Peter Beattie in the Executive Building. And within minutes of their meeting, Morris had extracted a public and private apology from the Premier. Mullan was reinstated. She never received a bill from Morris.

On any other day, the news tip from Morris about the Swiss bank scam would have been welcome.

'It looks like a cracking tale,' I told him, 'but I've got my hands full at the moment with Dr Death. Latest revelation is that he botched a surgery so badly, the young man was left impotent and urinating through his bottom.'

Still anxious to avoid a high profile judicial inquiry which might quickly spin out of control, Beattie had begun sending signals to Robert Needham, the Crime and Misconduct Commission's chairman, to run a self-contained mini-probe. 'People say there should be a royal commission – well that's what exists,' Beattie said. 'The CMC is a standing royal commission, that's their job and I fully support them conducting a full, open inquiry.'

There was only one problem. Needham had other ideas. When I telephoned him to ask about Beattie's proposal on Monday afternoon, Needham ruled it out, saying the anti-corruption body lacked the scope, powers and expertise for such a task. 'At this stage I'm not proposing to mount any inquiry,' he told me. 'I do not see any need for the CMC to become involved and cut across all areas that are best dealt with by the coroner or the homicide squad.' Needham believed the issues of possible criminal negligence were best left to Police Commissioner Bob Atkinson's officers, while the wide statutory powers of State Coroner Michael Barnes permitted him to exhume bodies and conduct forensic examinations.

When I relayed this information to Beattie's media adviser, Steve Bishop, he sounded surprised. It was unusual for the Premier's proposals to be publicly rejected by one of his own appointees. 'He will seek clarification himself from the CMC,' Bishop told me.

I began writing a comment piece for the next day's *Courier-Mail*:

Peter Beattie is shirking a core responsibility over issues of life and death affecting hundreds of thousands of Queenslanders.

By ducking and weaving around calls for a royal commission-style inquiry into the scandal over Queensland Health's appointment of a 'grossly negligent' surgeon to Bundaberg Hospital, he is playing politics with lives.

A broad inquiry into this systemic failure across Queensland's health and regulatory systems would be painful. But it would end with remedies for ills which plague Queensland Health's bureaucracy.

There are compelling reasons for one inquiry, led by an eminent retired judge with extensive powers, to pull together all the terrible threads of this scandal and investigate in its entirety.

If a racing industry in which nobody has controversially died or been injured justifies a royal commission, then so, too, do Queenslanders whose lives depend on our public hospitals. Mr Beattie needs to show that whatever the political fallout, he has the ticker to take his most serious crisis seriously.

54

The blowtorch

19 April 2005

PETER Beattie, master tactician, self-confessed media tart and consummate all-round politician, had nowhere to go. He had been boxed in by the Crime and Misconduct Commission's refusal to take up his suggestion about a limited inquiry. And now the calls for a full commission of inquiry were becoming louder.

The Jayant Patel scandal had made everything else Beattie was doing to boost Queensland seem trivial by comparison. The timing for his latest expensive promotional campaign, called 'Smart Queensland – Creating the future', could not have been worse, for when the copywriters polished their material for the Smart State full-page advertisements, Patel was not a household name. Beattie says in the advertisements: 'Our researchers, scientists and health professionals are internationally recognised. Now we must keep up the momentum. Smart Queensland is a blueprint for doing just that.'

It was dream material for the Opposition. A Smart State which did not know how to use Google. A Smart State which ignored repeated warnings about a negligent surgeon. Beattie hated being mocked, particularly by Lawrence Springborg, who said:

I can say to the parliament today that our health professionals are certainly attracting international attention and for all the wrong reasons.

This is only the tip of the iceberg. What we have seen at Bundaberg Base Hospital is potentially happening elsewhere around Queensland. What we have is a government which is covering it up. If you complain you will be castigated, you will be bullied, you will be demoted, you will be driven to the point of suicide.

That is what has happened to some of these people. You will be made the problem. The Premier and the minister are hoping that they will be able to keep the lid on this and that they might be able to contain it to the Bundaberg Base Hospital.

This Premier is presiding over stuff-up after stuff-up after stuff-up.

Turning to Nuttall, the Opposition leader went for the jugular: 'People have died because of his maladministration. He has blood on his hands. He should hang his head in shame.'

Beattie had spoken earlier to Robert Needham, who confirmed his reluctance to involve the CMC. Privately, Beattie was unimpressed, but publicly he said he accepted Needham's reasons.

At 9.40 am Beattie took the biggest risk of his political career. In his bravest and most selfless act of leadership, he started a process which could only result in excruciating political pain. He told Parliament he would set up a wide-ranging inquiry into the appointment and work of Dr Jayant Patel at Bundaberg Hospital with 'terms of reference to ensure that the inquiry is effective':

> On behalf of the government of Queensland, I apologise to the patients who have suffered as a result of Dr Patel's appointment and to their families.
>
> I will ensure that the inquiry has the power to investigate all aspects of the appointment of Dr Jayant Patel at Bundaberg Hospital and the treatment of patients he dealt with.
>
> The issue of extradition has been raised. I advise the House that we have a longstanding extradition treaty with the US. We have extradition arrangements with India. We will do everything within our power to ensure that justice is done here.

After condemning the inquiry as a 'damage control exercise', the Opposition focused its rage on Nuttall, who looked increasingly forlorn and friendless. 'I do not get any joy out of this at all,' Nuttall said. 'But the job that I have to do is to try to fix it. The job that I have to do is to try to look after the people of Bundaberg and to try to reassure the rest of the people of Queensland who are treated by Overseas Trained Doctors that those doctors are suitably qualified, and we will do that.'

The Queensland Nurses' Union had not initially supported the calls for a commission of inquiry, preferring instead a much weaker form of review. After Beattie said he would establish a powerful inquiry, the union's leader, Gay Hawksworth, urged wide powers to also investigate Queensland Health's 'secretive and dismissive corporate culture'. 'The so-called managerial practice of shooting the messenger is a common experience amongst Queensland Health employees, especially nurses, and has been for years,' she said.

Dr David Molloy, head of the Australian Medical Association in Queensland, was effusive. 'This is a once-in-a-lifetime opportunity for them to change the system,' he said. 'For 30 years they've been immune to reviews. That's part of the reason the management system is so bad now.'

Having promised to endow the multimillion-dollar inquiry with extraordinary powers, Peter Beattie faced another momentous decision. He needed a retired judge or lawyer to lead it. Someone who would work tirelessly, who would command respect. Someone with whom Beattie himself could build a rapport. But someone who would not be seen as a political stooge.

Although the inquiry's leaders would not be known for several days, Beattie wanted Tony Morris, QC, at the helm. Beattie had been impressed by the tact and efficiency of Morris when they met to hammer out a solution to the political embarrassment involving Teresa Mullan and her then Minister, Liddy Clark, over taking the bottle of wine to Lockhart River in 2004. Morris was a strong supporter of the Liberal Party; he had even given free legal advice to its federal minister, Tony Abbott. Under these circumstances it would be impossible for anyone to brand Morris a Labor stooge.

Elsewhere, Attorney-General Rod Welford and one of his former top staffers, barrister Justin Harper, scrambled to put together a short list of contenders, including the newly retired Court of Appeal Justice, Geoff Davies, QC, and his friend, retired Supreme Court Justice Bill Pincus, QC. During its compilation, Morris was not raised as a remote possibility. Should Beattie want a practising lawyer, the top two on the list were Peter Applegarth, SC, and David Boddice, SC.

But Beattie had made up his mind: with a truly serious crisis threatening to engulf the Labor Party, he made one of his typically audacious moves. Morris picked up a message to call the Premier's office after Beattie's speech in Parliament. He spoke with Rob Whiddon, the Premier's 'fixer'. Would Morris be available to meet Beattie at Parliament House during the dinner adjournment? When Morris asked what it was about, he was gently rebuffed. It would be better, Whiddon explained, not to talk about it over the phone.

Morris had no idea he was about to be wooed to head the inquiry. On the way down George Street, he pondered the possibilities. There was a vacancy for a solicitor-general. Perhaps, Beattie might be about to offer the key position. Judicial appointment was another possibility. But Morris thought it would be unusual for such an offer to come from Beattie rather than the Attorney-General. It occurred to the ambitious lawyer that he might be offered a role on a state authority. Or as a state representative on a federal body like the National Crime Commission or the Australian Securities and Investments Commission.

On arriving at Parliament House he was ushered into a room with Beattie, Deputy Premier Terry Mackenroth, Whiddon and Steve Bishop. There was no courtship. Beattie came right to the point. He said that he was well aware of the connections between Morris and the Liberal Party, but was deadly serious about wanting a tough inquiry. He wanted to be seen as deadly serious. He told Morris that he had been chosen as someone who was, and would be seen to be, fiercely independent.

When Mackenroth specifically said that he supported the nomination, Morris, unaware that others in the Beattie Government were nervous about the job offer, found the assurance curious.

Beattie mentioned that Sir Llew Edwards, a non-practising doctor and former Liberal Party deputy premier, had already agreed to be a deputy commissioner. Sir Llew had one proviso. He only wanted to be on the team if its leader was happy for him to be there. Morris immediately indicated that he would be happy to work with Sir Llew.

At that time, the third member of the inquiry had not been determined. With a lawyer leading it and a former politician and doctor as a deputy, Morris and Beattie agreed the other deputy should represent the nursing profession. Margaret Vider, the Director of Mission at Holy Spirit Northside and a former nurse surveyor on the Australian Council on Health Care Standards, would later accept the position.

Morris was keenly interested in the job. He told Beattie he would be happy to serve. He saw it as a unique opportunity to do some good for the community, something which, he often lamented, was never easy in his profession. He found the issues particularly interesting.

Like all senior barristers, Morris had also begun to consider the possibility of eventual judicial appointment. It struck him as a good 'test drive' – an opportunity to experience a semi-judicial role, to see if he suited the job, and if the job suited him. Before accepting, however, he said he would have to talk it over with his wife, Alice.

It was a dream appointment. There would be broad terms of reference, wide powers for forensic examination of the evidence, national and international media interest, independence from the Beattie Government and a chance for Morris to leave his mark on Queensland history. At the end of what Beattie hoped would be a short but highly effective inquisition into a sick health system, Morris had the potential to be the hero with the remedy. Recommendations of extra funding for hospitals, changes to the law, sackings, compensation for patients and prosecutions of the guilty or incompetent were all there for Morris to make.

His mentor was Tony Fitzgerald, QC, whose successful inquiry into rampant police corruption in Queensland in the late 1980s had revolutionised the political and criminal justice systems. The inquiry had made Fitzgerald a highly respected figure, admired for his courage and tenacity in exposing the truth about the corruption of the Police Commissioner, Sir Terence Lewis, and his coterie of bent cops.

In his first full-time job in the law, Morris had been an associate to Fitzgerald when he was a Federal Court judge. When Fitzgerald left the Bench to return to the Bar, Morris was in chambers with him for the period of the corruption inquiry. He had appeared before Fitzgerald at the inquiry on behalf of one of the parties. 'There is no inquiry anywhere in the country that does not take Fitzgerald as the precedent to work from,' Morris told me after accepting Beattie's offer. 'Just like the Fitzgerald inquiry two decades ago, the credibility of this Commission of Inquiry hangs from the gossamer thread of public opinion.'

There were, however, grave reservations about Morris. As a long-time friend of the Liberal Party, he greatly concerned Beattie's colleagues. Morris was regarded by some of his legal colleagues as too unpredictable to entrust with something as serious as a judicial inquiry. 'You watch, this will come back to bite Beattie,' predicted one of the Queensland Bar Association's office-bearers.

A Supreme Court judge postulated that there were few lawyers with more ability than Morris, a product of Church of England Grammar. But, he added, there were few who also had as much potential to blow the inquiry to smithereens. 'He is an unguided missile,' the judge told me.

In an interview in his office in the Executive Building a couple of days before the start of public hearings in late May, Beattie told me some in the Labor Party thought he was mad to pick Morris:

We are not dealing here with someone who is going to be snowed.

We are dealing with someone who will be absolutely ruthless in getting to the truth. This is potentially as damaging for a government as Fitzgerald.

It's not about corruption – we're an honest government – it's about health. Health is the most significant vote-changer of any issue. So in terms of politics, of course it's an enormous threat to us which is why there is nervousness around my appointment of Tony Morris.

I knew exactly what I was doing when I appointed him. I warned all our colleagues that there will be a lot of pain out of this. Politically, we will get bashed.

I asked Beattie about Queensland Health's reputation for secrecy and cover-up. He replied:

Tony Morris has the power to get anything he wants. There's no point going through the pain and the revelation unless at the end of this we end up with a better system. That's the whole purpose of having an inquiry.

The thing that annoys me more than anything about this, let me be very blunt, is that you could actually get on a bloody website and find out what happened – and the Medical Board couldn't. And that was the crucial point when I decided there was going to be an inquiry. This is about life and death. A government can't play with people's lives.

I'm appalled that this has occurred. But I'm more concerned about the patients. They are in many senses in a powerless position. And we have a moral obligation. We represent those people, they're Queenslanders, and we have an obligation to fix this up.

When you're dealing with health, you've got to remember where the Labor Party comes from. There are two things we're obsessive about – one is equal opportunities for education and the other is health services. But this wasn't a cynical exercise. It's a philosophical exercise in the sense that we had to get someone who would take the cleaners to the system.

Before the public hearings began, the Labor Party was invincible. Its lead over the Opposition looked unassailable. Beattie had never been more popular. Still, even in those early days, Beattie feared Patel and the health crisis would flatten his government. 'What we have to do is keep our nerve in a sense of saying, "what is our moral duty here? What is our obligation",' he told me. 'The problem has been around for a long time but all this happened on our watch. If in the end the people of Queensland are still unhappy with us, then they'll vote us out.'

Although the public inquiry would grab everyone's attention, Beattie had also ordered a separate review of the health system by his favourite public sector consultant, Peter Forster. Separately, Morris and

Forster would lead what Beattie described as 'the most significant and far-reaching examination of Queensland Health in living memory'.

I left his office pondering the pledges. He sounded sincere, although he had an innate ability to sound like whatever he wanted depending on the circumstances. His powerful charisma and charm, the remarkable need to be loved, the natural cunning and the political savvy had made him Australia's most popular leader. But he could, I knew, turn on invective and anger when it suited.

It had suited Beattie as I sat in the same chair in his office five years earlier to interview him about corrupt voting in Labor Party electoral battles. I had written several articles about the claims of corrupt conduct of Labor campaign workers, including those who had helped the then Federal Attorney-General, Michael Lavarch, to keep his job by winning his seat on Brisbane's northern outskirts. Although one of the campaign workers strongly doubted Lavarch had known about the alleged corruption, a fact that I prominently reported at the time, the articles greatly distressed Lavarch, his wife Linda, and Beattie, their longtime friend.

'You wrote a number of untested pieces that damaged a lot of people without them having an opportunity to reply,' a clearly angry Beattie told me in the tirade witnessed by the *Courier-Mail*'s then state political editor Mathew Franklin. 'I don't have any faith in what you will write. And to be frank with you it's a case of my concern about whether I will get a fair go about what you are writing.'

A few moments later, Beattie apologised. The storm had passed. He was conciliatory again. 'My sensitivity is about this – my integrity means something to me, it's about my honesty, and I will not compromise on these fucking things ever.'

Back in the office, Franklin reckoned it was pure Peter Beattie. Pure performance.

Ready, set, go

Late April 2005

IN the weeks before the start of the inquiry's public hearings, state-ments and strategies were being hastily drafted in the Brisbane offices and boardrooms of a coterie of solicitors and barristers. Weaknesses, strengths, points of law and proposed tactics needed careful analysis.

The lawyers, most of whom could look forward to months of generous funding from the public purse for their efforts, knew the greatest peril for a client at a commission of inquiry was perjury. A finding of negligence was far preferable to a referral to the Director of Public Prosecutions for lying under oath. In the other commission of inquiry I had covered, led by retired Supreme Court Justice Bill Carter, QC, into a police car-stealing racket in 1992, confident witnesses were exposed as shameless liars during cross-examination.

Toni Hoffman had no experience of courtrooms and clever legal questioning. Whenever she called me to talk about how her formal statement was going, I implored her to leave nothing out. She was still concerned her contact with me would be used against her.

'If they ask you in the inquiry about our contact, you have to tell them the truth. Tell them everything,' I said.

She had heard that Dr Jim Gaffield, the American plastic surgeon, was still supporting Jayant Patel, defending his surgery and refusing to accept the problems with the patients. I asked her, only half-jokingly, if she thought the inquiry would exonerate him. 'They can't,' she replied. 'Even the Chief Health Officer has talked about his complication and infection rates.'

As the hospital's key managers – Darren Keating, Peter Leck and Linda Mulligan – were on indefinite leave with full pay, they had a distinct advantage over other witnesses. They had the time to research and prepare documentation, weigh their options and finalise a detailed statement. 'Linda Mulligan has been saying, "I can't wait to get into this inquiry and see the truth come out",' Hoffman told me.

Leck, however, was in a dire state. He had been fragile before the truth about Patel's past came out in the *Courier-Mail*. As the revelations mounted in the days afterwards, Leck became withdrawn and deeply depressed. Friends feared he might even commit suicide. When a leading Brisbane psychiatrist, Dr Jeremy Butler, first saw him in May a fortnight before the inquiry started, Leck was suffering extreme anxiety and feelings of hopelessness. He told Butler he found it difficult to sleep. He was having trouble concentrating and remembering events. He looked haggard.

Hoffman was concerned that the lawyers for Leck, Keating and Mulligan would unite to target her and destroy her credibility. Hoffman's solicitor, Gavin Rebetzke, shared her concerns. He had asked her to ease up on the media interviews.

On the other side of Australia in Perth, her young niece scampered into the kitchen and told Toni's sister-in-law: 'I just saw Aunty Toni on the TV with her puppies.'

The little girl was scolded. 'Don't tell fibs,' said her mum, Leanne Hoffman. But the child was right. The West Australian media was running hard on the story. Toni's brother, Matthew, was in Hawaii with his Australian Defence Force submarine crew when he spotted his sister on the cover of the *Bulletin* magazine.

Claire Forster, one of the top producers of the ABC's *Australian Story*, had begun working on a documentary to depict the Bundaberg disaster. Not to be outdone, the Nine Network's *60 Minutes* invited Hoffman to fly to Oregon with reporter Paul Barry and crew to confront Patel near his home. She wanted nothing to do with the plan. So they asked instead about any identifying features of Patel. Did he wear jewellery?

Paul Barry planned to hire a private investigator who would need clues to track the surgeon. Apparently, his home address and swarthy

Indian appearance were not sufficient clues. Hoffman remembered his watch. A Rolex.

Jayant Patel was no longer answering the constantly ringing phone or opening the door at the family home in Portland. There would be no more interviews. A large sign reading 'Please, no media person, newspaper, radio or television, do not knock please' greeted visitors. Patel's chequered past in Oregon was an open book. The clamour for more information spanned the globe.

In Jamnagar, India, his former colleagues were shocked to learn about the wrongdoing of one of the town's most famous and successful exports. He had returned to Jamnagar near the Pakistani border many times since emigrating to the United States in 1977. On each visit he brought news of his successful career. Patel was clearly prospering. None of his friends suspected he had been in any trouble. 'I was shocked to hear the news. Dr Jayant Patel used to study with us and was a very bright student,' Dr Vikram Shah told an Indian television outlet.

Patel's elderly mother, Mrudulaben, meant only to support her favourite son when she told the *Express India* newspaper: 'I am proud that my family has 14 doctors – my children, grandchildren, nieces and nephews are all doctors. And Jayant is the best of them all.' Toni Hoffman light-heartedly told me: 'Quick. Find those other thirteen!'

For Hoffman and most of the other Intensive Care Unit nurses, the work at Bundaberg Base Hospital would not wait. She was also under enormous stress but received little help from Queensland Health.

Although a disaster counselling team had moved into the hospital to look after the staff, the ICU nurses who had borne the brunt of Patel's conduct were overlooked. 'Now everyone at the hospital is saying, "we need help, we need counselling",' Hoffman told me. 'Where were they when we needed help?'

Her father, Warwick, had advised her not to take any leave. 'While you're still there working you can see some of the knives coming,' he said.

At the same time Hoffman was under pressure from Rob Messenger. They had not seen each other since the fateful 18 March meeting at his electorate office. She feared that the parliamentarian had been pressed by his masters to wring more political mileage from the tragedy. 'He wants me to tell him it's okay to release my name as the person who gave him the material,' she told me. 'And he's trying to make me say things about the people on the inquiry – who is a crony and who isn't – and I don't know who is who, so I'm saying "no way".'

Hoffman had only a few regrets about going to Messenger. The material she had handed to him included a special identifying characteristic – a unique number, which was tagged with the name of a patient upon admission to hospital. Due to a misunderstanding, Messenger had not removed the number when he tabled the documents in State Parliament. The breach of patient confidentiality upset Hoffman and unnecessarily exposed her to potential punishment.

'I only gave those so that he would have some documentary back-up. I didn't think or imagine that he would release them with the UR numbers,' she said. 'But it was a matter of life and death – we were desperate, there were still procedures taking place, there were more than 16 complications after our written complaint. What else could we do?'

In the streets around Bundaberg, strangers stopped to shake her hand or kiss her cheek. 'Good on you, Toni!' became a familiar cry. But she could only shake her head after meeting Nita Cunningham, the Labor Party's Member for Bundaberg. When she mentioned to Cunningham the name of Queensland Health's chief, there was a blank stare from the politician. 'She didn't even know who Steve Buckland is. She said "Who's he?",' Hoffman told me. The local parliamentarian was happy to condemn Messenger for his disclosures, but she had no idea who ran the massive government department.

In her time of need, Hoffman drew comfort from the support of the nurses. Even those critical of her in the beginning realised how she had been prepared to sacrifice her job for the patients. At a meeting of the nurses, Hoffman told them: 'Look, I've never been in this situation before. Tell me what to do. If you think we should be doing this or that, please, just tell me.' But they didn't know either. Everyone was in uncharted waters.

Patel's surviving patients and their loved ones remained gravely worried. In a number of cases where wound sites were angry or infected, they feared the worst. Blame for ongoing pain after a Patel procedure was directed to the missing surgeon and Queensland Health.

Beryl Crosby worked around the clock, reassuring people who clung to the mushrooming support group and pushing Queensland Health to organise rapid appointments with specialists to assess the need for corrective surgery.

A team of nurses with experience in trauma counselling went to Bundaberg to soothe patients suffering physically and psychologically. These patients shared the anxiety of Mary Lee, whose stomach swelled with bile after a Patel procedure. 'Before I could enjoy things a little bit, but now when I try, later I feel sad and down. There's no day or night that I feel good about myself,' she said.

A quick fix was impossible. The hospital in Bourbong Street had been under intolerable strain before the Patel crisis. It would not cope with a sudden influx of former patients seeking urgent help. Almost 900 Patel patients received a 'Dear Patient' letter from Queensland Health to explain the work of a team of liaison officers who had converged on Bundaberg. Surgeons from the private sector were contracted to see patients referred by a senior hospital doctor. The plan involved corrective surgery in private hospitals. The option for care outside the public hospital system was welcomed by Beryl Crosby, who knew that the trust of many of the patients, and much of the community, had been shattered.

'I hope the people who have been involved in employing this so-called surgeon and the hierarchy who have swept these misconduct allegations under the carpet never sleep peacefully,' wrote Sharon Eggmolesse in a letter published by the *Bundaberg NewsMail*. 'My father-in-law, and my husband's uncle were victims of this incompetence and you have deprived our family of so much, not to mention all the families you have ripped to pieces.'

I had been wondering how Gerard and Lorraine Neville felt about the revelations. Nothing would bring their daughter Elise back, but it might comfort them to know her death was a catalyst for change. The stories I wrote about Elise back in July 2004 had motivated Toni Hoffman to contact me for the first time. In my talks with Hoffman since the Google search, we considered disclosing to Gerard and

Lorraine Neville the little-known but critical role Elise had played. I wanted to tell them how she had been vital to the Patel story and the reforms sure to follow. Hoffman wanted to disclose the truth too. But she decided it was too soon. She remained fearful of retribution.

Although Gerard and Lorraine had no knowledge of the chain of events, the still-grieving couple dashed off a letter. 'If our concerns about Queensland Health's internal investigation of our complaint had been taken seriously when first raised in 2002 and if those concerns had been investigated and reported publicly, we think it is quite possible that the culture of health complaints handling...might well have changed for the better,' they wrote. 'If so, the tragic events at Bundaberg Hospital might not have occurred or, at least, been so widespread.'

SUSAN Goldsmith, senior investigative reporter for the *Oregonian* newspaper, was determined to localise the Patel story running on the wires. She began making calls and received a tip-off that Dr Sally Ehlers, a surgeon in the township of Centralia in Washington State, about 140 kilometres north of Portland, had blown the whistle on Patel a decade earlier when they worked together for the Kaiser Permanente group. Ehlers had heard nothing of the scandal in Queensland.

'Just put Jayant Patel into Google. You'll see what I mean – he's Australia's Dr Death!' Goldsmith told her.

Maintain the rage

May 2005

AFTER an informant urged me to investigate the US background of one of Queensland Health's psychiatrists, I went to the same website which had revealed Jayant Patel's past. It took a few seconds for my computer to display the results from the State of New York's Department of Health. Dr Keith Muir, a prominent Queensland psychiatrist, was struck off in the US in 1995 for having sexual relations with two vulnerable patients.

The neighbouring New Jersey State Board of Medical Examiners had earlier cited Dr Muir for engaging in 'gross and repeated malpractice which clearly placed two patients at emotional risk and indeed caused them harm'. The New Jersey board ruled that he had preyed on the vulnerabilities of the patients and corrupted the therapeutic relationship by engaging in sexual relations for his own gratification while continuing to treat and prescribe antidepressants to the women. He had 'utterly failed to maintain an appropriate patient record. . .[and] he clearly knew or should have known of the patients' vulnerabilities and the likelihood that transference of the patients' feelings on to the therapist could occur'.

In Australia, Dr Muir had headed the mental health unit at Cairns Base Hospital for a decade and was acting deputy director at Nambour General Hospital. When I called him he told me he was the innocent victim of a gross injustice. He had left the US to work in Queensland when the proceedings against him were underway, adding that he was 'shocked but not entirely surprised' at the findings.

'It's like a bad dream that doesn't end, but comes back to haunt you,' he said. He accused the two women complainants, both of whom had been accepted by US health investigators as highly credible, of being 'in cahoots with each other and best friends'.

Unsurprisingly, the Medical Board of Queensland had been unaware of Dr Muir's background until the Patel case erupted. Had the Board known of the disciplinary proceedings, Dr Muir might not have been registered in Queensland.

My interviews with staff in Cairns disclosed that Dr Muir's conduct had troubled psychiatric nurses and patients for years. Another psychiatrist, Annette Johanssen, had formally complained to the Queensland Health Rights Commission about Dr Muir in 1995 – the same year New York State authorities revoked his licence to practise. After an investigation which somehow took four years to complete, the Health Rights Commission had decided Dr Muir was unfairly accused of sexual harassment. Its investigators did not bother checking his US background.

My articles about Dr Muir drew a hostile letter from the commission's head, David Kerslake. 'For the record, it is not, nor has it ever been the Health Rights Commission's role or responsibility to check the validity of a health practitioner's registration or whether a practitioner has been subject to disciplinary action in any other jurisdiction,' Kerslake wrote.

It struck me as classic bureaucratic buck-passing. Whatever happened to initiative? To thinking outside the square? Here was a case in which an investigative agency conducted an unbelievably prolonged inquiry into the goings-on in a public hospital mental health unit, headed by a psychiatrist who was also accused of sexual harassment of a colleague, Annette Johanssen. A cursory check to see if Dr Muir had a clean slate in his previous job would have been easy and conclusive. 'That is the sole preserve of registration boards, which is no doubt why they are so named,' Kerslake said. His absurd statement proved how utterly hopeless the various agencies were in uncovering basic facts, let alone fulfilling their statutory duties.

The public responses to the *Courier-Mail* after the revelations over the Dr Muir bungle were mostly angry. One of Dr Muir's patients, however, wrote about her life being positively transformed by the man. A former colleague attacked the public 'crucifixion' of him.

At a media conference, Beattie, still furious with the Medical Board for failing to check Jayant Patel's background, became angrier when asked about the *Courier-Mail*'s reports on Dr Muir. 'I've got to the stage where I'm sick to death of these allegations,' he said. 'And let me tell you as Premier, I've got to the stage with this where I'm looking forward to this Royal Commission getting to the bottom of how all these systems operate and coming up with some very clear medicine to fix it. I hope [Tony Morris] takes a scalpel to the whole process.'

The next day, Morris drove his car to the Gold Coast Hospital, 80 kilometres south of his George Street office, to deliver personally a summons for all documents related to the treatment by district management of doctors and specialists. He had been alerted to problems there in a letter received from Beattie. The top-level attention was a coup for the *Gold Coast Bulletin*, which had been campaigning on local health woes.

Morris held an urgent meeting with hospital management and handed over the summons, which would have cost the public purse about $30 for a functionary to deliver. The story improved when, on the way out, he and the *Bulletin*'s reporter, Ann Wason Moore, were told by security staff to leave the premises.

Morris had truly entered the arena. He was going to extravagant lengths to promote the inquiry and demonstrate his zeal. His actions afforded an early glimpse of his willingness to step across a line. Morris had no intention of sticking to an orthodox and conservative script.

Queensland Health staff, already severely rattled, were apoplectic. A few days later, Morris ordered Dr Steve Buckland, Queensland Health's Director-General, to hand over the report arising from a clinical review by two orthopaedic surgeons, Dr Peter Giblin and Dr John North. They had investigated orthopaedic services at Hervey Bay Hospital after my November 2003 stories on the two Fiji-trained doctors. Morris had received a tip-off that Queensland Health was trying to smother the scathing findings.

After perusing the document, Morris promptly released it to all media outlets and put it on the inquiry's website. In his accompanying 13-page ruling he disclosed that although the inquiry was still at an investigative stage, 'it has received a great deal of information suggesting that there is a culture of bullying within Queensland Health'. He referred to a practice of 'burying' adverse reports and of 'making life difficult' for anyone in the public health system who was seen to make complaints or criticisms of Queensland Health. He continued:

> All other considerations aside, it seems to me that the public of Queensland, and especially people who live in the Fraser Coast region, are entitled to know that – in the opinion of two eminent orthopaedic surgeons specifically appointed by Queensland Health to review the situation – patient safety is at severe risk.
>
> Public inquiries, like this one – which are conducted at the public expense in relation to issues of public interest and concern – should, in the absence of the strongest reasons to the contrary, be conducted in the full blaze of public scrutiny.
>
> Proceedings conducted behind closed doors, with secret exhibits and anonymous witnesses, are characteristic of organisations like the Star Chamber, the Spanish Inquisition, the Gestapo and the KGB, found in totalitarian dictatorships, rather than the institutions of a democratic society.

Morris had initially planned to restrict television cameras from the inquiry's hearing room, but he began to reconsider after hearing from the Nine Network's political editor, Spencer Jolly. Morris consulted Jolly's competitor, Seven's Patrick Condren, who added his enthusiastic assent.

'As you know, this is virtually unprecedented in Australia. But I can't really see any objection in principle, and there are some obvious advantages,' Morris told him. 'If people are given an opportunity to see and hear what goes on at the inquiry, I am optimistic that this will increase their confidence in the commission's independence from the government, including Queensland Health,' Morris said.

It seemed viewers were going to witness a televised real-life hospital drama beamed into their living rooms. The TV networks salivated. It would be great for ratings.

Meanwhile, the Patel story was widening every day. Public and political outrage followed the revelations of Queensland Health spending more than $3000 on a business class fare for Patel to leave the country in early April.

The number of deaths being formally investigated topped 80 because vascular surgeon Dr Peter Woodruff and the Queensland Health review team had instructions to examine the circumstances of every deceased patient who had any contact with Patel, no matter how limited. Chief Health Officer Dr Gerry FitzGerald, who remained in contact with the families, still believed that many of the seriously ill patients would have died anyway. He suspected Patel's intervention had hastened their demise and worsened their quality of life before the end. 'But until somebody crawls through all of these patients' files and determines if they would have died or not, it's pretty hard to say anything definitive about it,' he told me.

Well-placed informants emerged from obscurity every day to provide news tips about outrages in the health system. Pressure was building. The *Courier-Mail*'s editor, David Fagan, ensured generous space for the ongoing story. He was calling, in the newspaper's editorials, for the resignation of Health Minister Gordon Nuttall and his Director-General, Dr Steve Buckland.

Astute observers of power and politics – insiders such as the Beattie Government's top media strategists – knew it would only worsen when the inquiry's public hearings started. 'Three fundamental things hurt governments. Health, crime and education. Health moves votes. This has the potential to be incredibly destructive,' one told me. 'The problem here is the direct connection between government inaction and dead people. One of Peter Beattie's great capacities is his ability to stand up and say "we fucked it, we fixed it, now move on". But, in this, there are all sorts of horror stories coming out.' Nuttall's bureaucrats saw Morris as an unstoppable wrecking ball who threatened everything. They seethed over his powerful mandate to discover the truth. They would have preferred to limit damage from his inquiry by severely restricting certain information, such as the Hervey Bay review. The relentless lawyer, however, held all the cards. He had Peter Beattie's ear and the authority to 'take a scalpel' to the whole process.

Morris underlined his resolve in a 19 May statement which foreshadowed 'possibly sweeping changes in the administration of

Queensland Health'. He spoke of claims of 'concealment of bad news, obfuscation of the truth, use of creative or falsified statistics and use of spin to distract attention from adverse media reports'.

The doctors, nurses and allied health staff, who had known this for years, cheered. Toni Hoffman wrote to Fagan to thank his journalists and the public for their support. 'I had previously no contact with the media and, prior to my dealings with the *Courier-Mail*, I also was a sceptic,' she said. 'Please continue to help keep us honest, by reporting the truth and exposing the falsehoods. In a democratic state, this is what we should expect and accept nothing less. There is some very important work to be done in the coming weeks to ensure that what happened at Bundaberg never happens again.'

Hoffman and her colleagues saw in Morris a fearless lawyer wielding a new broom. He talked their language. He was rapidly winning public support. But old hands like some of the retired Supreme Court judges regarded Morris as a show pony obsessed with image and tipped the inquiry would fail.

'There will be a few more body-bags before it's over,' one judge told Nuttall.

57

Fasten seatbelts

23–25 May 2005

A WHINE in the elevator shaft of the Beattie Government's newest monument to law and order, the Magistrates Court Building on George Street, echoed around Court 34. A man marched in the lobby outside wearing a hand-painted shirt that read: 'I am a medical blunder victim.' In the minutes before the advertised starting time of 10 am, lawyers, journalists, onlookers and inquiry staff exchanged nervous glances. Folders of statements were passed across the wide tables reserved for the barristers and solicitors. Trolleys laden with legal documents were pushed back and forth.

Ralph Devlin, looking jaunty in an expensive suit and trademark bow-tie, met my gaze. A tenacious lawyer with much experience in commissions of inquiry, he was appearing for the Medical Board. I half-joked that he had been handed a poisoned chalice. 'Not at all,' he said confidently. 'We are only here to help.'

We awaited the entrance of Tony Morris, QC, and his deputies, Sir Llew Edwards and Margaret Vider, for day one of the Bundaberg Base Hospital Commission of Inquiry. After the inquiry's secretary, David Groth, had read aloud the inquiry's terms of reference, a succession of lawyers sought from Morris his permission to appear on behalf of their respective clients.

For the patients, there were Gerry Mullins and Justin Harper.

For Queensland Health, David Boddice, SC, Brad Farr and Chris Fitzpatrick.

For the Australian Medical Association Queensland, David Tait.

For the Queensland Nurses' Union, John Allen.

For the Medical Board, Ralph Devlin.

For Dr Darren Keating, Geoff Diehm.

For Peter Leck, Ron Ashton.

For the Health Rights Commission, Ross Perrett.

For senior clinicians, Raelene Kelly.

Morris made notes during the rollcall.

'And I don't know, I suppose, whether Dr Patel wishes to be present or heard?' he asked.

The room chuckled as the tension eased.

'I haven't heard that Dr Patel wishes to be heard,' David Andrews, SC, the senior counsel assisting Morris, replied dryly.

Morris and his staff had been overwhelmed by letters and calls from Queenslanders who wanted the inquiry to investigate the allegedly negligent care they or loved ones received in hospitals the length and breadth of the state. Morris wanted to nip in the bud any notion that such investigations would be feasible. 'It would be impossible for this inquiry to examine everyone who feels that they have a grudge or a complaint or a dissatisfaction with medical treatment received by themselves or by family members somewhere in Queensland,' he said. 'What we want to see is a short sharp lean investigation that gets to the facts, comes up with appropriate recommendations and puts in place systems and structures that ensure that the problems of the past don't happen again. Most importantly, we want to look to the future.'

Morris summarised some of the areas he had begun to consider for reform – areas such as protection for whistleblowers; the complaints handling systems in the public health sector; the recruitment and retention of medical staff; the burgeoning bureaucracy. He ended the opening speech with an anecdote related to him by a leading Queensland surgeon who had done his postgraduate training in Scotland. 'He mentioned that he has a registrar who's of Asian origin and, in fact, a second or third generation Australian. And a patient recently said to this surgeon, "Well, I don't want that foreign-trained doctor coming near me". And the surgeon said, "Well, I'm the foreign-trained doctor, I was trained in Edinburgh, so if you don't want a foreign trained doctor operating on you, you better have the registrar, who was trained exclusively in Australia".'

Morris wanted to quell the community tensions and racism that had arisen since the Patel revelations. For a number of Overseas Trained Doctors, the taunts had been too much to bear. 'Some of them have different coloured skin, some of them come from what might be regarded as non-traditional backgrounds for the medical practice in this state, but they are still extremely talented doctors,' Morris said.

A short time later, David Andrews, whose key role involved planning inquiry strategies and questioning the main witnesses, got down to business: 'Commissioner, I call Toni Hoffman.'

She walked tentatively to the table for witnesses, below and to the right of the bench where Morris and the deputies sat. The cameras clicked and flashed. Hoffman started nervously, responding to questions about her experience and training over the years as an intensive care unit nurse in London, Saudi Arabia and Australia, her Masters degree in bioethics and tertiary qualifications in management.

For most of that day and the next one, Hoffman recalled two years of agony at the hospital. At times she was tearful, describing the dysfunction of hospital management, the injuries and deaths of patients and the fears of reprisals against staff who complained. 'All the nurses in intensive care were seeing all these patients die and we could not do anything,' she said. 'We just thought, "what on earth can we do to stop this man?". We took to hiding patients and telling them they should ask to be sent to Brisbane; we were telling them things we shouldn't be saying.'

Hoffman painted an ugly picture of Patel's competence. Her sincerity and courage clearly made a strong impression on Morris. At 4.55 pm on day two, after adjourning for the day and telling Hoffman she would next be needed to give evidence at the Bundaberg sittings in June, he stepped down from the bench to approach her.

He extended an arm and shook Hoffman's hand. She was chuffed. But the lawyers who witnessed it were agog. They apprehended a bias. A predetermined view. Nobody had heard of a judge, or an inquiry commissioner, approaching a witness during the actual proceedings.

Like the rest of the community, Morris regarded Hoffman as a heroine. Accordingly, had he already decided that those who opposed her were villains? Morris had just sown the first seed for his inquiry's failure.

58

Human headlines

26 May to 3 June 2005

THE drama unfolding in Court 34 transfixed political junkies and everyday folk who saw a tragedy undergoing forensic scrutiny. Although Tony Morris, QC, was making few friends in the top layers of Queensland Health, his robust style won plaudits in the community.

Each morning, listeners to Steve Austin's ABC Radio 612 program in Queensland heard extended tracts of the proceedings. They heard clinicians such as Dr Peter Miach, the hospital's renal specialist and Director of Medicine who had stood up to Jayant Patel, speak of efforts to sideline the Director of Surgery: 'The advice I provided to everybody around me, I sort of said "Don't go anywhere near this chap, absolutely not". I mean, I told everybody. I insulated patients, I did my own audit, I submitted to the appropriate channels there were issues, there were problems there, they were identified. I stopped using him. I told everybody not to go near him,' Miach said. He recalled a conversation with Dr Darren Keating in the days after Patel's true past had been revealed:

> It was interesting, it was a strange meeting. I was in the renal unit, which is stuck to the medical ward, doing some procedures or talking or looking at patients.
>
> In fact, he came up one afternoon to that area, up in the ward, which was somewhat unusual because, as I mentioned before, he was rarely seen on the ward, and he sought me out and we sat in my little office and we just started talking in general terms about the Patel issue, and I wasn't quite sure what was

319

going on, what was the discussion about, where it was heading, all the rest of it.

But anyway, I talked, you know, about how unfortunate it is that patients have been hurt and the rest of it and I'm not quite sure what he wanted but part of it, at the end, in fact he made a comment which I regarded as a veiled threat. He sort of said 'you have to understand, what goes around comes around'. I was a bit lost for words and I said 'Darren, you and I see things very very differently', and that was it.

Miach spoke of another conversation in which Dr Keating described the hospital as a business. They were, indeed, poles apart.

Margaret Vider asked: 'I would have thought it was the business of a hospital to be looking after the sick. What would your interpretation then be of what is the business of the Bundaberg Base Hospital?'

Miach: 'To make money, to come in on budget. That's my interpretation of it, quite simply. Patients are a secondary consideration. And most physicians, most nurses, most people who work in fact, would see it 100 per cent differently.

'You can't run a hospital as a business, irrespective of what anybody tells you. In fact, the hospital is there to serve a community. Patients don't come in with a sign on their forehead, you know, "Heart Attack". When they come in, in fact, they have hundreds of other things you have to tackle. So that's my interpretation of it. It has to do with money, which I think is a pity. I think it is totally wrong.'

Before Miach had given his powerful evidence about the gulf between clinicians and administrators, and the abyss into which patients could fall in a sick and fractured health system, the inquiry's staff had planned for Dr Keating and Peter Leck to be called as witnesses in June. Immediately after Miach had finished, however, Morris asked his senior counsel David Andrews, to join him and the two deputy commissioners for a brief meeting.

Jarrod Cowley-Grimmond, a Crown Law officer seconded to the inquiry's staff to conduct investigations and interview witnesses, was handed a note from Morris with instructions to contact Leck's solicitors and his barrister, Ron Ashton, and ask that they be present in the hearing room before the lunch break. When Ashton arrived about 12.30 pm, Morris asked the whereabouts of Leck. Ashton, who had little experience as a barrister after a long career as a solicitor, sounded taken aback. 'Well, he is in the city. I mean, he is in the City of Brisbane,' Ashton said.

'Well, will you convey to him that we will want him present after the lunch break to go into the witness box,' Morris said.

Leck's solicitor, Patricia Feeney, a longtime professional acquaintance of Ashton's, was shocked. At the lunch break she asked Andrews if he was able to explain why Leck was required to give evidence at such short notice. Andrews said he could not.

Feeney called Leck on his mobile phone. He had been in the city, walking, and did not have time to return home to change into a coat and tie.

Although Ashton and Feeney could have strongly protested on the record that the position suddenly adopted by Morris was unfair, they remained silent. Leck was duly sworn and, for most of the next 100 minutes, sat hunched at the witness table. He endured a scathing examination conducted almost solely by Morris, who did not know that Leck was being treated for a psychiatric condition.

Watching from behind a glass partition, I winced at the severity of the interrogation. Leck looked like a whipped dog who wanted to roll himself into a ball to make the smallest possible target. His lawyers, who raised scant objection at the time, would later speak of him being 'lacerated'.

At times Morris seemed incensed.

Morris: It doesn't worry you that patients might be dying or that 15-year-old boys might be losing their legs? It's not your role to see where there might be some truth in these allegations?

Leck: It's the role of the Director of Medical Services in terms of clinical issues. I'm not a clinician.

Morris: Did you talk to anyone who, you know, actually works in the hospital seeing patients? Why doesn't someone get out of the office occasionally and go down and say, 'Nurse Hoffman, we hear you have a bit of a problem with Dr Patel and that you are not talking to one another. Can we sort it out?' Instead of all this nonsense about mediation, and fixing meetings, and scheduling things, and going on for months and months while patients are literally dying in the ICU. What have you done since you were first told about this problem in October to achieve anything to save the lives of the patients who are being killed by Dr Patel?

Ashton: With respect, Commissioner, can I say, with the greatest respect, rhetorical questions of that kind are unfair to the witness.

Morris was only warming up. He told Leck that, historically, doctors ran hospitals and performed operations with a minimum of 'pen-pushers' or bureaucrats.

Near the end, Ashton told Morris: 'May I hasten to say, respect-fully, we do not for a moment complain about – certainly don't dissent for a moment about your authority and power to require him to give evidence today and we don't complain about your decision to do so but I simply respectfully ask that it be understood by all the disadvan-tage under which he labours in those circumstances.'

At 4.05 pm, Darren Keating, who had taken a seat each day to follow the inquiry evidence, heard for the first time that he would be up next. Morris put to Dr Keating that if he'd 'spent a bit more time in the operational parts of the hospital rather than in your office', he might have discovered that 'nurses were hiding patients from Dr Patel so he couldn't operate on them' and that 'senior medical staff were rec-ommending to patients that they seek transfer to Brisbane rather than go under the knife of Dr Patel'.

Morris: What needs to be done to ensure this sort of tragedy doesn't happen again...relating to the people that died, the boy who had his leg amputated, the woman who had her breast cancer passed over by Dr Patel, all of these tragic circumstances that we've heard over the last four days? Would it be a good start to have hospitals run by doctors who are real doctors who see patients and know what goes on from day-to-day in the operating theatre and the ward rooms?

Keating: Not necessarily.

The replay of the evidence on the evening TV news further shredded the public reputations of the two men. Leck and Keating were humiliated. Their lawyers were livid.

The previous day in State Parliament, Beattie and his team were taunted by the National Party's hit man, Jeff Seeney, who carried a sign 'Labor Killing Queenslanders – 87', a reference to the number of patients who had died after contact with Patel. 'I've had to deal with a number of their families. I've found that to be very distressing, and I didn't want to let the spin doctors carry the issue forward,' Seeney, who was ejected, explained.

Over the weekend there were rumours that Morris had dangerously exposed the inquiry to a potential Supreme Court legal challenge by Leck and Keating for apprehended bias. Even some of the inquiry's staff were concerned that if Morris overplayed his hand, the inquiry would be shut down. Damien Atkinson, one of the two junior counsel assisting Morris, had little sympathy for Leck or Keating, but he was anxious for the inquiry to reach findings after a fair fight.

In the court of public opinion and amongst the patients and their loved ones, however, Morris was cheered. People saw him illuminating matters of life and death in a system which relied on secrecy and distortion of the truth to hide mistakes and negligence. The pain and embarrassment of a couple of bureaucrats paled into insignificance compared with the carnage at the hospital and the grief and loss of relatives. As veteran newspaper reporter Peter Cameron told me on the way down George Street: 'Nobody ever made a great omelette without cracking a few eggs.' But Morris had sown two further seeds for the inquiry's failure.

By the end of the following week, Ron Ashton had adopted a new approach. He sought to reverse his acquiescence over the handling of his client, Peter Leck, by Morris on day four. If Leck should decide at some point to attempt to shut down the inquiry for apprehended bias, his lawyers would have a difficult time explaining to the Supreme Court why they had been happy to go along with Morris at first. Accordingly, Ashton rowed into day nine on a different boat and described the process of calling and questioning Leck 'unfair, unnecessary, unexplained and, in the context of the treatment of witnesses in the commission so far, essentially unique to our client'. It was a pointer to the potential for a future challenge.

But the evidence of most interest to me on day nine came from Dr Denis Lennox, the author of the Queensland Health report on Overseas Trained Doctors which had been leaked to me in late 2003. Lennox had suffered because of the leak. He was not even the leaker. He told Morris of the bureaucracy's bullying, secrecy, practice of suppressing reports and shoot-the-messenger culture.

Lennox also rejected the spin peddled back in November 2003 by health minister Wendy Edmond and her new chief, Steve Buckland, about the report being a 'draft' with no official status.

He lamented a health system which lacked transparency and sold out its staff.

After Lennox ended his testimony, it became apparent that my proposed evidence was being rejected by one of the key parties at risk of being punished by the inquiry.

I was leaked a confidential letter written by Paul McCowan, a solicitor for the Medical Board, in which he attacked my formal statement. 'We are concerned that a draft proof of evidence has been produced and circulated, which is directly, or impliedly, critical of our clients, in particular Mr O'Dempsey and the Medical Board of Queensland,' the letter to the inquiry states.

The Board's hide took my breath away. When it became clear that my statement would not be formally tendered as evidence, I thought I knew how Lennox felt when his report was buried.

Meanwhile, Beattie's book, *Making a Difference: Life, Leadership and Politics*, flopped on its release. Written before the Patel story broke, he nominates one of his top ten achievements as: 'Providing the systems and budget to enable doctors, nurses and health workers to cut waiting times for public hospital operations to the best on record, in a health system which has been judged the most effective in Australia.'

59

Bring him back

9–11 June 2005

TONI Hoffman felt like a supporting actor in a horror film that had received worldwide attention. The heroine's screams had finally been heard, but where, she asked, was the lead performer? Where was Jayant Patel? 'Lisette, my friend from Sweden, reckons he's put on a turban and is riding the Jammu express,' she told me.

Hoffman's close friend, who lived in Gothenburg where the Patel story had just made the front page, recalled fond memories of their travels in India when both were young nurses. Except for some hair-raising experiences on the Jammu express.

Before public hearings moved from Brisbane to Bundaberg on 20 June, I wanted to visit Patel's hometown in Gujarat Province in south-west India to talk to his friends and former colleagues. There was a new urgency. On 10 June, two days before photographer John Wilson and I boarded a Qantas flight to Bombay, a New Delhi-based friend, Rahul Bedi, sent me one of many stories running prominently in India.

> An Indian-trained surgeon linked by health officials to the deaths of at least 87 patients in Australia over two years should be charged with murder, a government inquiry recommended on Friday.
>
> The Commission of Inquiry investigating Patel's practice at the Bundaberg Hospital recommended in an interim report on Friday that he be charged with murder in the death of James Edward Phillips, who died five days after Patel surgically removed part of his oesophagus.

In recommending the murder charge, the report said there was no doubt 'that the surgical procedure undertaken by Patel – an oesophagectomy – was, objectively, likely to endanger human life'.

The inquiry also recommended that Patel – dubbed 'Dr. Death' by the Australian media – be charged with negligence for causing bodily harm in relation to an Aboriginal patient, Marilyn Daisy, who developed gangrene in her leg after she was allegedly left without treatment for several weeks following an amputation performed by Patel.

Patel has also been accused of making false representations and fraud for allegedly falsifying his application to practice medicine in Australia by removing any mention of his disciplinary history in the United States.

If prosecutors decide to file a murder charge against Patel, he could face extradition to Australia under a 1974 treaty between the two countries. If tried and convicted under Australian law, Patel could face a maximum sentence of life in prison. However, some media reports have suggested Patel may have returned to India, which has no extradition treaty with Australia. Patel's Oregon-based lawyer, Stephen Houze, refused to comment about his client's whereabouts.

'I have just received the interim report and I intend to give it very close scrutiny, but will not be able to make any public comments about the matter until I have reviewed it carefully,' Houze said.

THE picture opportunity is usually a predictable set-up in which the participants shamelessly exploit an artificial moment and each other for mutual benefit. Peter Beattie orchestrated picture opportunities every day. They were a lot cheaper than paid advertising. After nine days of public hearings involving evidence from 13 witnesses, four of whom were from Bundaberg Base Hospital (Toni Hoffman, Peter Miach, Darren Keating and Peter Leck), Tony Morris believed he had heard enough to give Beattie an interim report. Their meeting meant a picture opportunity.

Meanwhile, both Beattie and I had penned separate letters to Jayant Patel. Mine went to his hotmail address. It said in part: 'Perhaps you are following the evidence in the Commission of Inquiry, as well as the media's reporting. If you would like to put any part of your side of the story or make any comment, feel free to email me...I assure you that anything you want to say will be reported.'

Beattie tabled his letter to Patel in State Parliament, posted it on the Smart State's website and sent it to the media in Oregon. It was unsubtle. 'If you maintain, as members of your family have reportedly stated, that you are an excellent doctor who provided quality care to your patients, you also owe it to yourself to come forward and defend your actions,' Beattie wrote. He urged Patel to 'return to Queensland as soon as possible to explain your actions in relation to the treatment received by patients of the Bundaberg Base Hospital'. As part of the enticement, Beattie offered a one-way economy class airfare to Brisbane. It was a far cry from Patel's last flight funded by the Beattie Government, in April, when he fled Queensland with a one-way business class fare to Portland.

The letter was meant to be seen as deadly serious, but it looked like a childish stunt. Nobody should have been surprised when Patel did not hop on the next available flight to Australia, although Beattie became momentarily excited when the government's website man-agers noted his letter had attracted a 'hit' from someone in Portland, Oregon. Beattie publicly tipped that Patel was paying attention and considering the offer. His hopes were dashed by Opposition leader Lawrence Springborg, who identified the real cyber-visitor – an inquis-itive Portland practitioner, Dr Russ Faria. 'The Premier and his spin doctors need to be more careful in the future when they go about wildly speculating in the media as to how close they are to capturing Dr Patel,' Springborg gloated.

My missive to Patel went unanswered, too. Morris had been doing his bit to encourage Patel's return to Australia. He approved a letter to the surgeon's Portland lawyer, Stephen Houze, to establish 'whether Patel is prepared to return to Queensland to participate in the inquiry, and, if so, what conditions (such as payment of travelling and accom-modation expenses, or even an indemnity from prosecution) might be required by Patel in order to secure his return'. 'Those communications have attracted no response whatsoever,' Morris said.

The suggestion of an indemnity was surprising. The outcry from the people of Queensland, had one been granted, would have been deafening.

Morris was approached before the start of the inquiry by Perth lawyer Tom Percy, QC, who offered to represent Patel. When Percy did not turn up at the public hearings, Morris decided that Patel, having chosen not to avail himself of the opportunity to participate in the inquiry, had waived an entitlement to challenge the evidence of his accusers or to introduce his own.

Accordingly, Morris recommended a multitude of criminal charges in his interim report. He went further than anyone expected by proposing 'felony murder' charges as an alternative to manslaughter. 'It has traditionally been applied where death results from an act of violence or negligence committed in the course of a violent offence, such as a rape or an armed robbery,' Morris said. So long as the 'act', done unlawfully, is 'likely to endanger human life', the charge could be justified.

Morris provided a helpful example: if a pedestrian is knocked down and killed by the reckless driving of a getaway car used by bank robbers, a 'felony murder' charge could be brought – because the reckless driving of the car was likely to endanger human life. 'Ordinarily, even the grossest negligence on the part of a medical practitioner would not attract a murder conviction, unless the jury could be satisfied beyond a reasonable doubt that the degree of negligence was inconsistent with any state of mind other than a positive intention to kill,' Morris explained. 'But very different considerations apply where, for example, an impostor pretends to be a medical practitioner, and kills a patient whilst attempting to perform a surgical procedure.'

Although Patel had medical training and qualifications, his efforts in Bundaberg and the outcomes for the patients were the result of his deceptions. Put simply, as he was operating unlawfully, he had forfeited the usual protections afforded to doctors.

Beattie, who commended every word of the interim report from Morris, rammed through more legislative changes to tighten the registration system for doctors and increase the penalties for impostors. 'This is terrible, this happened on our watch,' he said. 'This will be a matter on our consciences until the day we die. What we have to do in those circumstances is to ensure that the perpetrator is brought to justice and the system is improved so it never happens again, and that's what we're doing with the legislation today.'

The promotion by Morris of the idea that a surgeon could be charged with murder caused grave concern outside the political arena. Some lawyers believed he was grandstanding again and had gone too far. The interim report gave Ron Ashton and Geoff Diehm, the lawyers for Peter Leck and Dr Darren Keating respectively, another potential legal argument in any Supreme Court challenge. They would be able to argue that Morris had made up his mind before witnesses were cross-examined.

Morris had made secondary recommendations for the provisional arrest of Patel and his extradition. But extradition from where? Where do you hide or reside, never mind work, when thousands of Internet sites around the world have posted your photograph and name under the heading 'Dr Death'? For someone accustomed to living the high life, flying up the front of the aircraft, enjoying the financial spoils of surgery and the ego-stroking, Patel's predicament was difficult to imagine.

The news had travelled quickly to India and the United States where reporters and TV crews began staking out Patel's home again. Bloggers and media conglomerates alike, from one-person outfits to the New York Times and its worldwide subscribers, were zeroing in on him as surely as law enforcement officials. His name, image and home address were known to millions of people. Thanks to evidence at the inquiry, we even had details of his US passport. Issued shortly before he came to Australia, it bore the number 207556040 and was due to expire on 17 December 2012.

If he used his credit card (American Express), police would know about it.

60

Ego analysis

13–20 June 2005

THE journey from Brisbane to Jayant Patel's home town took us through Mumbai, Ahmedabad and on a 5-hour bone-rattling ride through Gujarat province to the town of Jamnagar. Our friend and escort, Rahul Bedi, decided he knew just where he would go if he were in Jayant Patel's shoes. We were crossing the south-west corner of a country where as many as 300 million people earned a dollar a day. In India, medical treatment is largely for the wealthy and doctors, even those who should not have been trusted with a pocket knife, revered unquestioningly.

Bedi decided that if Patel felt threatened, he would return to Jamnagar where he grew up and enjoyed an education. and where his family retained strong caste ties. Patel could even start a clinic to complement the hospital where he first performed surgery. His troubles in the US and Australia would be of little consequence in India, according to Bedi. 'Because life is very cheap here. It's not such a big deal,' he explained. We left Ahmedabad at dawn, and were in Jamnagar by noon.

India's poverty made it difficult to put the Patel scandal into perspective. My First World standards and values worked well in Australia. These same standards and values could not withstand the sight and smell of needy children in rags, lying with their parents in the dust and rubbish beside the road as we sped past in an air-conditioned four-wheel drive emblazoned with the insignia of one of Gujarat's most luxurious hotels, the Taj. Our room rate of US$170 a night plus taxes would have taken a low-caste Gujarati labourer half a year of back-breaking toil to earn.

At dusk in Jamnagar, the potholed road to the Guru Govindsingh Hospital heaved with a chaotic jumble of cars, trucks, motorcycles and cabs, weaving noisy paths around street urchins and pedestrians alike. By nightfall, casualties from several accidents had been dropped at the hospital for patching up. Some, like the man we saw wheeled out of the surgery ward on a decrepit trolley at sundown, would not survive.

The equipment in the surgery ward looked decades old. If a hammer and anvil had been in one of the cupboards, I would not have been surprised. There was no air conditioning to offer relief from the near-40 degree Celsius summer heatwave. No electronic lifesaving devices monitored the vital signs of patients fallen on hard times with failing health. The ward was quiet apart from the swishing of overhead fans.

'Dr Patel was a resident here with me – we worked together in these wards,' Dr Mansurali Mamdani told me during a tour. 'We did general surgery including neck, abdomen, hernia, breast lump and thyroid. Many times he operated and I assisted, or he assisted me.'

An old hand-painted sign above the dusty entrance to the adjoining MP Shah Medical College, the teaching showpiece for every privileged Gujarati wanting to study to be a doctor, implores students to leave their arrogance behind. 'Be teachable – always assume that there is vital information you still need to learn,' it says.

Little had changed at the college whose graduates three decades ago still remembered their confident classmate, Jayant Patel. His regular visits back to Jamnagar, population about 500 000, from the US and Australia were always warmly received. Their most illustrious export had become their most disgraced.

Dr Mamdani walked me into the college's student branch to seek old files proving Patel's original enrolment and grades. For those who knew him as a medical student and then a resident doctor in Jamnagar, and who stayed in touch during his career as a surgeon in the US, there was a shared view. The doctors I spoke to agreed that Patel had abnormal self-belief. He never accepted he was wrong. Mamdani described this personality trait as the key to understanding Patel's downfall. Patel, whose deception and pride meant nobody in Jamnagar knew of the bans and disciplinary action against him in the US, was always dangerously confident in his own abilities. Mamdani continued:

He saw no need for consultation – colleagues with alternative solutions to surgical or medical questions were deficient. He had a very different type of personality. He is arrogant. He thinks that whatever he says is the word of God. He doesn't like to hear anyone's challenge. He's very intelligent but he is autocratic. He feels he is the superior doctor and he knows everything, and that there is no need for him to have any supervision.

He would not like to consult. He was final. He was never prepared to accept whatever he has done wrong. Suppose he was having a discussion about surgery and there were questions about his responses – his answer was always, 'No, whatever I say is true'. Then he would refuse to discuss it. We saw this in the teaching program. Whatever answer he gave, he said, was always right. That is the root cause, I think. The autocratic personality will ruin your life. This trouble he's facing now is the result. He could have found peace doing something else. But Jayant Patel would never believe that such things should happen to him.

I'm not against him – he has done nothing wrong to me. His wife, Kishoree, and my wife are closely associated. We have had many family dinners. The medical negligence he can fight – this is a professional thing and we say to him, 'We can help you'. But as far as the other things are concerned, with the fraud and misrepresentation, this is not something we can help with. He will have to face the consequences.

As we chatted, a small group of medical students gathered around Mamdani, the associate professor of the college for a decade. He patiently explained the reason for our presence.

During a meeting with Dr Subhash Patel in his nearby gastroen-terology clinic, I understood the disappointment so keenly felt by Jayant's closest Jamnagar friends.

They are not related, but Subhash and Jayant were childhood play-mates, college classmates and professional colleagues. In the years since Patel had emigrated to the United States, they remained friends. Subhash had fretted every day for weeks about whether to pick up the telephone to offer support. 'He always decided against it. Patel, says

Subhash, was not someone who could take the call in the spirit in which it was intended. He would think it offensive or in bad taste. He has always been like that. He has never liked anything negative said about himself,' Subhash told me. 'He is very strong-willed and ambitious; he has always been very sure about himself. All of us are very worried about him, but we do not want to hurt his feelings. He has been branded "Dr Death". His career is doomed. It is something very tragic for someone who has had such an illustrious medical career.'

Until Patel left the antiquated and cash-starved Guru Govindsingh Hospital to make his fortune and improve his qualifications in the US, he and Subhash had something else in common. They grew up together as the privileged progeny of well-off families.

In the campus cafe, the manager, Vinu Bhai, recalled Patel as a 'son of royalty', and indeed Jayant Patel's grandfather, a former deputy chief minister of Gujarat State during the pre-independence era of fellow Gujarati Mahatma Gandhi, was once treated like royalty. The prominent politician's son became a successful and influential oil mill businessman. Jayant's father trusted one doctor in Jamnagar to look after his health: the father of Dr Subhash Patel. The bonds, loyalties and recognition of clan and caste are far-reaching, particularly among Patels, in this traders' town with its strategic military interests near the Pakistan border. Whenever Patel visited Jamnagar, he would make a point of meeting Subhash, who told me:

> He came from Australia one time and said he was commissioned
> by the US Government and an institute in Australia to set up a
> surgical facility. He took it as a challenge; that's what he told me.
> I am now learning of matters that I didn't know about before
> – we knew nothing about his Oregon and New York history.
>
> He would come to visit me here and said nothing of his
> trouble. But on the Internet now there are 1500 references to
> him. We can only hope that some good comes of all this, if only
> that doctors will think twice before indulging in such things in
> future.

Patel's old mentor and teacher, Dr Rudhresh Mehta, now retired, led me to the roof garden above his flat. There was still no sign of the monsoon rains needed to rejuvenate the land and ensure a harvest to ward off famine. Mehta looked crestfallen. He had regarded Patel as almost infallible; a most brilliant product of the MP Shah Medical College to which Mehta had devoted most of his working life. Indeed, Mehta had taken credit for Patel's apparent success. His wife was also fond of Patel's wife, Kishoree, a junior gynaecologist at a Jamnagar private hospital before the move to the United States.

A fortnight before our visit, Patel had telephoned Mehta. 'I said to him, "What is all this?" I asked him, "Where are you?" I told him that people are looking for him, that's what the TV says,' Mehta said.

Mehta listened incredulously as his former student made light of the problems. Patel insisted to his old teacher he had done nothing wrong. It was a misunderstanding. 'He said "it's nothing that serious". He said "A surgeon never operates to kill – and cancer patients can die". He was upset in the beginning but I found him very calm and composed. It was a serious talk. He said he was waiting for Australia's movements.

'For 50 years we have been giving excellent teachers to the US. I feel very bad. What is the real story? Will we ever know? He could have talked to me earlier. Unless one recognises one's own mistakes, one never improves.'

Some of the other doctors we interviewed in Jamnagar suggested that Mehta's overt favouritism of Patel as a student had unhealthily fed the understudy's ego.

Down a rubble-and-rubbish-strewn alley close to the town hub, the Patel family's Mukund Villa, where he grew up, stood desolate and uninviting. His mother was living with her daughter in a nearby town.

Gujarat police inspector Shri BB Mohite doubted the issue would ever excite his jurisdiction's interest. 'This is very big news in Australia where life has more value, but it is of less interest here,' he told me.

IT was a different story in Portland, Oregon, where my colleague Tuck Thompson competed with Australia's *60 Minutes*, US TV crews and journalists representing newspapers and radio outlets along the West Coast. He went to Patel's neighbourhood with 'neat front gardens and double-fronted two-storey houses evoking notions of prosperity and solid family values'. Patel was holed up inside the house as Mexicans tended the garden. His wife, Kishoree, played cat-and-mouse with the media crews on her drive to work. Thompson spoke to doctors and Patel's former patients who described a 'sociopathic personality and a monumental ego'. 'You don't want a doctor with a God complex,' Lindy Davis, an Oregon medical technical assistant whose right arm was partially paralysed when Patel severed three nerves in her neck while removing a lump, told Thompson. Davis was one of Patel's last surgical cases in Oregon in 2001 before the Kaiser Permanente health-care group finally forced him to quit. She had been referred by Patel's wife, Kishoree.

'My hand and shoulder went instantly numb. He said not to worry about it. It was common. The medical oath says, "first do no harm". He has done harm and he should be held accountable for that,' Davis said. 'I'm upset with the regulators. They protect the doctors and the organisations. There's a brotherhood of doctors who don't want to let anything out. They think they are gods.'

When Tuck Thompson contacted the American doctors who had lauded Patel in the references that helped him win the job in Bundaberg, none would defend their earlier favourable assessments. He was scolded for having the temerity to bother them.

Oregon Medical Association CEO Jim Kronenberg said that 'to be a good surgeon, you need to understand how to navigate anatomy, you need good eye-hand coordination and you need good surgical judgement, when to operate and when not to, and what to do and what not to do'. 'This guy was lousy technically and had terrible surgical judgement. This is a remarkable case. In 30 years, I've never seen anything like it. He doesn't understand consequences. He does what he does and he doesn't care,' Kronenberg said.

As top Queensland Government lawyers in Brisbane held confidential talks with Patel's Australian barrister, Tom Percy, and newly hired solicitor Damian Scattini, the surgeon's Portland lawyer, Stephen Houze, was also holding a closed-door meeting in Oregon.

Peter Beattie, embarking on a trade and investment mission to the United States and Italy, had ordered his Director-General Leo Keliher and State Development Minister Tony McGrady, who were in the US for a biotechnology conference and trade mission, to make a very public appearance in Oregon. 'Every Queenslander thinks Dr Patel should return,' McGrady told an airport press conference in Portland.

Thompson described a dishevelled Keliher 'looking like he came down the luggage chute'. But McGrady had designs on stardom. Descending the escalator to the baggage claim area, Thompson watched a passer-by ask McGrady why he was so important; why the media horde? 'I'm a movie star. Tom Cruise,' he quipped.

Later, in Houze's high-rise law office on the 11th floor of the PacWest Center, the talks went nowhere. Houze regarded his visitors from Brisbane with disdain. When McGrady taped an interview with the ABC's *Stateline* host, Kirrin McKechnie, shortly after the hopeless meeting with Houze, the politician sounded pleased with himself. McGrady spoke of generating 'massive coverage of our trip'. He empha-sised the turnout at his morning media conference and boasted that the coverage went across the US. It raised the question: was his mission more to do with hogging the news or seeking the return of a surgeon?

> Kirrin McKechnie: Given all of these media conferences that you and the Premier are doing, I mean is this just a media stunt, because you know that you have very little hope of extraditing Dr Patel?
>
> Tony McGrady: Now I get a little angry when people suggest that this is some sort of a political stunt. I mean, that's the sort of nonsense you hear from the Opposition all of the time. The reality is that we are determined, we are determined to do everything we can to get Dr Patel to return to Queensland to face the inquiry.

Meanwhile, Beattie had held another media conference, this time at Los Angeles airport. Just in case anyone missed the earlier coverage. 'What we're trying to do is create a set of circumstances where Mr

Patel can't practise medicine anywhere in the world unless he comes home to Queensland, or to Brisbane, to give evidence to the inquiry,' Beattie said.

Dr Bruce Flegg, the Liberal Party's hardworking politician with ambitions to succeed Beattie, condemned the travelling circus: 'The Beattie–McGrady publicity stunt in America is bizarre. It's got to be one of the strangest activities in a criminal pursuit in Australian history. Thinking people understand that a criminal pursuit is a matter for legal authorities and not for politicians looking for a media headline.'

Tony Morris took some of the credit for the international ruckus: 'One of the purposes of the Commission of Inquiry, when it decided to release the interim report last Friday containing recommendations for Patel's prosecution, was to flush out Patel and his legal representatives.'

Scattini and Houze stayed in regular telephone and email contact, comparing notes from their respective meetings. In the two hours Scattini had spent in talks with Crown Law officials, it appeared possible, under certain conditions, that Patel would come back to Brisbane.

'He is interested in returning to Australia to give some account of how he managed things in Bundaberg,' Attorney-General Rod Welford said. But the terms were unacceptable. Patel asked for an indemnity from prosecution. Beattie was prepared to pay the economy fare, organise safe accommodation, and even fund a portion of the legal expenses. The indemnity was unthinkable. By the end of the week, Scattini, Houze and Patel were all agreed. He would definitely not be returning voluntarily to Queensland. Not under any circumstances.

I was surprised that Scattini, a fierce critic of Queensland Health who had made his name and money by suing doctors for negligence, wanted Patel as a client. If Scattini had been leading the legal fight on behalf of the patients for compensation and corrective surgery, nobody would have batted an eyelid. When the Patel furore erupted two months earlier, Scattini had been one of the first to express alarm and to encourage follow-up articles. 'Congratulations. It beggars belief. I can think of another regional hospital with guest doctors that bears scrutiny as well,' Scattini had emailed me.

The dry-humoured son of an agricultural scientist, Scattini had always struck me as honest and ethical. His reputation among his peers was excellent. He genuinely believed that Patel was being unfairly treated, but some of the staff in his own firm, Quinn & Scattini, were uncomfortable about the decision to act for the surgeon.

Scattini stayed back at his desk to compose an appropriate explanation, then sent round an internal memo:

> Probably many of you have had friends or relatives ask you how we can represent such a person. The practice of law is not a popularity contest. Sometimes our clients will be unpopular. Sometimes, such as now, they will be actually hated by large numbers of people, who like the rest of us only know what they have been told to believe.

Houze, however, was well suited to one of his toughest legal assignments. He had been making headlines in Oregon for years. I found a revealing profile from August 2003 in *The Oregonian* newspaper. It was headlined, 'Champion of the unpopular causes: Attorney Stephen Houze'. Reporter Robin Franze describes him as a short, unassuming, publicity-shy criminal lawyer who pursues justice for the most publicity-prone clients.

> Friends say he often takes cases where he sees the possibility of redemption. And he tells clients facing lengthy prison sentences that the best measure of a man is what he does after he stumbles.
>
> Those who know him well – attorneys, prosecutors, judges and private investigators – say he's a complex man: highly principled, intelligent, and driven by a ferocious energy that intimidates his adversaries in the courtroom.
>
> 'I think winning was everything he ever thought about,' says Pat Mancuso, Houze's high school football coach in Ohio. Despite his small size, Houze played quarterback and defensive back. 'And what he lacked in size, he made up for with determination. He was a scrapper, a fighter... all go-go-go'.

With Houze in Oregon and Scattini in Brisbane, the Beattie Government had met its match.

61

Wound feuds

20 June 2005

JODIE Hillier could stand it no longer. Shantu Shah, one of Jayant Patel's acquaintances in Portland, had described cancer as 'a punishment of God for the past and present life deeds of a person'. Patel was 'a Dr Life and a hero who helped cure thousands', according to Shah. On the TV news, Hillier had also heard one of Jayant Patel's Oregon neighbours extolling the surgeon's friendly virtues. The sympathy infuriated Hillier. She had felt a burning hatred. Her mother, who also had cancer, Doris, had suffered greatly as one of Patel's patients. They wanted to throttle Patel.

For many of the traumatised patients and their relatives in Bundaberg, the start of public hearings in the sugar town meant the reopening of angry wounds.

The story was still dominating the news agenda. The private investigator retained by reporter Paul Barry and *60 Minutes* had earned his fee for some old-fashioned covert surveillance. Several million Australians saw Patel, looking harried and drawing deeply on a cigarette near his Portland mansion, on the top-rating current affairs program. 'This is his third stop at the video store,' the private investigator, a former FBI agent, tells Barry. The reporter strides to the front door of Patel's home and starts knocking. 'Dr Patel? Dr Patel, we know you're in there,' he says.

There was even talk of a dramatic movie. W Lance Reynolds, President of Atlantic Films and Television in New York, wanted a few key figures to consider an offer for film rights.

The same day, the *New York Times* published a lengthy front page essay by correspondent Ray Bonner, headlined 'Deaths and a Doctor's

Past Transfix Australians'. Patel's celebrity lawyer, Stephen Houze, told the world's most influential newspaper: 'We have very grave concerns about this drumbeat of incessant and prejudicial publicity that is saturating all of Queensland, and indeed all of Australia.'

Houze and his new-found legal colleague in Brisbane, Damian Scattini, were running hard on a line that the publicity meant Patel would never receive a fair trial. I was reminded of one of the most notorious accused killers in the United States, OJ Simpson, who was televised live-to-air in a freeway chase after the murder of his wife, Nicole, and a friend. In high-profile cases involving multiple deaths, overwhelming publicity was inevitable. The more heinous or sensational, the louder the drumbeat. If society adopted Houze's philosophy, the most wicked alleged offenders would never be brought to trial. Nor did it necessarily follow that sensational publicity led to a guilty verdict. Simpson was acquitted despite overwhelming DNA evidence.

When I trawled the Internet to try to understand more about Houze, I noted his earlier, seemingly contradictory, comments to his own professional association, the Oregon State Bar. 'I've observed that crime news coverage is a huge phenomenon in this country [USA],' Houze told the May 2004 Bar Bulletin. Despite that, Houze said he had been 'pleasantly surprised by the relatively minimal impact media coverage seems to have on prospective jurors'. 'The saturation of the media is not as great as we think,' Houze said. 'It's not as bad as we think in terms of tainting the process. Which is good, because it's very, very difficult to get a change of venue.'

When Terry O'Gorman, a Brisbane criminal lawyer and Queensland president of the Council for Civil Liberties, said there was a high risk that Patel, if extradited, would not get a fair trial, Peter Beattie denounced the theory as 'absolute rot'. 'It is just taking civil liberties to an absolute absurd position,' he said. At last, Beattie had found favour with Jodie Hillier, who commented:

We have people saying that this man won't have a fair trial and that he can have all the media and patients for defamation for his new name that suits him so well, Dr Death. What would he like us to call him? God? Does he expect us to thank him for the hell that he has put so many people through? How can this man get away with it? How on earth are people ever going to feel the same again about going to a public hospital?

I hope to God that he is prosecuted for every single person that he touched with his hands of death. I hope that he suffers like all his patients have and I hope to God that he will never be able to pick up his scalpel again. But if he ever does, he can use it on himself.

Her mother told how she had been 'left for five days with a horrific flesh-eating disease feasting out on my body'. Doris Hillier blamed Patel for a botched operation and subsequent complications. She urged anyone upset at the treatment of Patel to travel to Bundaberg 'and sit in on one of our support group meetings and listen and see what this barbaric animal has done to us all'.

Detectives from the homicide squad, who had kept a low profile in Brisbane while downloading transcripts and exhibits from the inquiry's website, were seconded to Bundaberg to take statements and attend the inquiry's public hearings in the lecture hall of a local education centre. Two detectives went to Portland and New York to gather formal documentation about the disciplinary actions by the respective regulatory bodies. It was the same documentation we had discovered on the websites.

Police Commissioner Bob Atkinson had already parted company with Tony Morris on the extradition issue. Atkinson favoured a slow-burn approach: a laborious investigation by a handful of experienced detectives, hundreds of interviews, a panel of medical experts, thorough reviews by the Director of Public Prosecutions. Finally, an approach to the Federal Justice Minister to trigger a formal extradition application and the arrest of Patel by US Federal Marshals. There were risks in this strategy, too, the most obvious being a move by Patel to India, which does not share an extradition treaty with Australia.

Morris firmly believed there was more than enough evidence already for a prima facie case for fraud, manslaughter and grievous bodily harm. Patel should not have been practising in Australia, full stop. Any adverse outcomes arising from his deception were, therefore, criminal. The Morris view seemed plausible, particularly after a leading US criminal lawyer who specialised in extradition, Douglas McNabb, contacted me to query why the Queensland police had not moved swiftly. McNabb said Patel should have been arrested immediately.

I thought it unlikely that the American justice system would wage a battle to prevent Patel being extradited. He had been blamed by independent US medical investigators for the deaths of Americans before he came to Australia. We were not dealing with a blue-eyed all-American hero with no blood on his hands. Patel was drenched in it.

62

Sound bites

20 June to 1 July 2005

GAIL Aylmer felt uncomfortable about being filmed in the cavernous inquiry venue, a short walk from the shopping malls in Bundaberg's commercial heart. She exercised her right to have the cameras turned off during her evidence. In a makeshift office strewn with TV cables, screens and film-editing equipment, the journalists and their crews collectively groaned. They needed dramatic footage. It would be a lot harder to package a story bereft of pictures.

As the first witness called onto the stage for the start of the hearings in Bundaberg, Aylmer painted a sorry portrait of Jayant Patel and his contact with the patients. She recounted the efforts to persuade Patel to wash his hands and wear gloves, and his stubborn reluctance to observe basic hygiene.

> David Andrews, SC: Now, can you explain – was this simply a matter of principle or was there something significant? Was Dr Patel simply touching patients on the head?
>
> Aylmer: Oh no, he was touching their wounds, pulling off dressings to have a look to see how the wound is going, poking around the wound. He was actually really touching the wounds, where I felt that there was a risk to the patient and to the next patient that he went to as well.

It explained why many wounds had become infected and broken open. The evidence of nurses, patients and doctors over the days and weeks was tragically spellbinding. Aylmer was followed by other senior nurses, Lindsay Druce, Robyn Pollock and Jenny White who all gave damning evidence.

Dr Darren Keating sat impassively for most of the Bundaberg sittings, 21 days in all, staring ahead at the stage as patients glared at him. Was he taking in every word of testimony? Would he seek redemption for his failings as a manager?

Amanda Watt, my friend and reporting colleague from the *Courier-Mail*, doubted Keating had accepted responsibility. She suspected he was coming each day out of arrogance and the need to absorb as much detail as possible to better brief his lawyer, Geoff Diehm. Keating was not going down without a fight. He won grudging respect for his stance.

Jane Hodgkinson, Channel 9's senior reporter, boiled the complexities and tensions down to a succinct sound bite. 'This is about heroes and villains,' she told me.

Sitting in the front row of the second tier of the lecture hall and hearing the testimony of nurses, doctors and patients, it was clear Morris still enjoyed public approval. People were speaking their mind about serious matters that in the past they had felt compelled to bury. The administrators and bureaucrats, who had been accustomed to turning bad news into a series of bumps under the carpet and overriding doctors and nurses on what was good for the patients, were ducking for cover.

Morris had also begun to herald bad news for the Beattie Government. He was broadening the inquiry's focus from a dysfunctional hospital and a deadly surgeon to a sick system replete with cover-ups and negligence. Inevitably, this would cause heartache for Labor politicians in electorates across the state. We were seeing the stirrings of a potential revolution in health and politics. On the other hand, reputations were being damaged. Some were to be damaged irreparably.

One afternoon outside the lecture hall, I stopped briefly to talk to Patricia Feeney, the solicitor for Peter Leck. She looked distressed. 'It's so unfair,' she said.

Although at the time it was a closely guarded secret, Feeney had received further advice from Leck's psychiatrist about his worsening mental state. Dr Jeremy Butler told her the principal factor in Leck's declining condition was his unexpected appearance at the inquiry in

Brisbane when he endured the withering examination by Morris. Leck subsequently exhibited 'significant psychiatric symptoms indicating a fragile mental state'. Butler warned that if Leck appeared at the inquiry in Bundaberg, his condition would further deteriorate.

Toni Hoffman, meanwhile, needed to finish her evidence. She knew the lawyers for Leck, Keating and the Director of Nursing, Linda Mulligan, wanted to discredit much of what she had already told the inquiry. Hoffman feared that she would be singled out and have her motives questioned, yet the doctors who had done little or nothing would emerge unscathed.

Even the highly experienced and authoritative Dr Peter Miach, the strongest critic of Patel throughout his reign, had not taken an opportunity to report his concerns to the Director-General or the Medical Board or the Health Rights Commission or the AMA or the Coroner. He looked uncomfortable when Justin Harper, one of the lawyers for the patients, pointedly illustrated the many avenues Miach had not taken.

Miach: I'm not an ombudsman in a surgical ward. I don't de facto become sort of a policeman for the surgical unit.

Harper: If I put to you an assertion that there is a culture within the hospital that you keep the reports within the system and that you don't go outside the system, would that be a fair reflection of the culture of the Bundaberg Hospital and the associated medical profession surrounding it?

Miach: I think that's probably accurate, yes. I mean, it's well known that if you go outside 'the system' you get into trouble.

As a senior nurse, Deputy Commissioner Margaret Vider understood the culture and hierarchy in hospitals. 'Was it difficult for you to advance your concerns factually without the support of Dr [Martin] Carter, given the culture in which doctors and nurses clinically operate?' she asked Hoffman.

'I think one of the hardest things is, in the unit, Dr Carter would verbalise how terrible he thought Dr Patel was,' Hoffman replied. 'He was the doctor who, you know, coined the phrase Dr Death...but when the chips were down he wouldn't – he was not willing to make a complaint or come with me or support me. He would talk about it to all of us in the ICU about how terrible he was and openly, you know, say, you know, "don't let him near me"...'

Linda Mulligan's barrister, Phil Morrison, QC, who was not in the least intimidated by Morris, launched himself at Hoffman. He accused the local hero of withholding information from Mulligan and of wanting to see her sacked:

Morrison: You were setting her up for a fall, weren't you? And you still are, aren't you?

Hoffman: No, I had one intention.

Morrison: To fix the system?

Hoffman: Not to fix the system. If we can fix the system, that would be wonderful. I had one intention and that was to stop Dr Patel from operating on any more patients. That was my intention, to try and save just one life, just one more life.

When Morrison tried to interrupt, Hoffman was having none of it. She was shouting and tearful: 'No, I will finish now! And that is what my only intention was. This was never about them and us. This was never about Executive and myself. I thought Executive would be glad to try and save some of these patients' lives, and I thought Queensland Health would be supporting me in that, but instead that is not the case and it has become a them and us situation.'

Morris had become fed up with what he saw as the bureaucracy's attempts to thwart his inquiry. He was convinced that the administrators were out of control. 'The evidence suggests a situation within QH which is rapidly approaching what might be termed "bureaucratic gridlock": there are so many bureaucrats writing memoranda to one another, reading memoranda from one another, and attending meetings with one another, that nobody has any time left to actually get anything done,' Morris said.

But on 29 June, Morris and the inquiry would 'self-destruct', as lawyer Robert Mulholland, QC, later argued to the Supreme Court. It happened during a penetrating cross-examination of Miach by Geoff Diehm, Keating's resourceful and quietly effective lawyer. Morris, unhappy at the tarnishing of one of his key witnesses, crossly asked Diehm if Keating had instructed him to attack Miach. The inquiry commissioner said he wanted 'everyone at the Bar table to understand that one of the issues that's clearly being raised is this shoot the messenger attitude, and if it comes to our attention that anyone from the Director-General of Queensland Health down has given instructions for a witness like Dr Miach to be attacked, then that will be an appropriate foundation for us to make findings at the end of the proceedings'.

Diehm, astonished, held his ground. How could he defend Keating without exploiting weaknesses in Miach's version of events at the hospital? Keating's solicitor in Brisbane, David Watt, sent an urgent letter to Queensland Health. Thus far, all of Keating's legal expenses totalling almost $5000 a day had been funded by the public purse. Watt wanted to know if the public purse would also pick up the tab for extra costs 'in the event that Dr Keating was advised to bring an application to have the proceedings of the Commission of Inquiry stayed due to the lack of natural justice'.

The confidential response from Queensland Health lawyers Kate Curnow and Peter Crofts heartened Keating. The taxpayers had funded the inquiry. And the taxpayers would fund an attempt to obliterate the inquiry.

I had missed the exchange involving Miach, but was similarly angry about a 'shoot the messenger' attitude over a story I had published that day. The story gave a sneak preview of the just-completed clinical review, which found Patel culpable in up to 16 deaths. Eight of these were definite. A further eight were probable, though inconclusive, according to Dr Peter Woodruff.

As the review had not yet been handed to either Peter Beattie or Tony Morris, both were miffed. When Beattie flew into a rage, my major concern was to protect sources. As if there were not enough inquiries underway, Beattie demanded another. Queensland Health's internal investigator, Rebecca McMahon, was ordered to try to identify the source. She worked hard, wasting valuable time – hers and others' – to produce a 'Strictly Confidential' 185-page inconclusive report.

'Doesn't Beattie understand what has been going on?' I asked my wife, Ruth, who had moved to Bundaberg with the children so we could stay together for the hearings. She encouraged me to make the point in my column, which was written in anger and criticised Beattie for losing the plot. The political hypocrisy was breathtaking. When it suited the politicians, they leaked like sieves to promote themselves. But when well-intentioned public servants leaked matters of great public interest, all hell broke loose. If it had not been for leaks by Toni Hoffman in Bundaberg, the Jayant Patel scandal would have been swept under the carpet. All the far-reaching reforms and funds being promised to make hospitals safer would not be on the agenda. All the critical lessons would not be learned. Beattie still did not get it. He looked, I wrote, like 'a tin-pot dictator fermenting the very culture that has helped to produce the disaster in his health system'.

I wished he had met Dr Brian Thiele, a clinical professor of surgery who had been Bundaberg's highly effective and respected Director of Medical Services until the bureaucracy and the political games wore him out. 'I really do believe this was waiting to happen,' said Thiele, describing a system which through steady decline and corporate bastardry was no longer sensitive to patient needs. Thiele had become disillusioned because he saw political sensitivities, not patients, being the priority for administrators. He railed against their overly zealous controls:

> Bureaucratic administrators do not like to hear bad news. They do not like to be exposed to criticism. Many present problems are symptomatic of a culture of avoiding or burying criticism. The government has the view that health cannot win you an election but can lose you one. Against this background, it has not been keen to hear anything bad about health.
>
> It's a control-freak mentality that permeates the system. There is a desire to control which, to me, is almost pathological.

It discourages critical commentary. And it leads to a system which walks around with its head down and not a great deal of self-respect. It gradually erodes the importance of the individual contribution within the amorphous system. Goodwill has disappeared from the system. And, unfortunately, it has gone forever.

63

Kill it

Early July 2005

THE rumours were right. On 4 July, a Monday, David Groth, the inquiry's official Secretary, sat back in his chair. 'Holy snap!' he said.

The letter from Peter Leck's solicitor, Patricia Feeney, fresh out of the facsimile machine, was brief and to the point. 'We confirm our instructions to bring an application to the Supreme Court to have the chairperson, Mr Morris QC, disqualified from further proceedings in the Bundaberg Hospital Commission of Inquiry on the basis that he has demonstrated apprehended bias against our client in respect of matters arising under the inquiry,' Feeney wrote.

At 10.02 am the next day, 5 July, Morris started day 18 of public hearings in Bundaberg by disclosing the letter and the inquiry's fight for survival. I looked over to the tireless advocate for the patients, Beryl Crosby. She was slowly shaking her head in disbelief. As Morris asked Feeney for more information, Geoff Diehm, the lawyer for Dr Darren Keating, signalled his intention to join the challenge.

The financial, political and emotional cost of the inquiry so far had been enormous. Morris was determined to finish the work and ensure his place in history. He blinked. He held out an olive branch: 'One solution would be if – if there were a substantial case for bias or something of that nature, would be simply to say, "well, we'll make no findings with respect to your client, adverse findings". We might not say nice things about him; we won't make adverse findings. Would that address your client's concerns?'

For 40 minutes at the morning break, the patients – angry, bewildered and fearful – sought answers from their lawyer, Gerry Mullins.

'Are they allowed to do that?' asked Tess Bramich, who had been enduring almost every day of evidence with her daughter.

'So it's a cop-out,' said Crosby.

Ian Fleming volunteered that it was his own evidence the previous week – 'bullet-proof and ironclad' – of his complaint to Keating about Patel which had triggered the challenge. 'Where was the natural justice when we were suffering in that hospital?' he asked. 'When they were slicing me open like an animal, where was my justice? It was us together that got something done. This is unbelievable.'

Doris Hillier was so angry she looked ready to strike someone. 'How can they do what they are doing?' she demanded. 'Don't they give a damn about what we went through in the hospital?'

'I think Tony Morris is the most understanding and compassionate man,' said fellow patient Lisa Hooper. 'I don't believe for one minute that he's biased. How can they say that about him? It's so unfair.'

Toni Hoffman called my mobile telephone from the hospital's Intensive Care Unit to find out what was happening. The nurses were dealing with patient crises but the news from the nearby inquiry room was already racing around the ICU.

'There has been a bus accident, a triple a [abdominal aortic aneurism], a woman with a detached placenta – and now this!' Hoffman told me.

Keating, usually expressionless and unemotional, smiled broadly. Two days later, on 7 July, his legal documentation designed to sack Morris was filed in the Supreme Court. He started to giggle as he made his way to the exit of the Bundaberg inquiry room.

'You look very happy, Dr Keating,' I said.

He nodded in agreement. 'I haven't had much to be happy about until now,' he replied.

The witnesses – doctors, nurses, patients and their loved ones – soldiered on valiantly to give evidence in the days that followed. Morris rejected submissions to down tools pending a resolution. It would take weeks or months, Morris reasoned, for the Supreme Court to hear the legal arguments and reach a view. The stakes were enormous; the inquiry had become a lightning rod for change in the health system.

On the other hand, the most senior bureaucrats in Queensland Health, yet to give their evidence, wanted Morris to fail. They had given their blessing for Keating and Leck to rely on the public purse to fund the legal challenge. So, too, had the Crown Solicitor, Conrad Lohe, and his deputy Robert Campbell.

When Peter Beattie and Attorney-General Rod Welford were briefed, the agreement to fund Leck and Keating in their Supreme Court challenge was reversed. Just 24 hours after Keating's solicitor David Watt had heard of the generosity of the Queensland public purse, he received a letter from an embarrassed Dr Steve Buckland. 'I have been directed by the Premier to inform you that Queensland Health will not authorise the expenditure of public funds for the purpose of legal representation beyond that approved solely for your client's appearance at the Bundaberg Hospital Commission of Inquiry,' Buckland wrote.

Peter Beattie pledged his backing for the inquiry process, whatever happened.

Over a drink with the patients' lawyer Gerry Mullins at Bargara Beach, Keating's lawyer, Geoff Diehm, navigating a perilous legal course while managing to remain friends with everyone, said: 'You know, there will be only one person to blame if the inquiry falls over: Morris. You can't be accused of showing bias if you remain silent on the evidence. He will be the only person who can be held responsible.'

Payback

July 2005

THE evidence at the hearings in Bundaberg had been tragic, gruelling and, at times, gratuitously graphic. Bloody wounds. Cover-ups. Perforated bowels. Maladministration. Oozing pus. Missed opportunities. All of it amid tension and uncertainty raised by the looming Supreme Court challenge by Darren Keating and Peter Leck. If the challenge should succeed in bringing about the abolition of the inquiry, we feared it would all have been for nothing.

In declaring himself unbiased, Tony Morris had made an impassioned speech about the ramifications of his ousting. It would, he explained, 'have very grave personal consequences for the individuals who wish to see an outcome to this, and the thing that presses most upon my mind is the gruesome stories that we've heard over the past three or four weeks'. He omitted mention of the grave personal consequences for himself.

For most of the inquiry staff, journalists and support crew, it was almost time to return to families in Brisbane. We had been based in Bundaberg for a month. In the lecture hall in the education centre where the evidence was being heard, some of the reporters began planning a fitting farewell to Bundaberg: a dinner party at the Indian Curry Bazaar Restaurant, Jayant Patel's favourite. Jane Hodgkinson, the Nine Network's senior reporter, showed me a list of mock awards. They were directed mostly at the media, a few lawyers and the inquiry staff. We hoped they would raise a laugh. For being mentioned from time to time by Tony Morris, who had that day referred to me as 'the most reliable oracle' while clarifying something I had misreported, I would receive the 'Teacher's Pet' gong. Sean Parnell, whose articles in the *Australian* had caused Morris heartburn, was 'Best Ghost Writer' – for his absence from an inquiry he kept writing about.

There were a couple of gongs for the patients. For lifting his shirt to show his wound to journalists, and for asking the inquiry staff to post, on its official website, several photographs of his swollen and split abdomen, Ian Fleming would receive a 'Show Me Your Wound' award. One of our favourite patients, Beryl Crosby, the indefatigable chain-smoking leader of the support group, would be blessed with a 'Dirty Ashtray' award.

Geoff Diehm, the lawyer for Darren Keating, would be flattered by his special mention: an award for 'Courage Under Fire'. Similarly, John Allen, the tough but eminently fair lawyer for the nurses, would receive a glowing tribute. Hodgkinson together with Channel 10's Danielle Isdale, Channel 7's Cathy Weis and myself expanded the list. Word of our plans to party soon reached the inquiry staff, who were all welcome. The affable senior counsel assisting, David Andrews, was determined to make it a success. He volunteered to bring plenty of wine.

Before we left for the day, Linda Mulligan, the hospital's former director of nursing whose management style was criticised by Toni Hoffman and other nurses, gave her evidence.

Morris looked and sounded agitated. He regarded Mulligan's answers as unsatisfactory. 'What I read in your statement is that every time there's a problem you give the textbook bureaucratic answer, "you need more training, you need mediation, you need skills development, you've got communications problems", all those textbook bureaucratic answers rather than the natural reaction from a senior nurse which is to go and support her staff, see what they're saying, provide them with the comfort they need, ascertain the facts for herself and deal with the problem in a hands-on way,' Morris said.

Mulligan's reply – that she had suggested everyone sit down together – did not placate Morris.

The next witness, George Connelly, a white-haired and frighten-ingly frail 67-year-old, needed help to reach the stand. He took small steps while pushing along a large bottle of oxygen and other lifesaving paraphernalia. Just drawing breath was an effort for Connelly, who suffered from a collapsed lung and emphysema. He was gravely ill. He wanted to talk about the death of his wife, Doreen, after a hospital bungle. Morris gave the widower a sympathetic hearing.

Connelly asked to be able to say something in closing. With great effort the emaciated pensioner slowly rose to his feet. 'Today and over the last weeks we have heard a man carry out an inquiry under enormous strain,' Connelly said in his rasping voice. He raised it to ensure nobody misheard. The TV reporters knew even then that this grab would lead their report for the evening news. 'He's been pushed by the government, he's been pushed by everyone else under the sun, the hospital's taken him to court and everything. I have nothing but more appreciation for that man, Mr Morris, for standing up and showing guts and standing up and fighting our health system. And I'd like everyone now to stand up, put their hands together for Mr Morris.'

Those in the public gallery stood and gave Morris a rousing standing ovation. The lawyers and the journalists remained seated. Morris looked deeply touched.

'Thank you, Mr Connelly. We will take a ten-minute break.'

After Connelly shuffled away and news editors in Brisbane rewrote the bulletin, the hits kept coming for Mulligan. Her weighty written statement was likened by Morris to a telephone book. Mulligan's barrister, Alan MacSporran, told Morris that his questioning was 'objectionable'. 'You have entered the arena, taken an active role to denigrate this witness and, in my submission, quite unfairly,' MacSporran charged.

'Is there any reason why I can't use appropriate forensic resources to get at the truth?' Morris replied.

'Well, no one is objecting to you conducting yourself and conducting the inquiry appropriately,' MacSporran said.

'Well, Mr Leck is. He is taking me to the Supreme Court,' Morris countered.

A few hours later at the restaurant, about 35 of us headed upstairs to a special table setting organised by Pam Samra, who used to look forward to Patel's visits. We had most of the dining room to ourselves. The only other diners were at a table on the far side. About 10 pm

Hodgkinson asked me to join her in announcing the mock awards. Halfway into the announcements, the diners on the far side arose to leave.

On her way across the room, one woman, Pat Matthews, spoke sharply: 'Oh very nice. I'm sure the patients would love to hear that,' Matthews said.

We groaned when we discovered later that she was head of the patient liaison service for Queensland Health. Her words had cut the jovial atmosphere to ribbons. The banter was muted in the hour before we headed back to our accommodation.

The next morning, David Andrews, chipper as ever despite his sore head, joined Tony Morris and the deputy commissioners on a visit to the hospital. Andrews recognised the district manager, Monica Seth, who had taken over from Peter Leck as the hospital's manager in these trying times. She had been in the group with Pat Matthews at the restaurant.

On the last day of evidence in Bundaberg, other Queensland Health staff took time out to visit the inquiry. They jotted notes while scanning the public gallery to identify journalists and inquiry staff. Then they went back to work to swear statutory affidavits accusing us of lampooning the patients. In clinical episodes involving harm to patients, Queensland Health staff had moved like aged sloths. They took an eternity to investigate even where lives were at risk. But within 12 hours of last drinks at the Indian Curry Bazaar, the acting head of Queensland Health, Dr John Scott, was relaying to Premier Peter Beattie a dozen affidavits from the staff in Bundaberg.

Oblivious to the gathering storm, many of the reporters in the inquiry room were visibly moved by widow Tess Bramich. She told Morris and his two deputies: 'The only comfort for me to let my husband and soul mate go, is to think the health system will be fixed...I thank you on behalf of our children and all the rest of Desmond's family.'

In Brisbane, John Scott raised with Beattie whether our antics at the Indian Curry Bazaar might constitute official misconduct – a criminal offence. Beattie wrote to Robert Needham, the head of Queensland's anti-corruption body, the Crime and Misconduct Commission. As we boarded the last flight from Bundaberg that Thursday afternoon, Morris already knew Beattie had a bee in his bonnet about the previous night.

Jane Hodgkinson and I swapped intelligence on what we had heard might be brewing. We knew that something had been leaked to Sean Parnell at the *Australian*. I felt sure that if Parnell planned to write anything, he would call me first to check on the claims, or to seek comment. David Andrews was unworried as the aircraft left Bundaberg behind. 'Nobody did anything wrong. It's a nonsense,' Andrews said.

I seethed the next morning while reading the *Australian*'s on-line edition.

> A raucous dinner involving barristers for the so-called Dr Death inquiry and journalists covering the proceedings has sparked a scandal in the central Queensland sugar town of Bundaberg.
>
> Premier Peter Beattie will be asked to take action over the dinner at Bundaberg's Indian Curry Bazaar, which was attended by 33 people and featured a mock awards ceremony.
>
> The complaints to Mr Beattie raise the prospect of an official misconduct investigation, which could only be done by the Crime and Misconduct Commission.
>
> The *Australian* has learned the barristers assisting the $4 million inquiry, David Andrews SC and Errol Morzone, and other commission staff were present at the dinner on Wednesday night.
>
> On the eve of the completion of the inquiry's Bundaberg sittings, two journalists presented a series of awards to those present at the dinner, seemingly unaware that a group of health staff were seated at a nearby table.

The story went on to smear the inquiry staff, none of whom had any prior knowledge of the mock awards. Surprisingly, none of the inquiry staff or the journalists had been contacted for an on-the-record comment. The story cut us deeply. The mock awards were poking fun at ourselves. Where the patients were mentioned, it was good humoured.

To me the Patel story was simple: negligent health system introduces negligent surgeon to unwitting patients, resulting in very poor outcomes. I saw Patel as part of a big picture: the catalyst for overdue reform. Sean Parnell took a generally contrary approach. To his great credit he had identified major flaws in the conduct of Morris. The explanation of these flaws was a recurring theme in his articles. But it seemed to me that in playing Morris the man harder than the ball, he focused less on the serious systemic issues of the health system. This had the effect of immunising the political leadership and Queensland Health's chieftains. The conduct of Morris paled into insignificance compared with the plight of those patients unnecessarily dying or being maimed in hospitals because of unsafe or inadequate care.

The awards night triggered farce. Beattie and his staff began to flood media outlets with copies of the affidavits. He ordered the State Government jet to Bundaberg to meet patient Ian Fleming on the tarmac and, in one of his most repugnant performances of 2005, hugged him like a long-lost brother while apologising repeatedly. Danielle Isdale and the ABC's reporter, Alex Graham, both of whom witnessed the embrace and the platitudes, were disgusted. Fleming appeared to be crying.

When Graham asked Beattie at an impromptu press conference on the airport tarmac whether his calls for a Crime and Misconduct Commission inquiry, his apparent outrage and his use of public funds to divert the jet to Bundaberg for the photo opportunity with Fleming were desperate attempts to divert attention from the crisis plaguing his government, Beattie turned on the aggression. As Graham had been at the restaurant, Beattie angrily declared to her that she had no right to be asking him about his responses. Graham showed great composure and commonsense. She turned to an ABC colleague and asked him to repeat the question.

Beattie wanted the reporters who had been 'ring-leaders' at the awards night banned from covering the inquiry. He wanted me taken off the assignment, if not fired. It was the ultimate get-square. His staff sent the affidavits to David Fagan, the editor. 'The major players in this shouldn't cover the inquiry anymore,' Beattie thundered.

Back in his chambers at George Street, Tony Morris was almost apoplectic with fury. He had the *Australian* in his sights in a 10 am media release and a subsequent fiery media conference. 'The story written by Sean Parnell is a monstrous beat-up, and calls into serious question the author's motives – if not his journalistic ethics and professionalism,' Morris said. He accused Parnell of acting as 'unofficial press correspondent for the senior bureaucracy at Queensland Health' and of failing to consult others at the dinner to ascertain what it was all about.

At his media conference, Morris and the *Australian*'s Queensland bureau chief, Sid Maher, slugged it out. Maher, a staunch and loyal defender of his colleague, was not going to stand by in silence as Morris continued the tirade. When Maher started asking Morris tough questions, the lawyer cross-examined Maher on Parnell's actions and ethics. It was pure theatre. 'I'm under no illusion that Sean Parnell is being used by senior bureaucrats in Queensland Health to disseminate stories like this,' Morris said.

Beattie and his staff worked to fan the flames. It was the first sign of dissent between the Premier and Morris, who had not attended the infamous dinner. The Crime and Misconduct Commission decided to leave it well alone. One of their staff had been among the dinner party.

Beryl Crosby reckoned the awards were a harmless hoot. She knew we were letting our hair down and she appreciated how hard the media had worked. She embarrassed Beattie by revealing she had been trying to have him visit Bundaberg to address the victims for weeks – yet it was the opportunity to shoot the messengers which finally brought him to the town. On hearing of her 'award', Crosby had just one request: 'Can I have the ashtray?'

Public opinion was not with Beattie. Most people saw through the mock indignation. He let it go after a couple of days. 'I don't want to pursue the matter anymore – I've made my point about it,' he said.

The stoush between Morris and Sean Parnell was inevitable. Conflict had been simmering for weeks. Parnell, who had enjoyed a close working relationship with health chiefs over several years, angered Morris by wrongly reporting that Patel was within error rates and that none of the disciplinary action previously taken in the US would have prevented him doing procedures for which he was being investigated. After one of his reports stated Patel was linked to 'only eight deaths',

Morris sarcastically mused whether a century ago Parnell might have written 'Jack the Ripper linked with only eight deaths'.

MY mother, Diana, had been troubled by chronic back pain for a long time. She was losing weight and looked pale and frail, but she soldiered on without fuss, and looked forward to another overseas jaunt she might afford only in her dreams.

On the day the story about the awards at the Indian restaurant in Bundaberg gave Beattie an opportunity to call for scalps, Mum's underlying illness prompted drastic action. It was the first indication of something serious.

My older sister, Peta, sent me a text message just before noon: 'Mum is going to hospital for a lengthy stay. She is not in good shape. Will call with more news.' Our youngest sister, Kate, was giving birth to her daughter Mia in Sydney that day, and Mum was upset at being unable to be there for the arrival of another grandchild, her ninth.

The kids called her Mo, never Granny, and if you knew my mother you would understand why. She saw herself as being more youthful than her own four children. In some ways she was. A tall, beautiful and still-willowy blonde, she carried herself proudly in the latest designer-ripped denims, or an expensive Italian suit. Hospitals gowns were not for her. In her sixties, she had taken herself off to Italy, where she spent a year learning the language and immersing herself in village life.

She was admitted to a ward on the eighth floor at the Gold Coast Hospital after her heart specialist expressed alarm at worsening symptoms. Mum was gasping for breath. Her pulse raced. Her back pain had become excruciating. 'I can't believe that you're still walking around,' the specialist told her. As Mum rolled her eyes at being moved from floor to floor in the overcrowded public hospital, gossiped with my younger sister Rebecca, and leafed through power-of-positive-thinking books, the doctors ran tests.

The elevator carried a notice warning patients and visitors that unfair criticism and racist slurs against the hospital's Overseas Trained Doctors would not be tolerated. They had been copping a hard time since the Patel scandal erupted.

The doctors knew Mum had stomach ulcers and an internal bleed, but there was something else. A tumour. It was on her adrenal gland, silently squeezing life from a woman who, at 65, still had grand plans.

TWELVE days after the infamous awards night, Morris wrote to Buckland and pointedly condemned what he described as 'a concerted campaign of disinformation being orchestrated from within Queensland Health, apparently designed to discredit and derail this Commission of Inquiry, characterised by the strategic "leaking" of information to Sean Parnell of *The Australian*'. But in most respects, Parnell's reporting was courageous. He went against popular opinion to expose serious chinks in the armour of the inquiry chief. He pulled no punches in criticising Morris, who was obsessed with the media. The more his unorthodox handling of the inquiry was highlighted, the more Morris reacted. In my view, in his zeal to please everyone, he had jeopardised the inquiry.

Meanwhile, Buckland and Scott were doomed. Their organisation was in disarray. They were at loggerheads with their minister, Gordon Nuttall. They had lost Beattie's confidence. And the waiting lists for surgery in the public hospitals were growing.

In late July, Nuttall was sacked as Health Minister. 'Minister Nuttall is of the view – and I agree with him – that we need a fresh start to enable health reform so that Queenslanders have confidence that their health system is second to none in the world,' Beattie said.

Buckland was axed a few days later. The State Government's top public servant, Leo Keliher, told Buckland that Beattie no longer had confidence in him. He was given no reasons. 'It is with great sadness that I let you know I will be leaving Queensland Health as Director-General effective at midday today,' Buckland told staff on 26 July. 'I am incredibly proud of the journey we began 18 months ago to reform public health care.' Buckland's friend and loyal deputy, Scott, was the next to go.

When Karen Jenner heard about Buckland's sacking, she recalled his fateful 7 April visit to the hospital when she asked him why there would be no proper investigation into Dr Patel. And she recalled his demeaning answer: 'What part of "there's going to be no inquiry", don't you understand?' Buckland had asked her in the crowded room that day.

Now, the tables were turned. Jenner sent Buckland a message on the day he was told to clear out his office. 'What part of SACKED don't you understand?' she asked.

65

On the bench

Early August 2005

MARTIN Moynihan, the Supreme Court Justice with the unenviable task of determining if the Morris inquiry needed euthanasing, corrective surgery or a clean bill of health, dropped a few clues to his views during three days of legal argument in Brisbane. If Morris was dumped, Moynihan mused, the victims of Jayant Patel and a sick system might have to go through another painful legal process. 'The fact is what happened was devastating for them, and to have to repeat it would be even more devastating,' Moynihan said.

Senior lawyers told me Moynihan would not be influenced by the public and political support for Morris. The experienced judge looked forward to retirement and had nothing to gain or lose from whatever he pronounced. His judgement on Morris would be his most momentous.

Moynihan's bushy eyebrows arched as he read portions of transcript from the inquiry. Pressing the advantage for Peter Leck and Darren Keating were two of the more experienced Brisbane lawyers money could buy, David Jackson, QC, and Robert Mulholland, QC. They characterised Morris as a sarcastic and unfair bully who had two categories of witnesses: heroes and villains. White hats and black hats.

Moynihan was taken to two passages from the record of the questioning by Morris. The interrogation was likened to a 'laceration' in Leck's case; an 'ambush' in Keating's.

'Dr Miach was a doctor who actually deals with patients, not a bureaucrat.' 'Would it be a good start to have hospitals run by doctors who were real doctors?'

Moynihan: 'Well, they're not questions really, are they? They're assertions which the witness has little room to manoeuvre in terms of accepting or rejecting, I mean, in the circumstances in which he's found himself.'

Mulholland: 'Yes. It's really abuse, we'd say. At the very least, your Honour, it's grossly discourteous.'

Thanks to the decision of Morris to permit cameras into the inquiry, Leck and Keating had the benefit of DVDs, obtained under subpoena from the TV stations. The footage provided glimpses of the hostility Morris at times showed. It featured him shaking Hoffman's hand, a moment described by Jackson as 'almost surreal'. The pictures painted a thousand words. Hundreds of black and white pages of transcript were not as powerful as one or two DVDs.

For Leck and Keating to succeed, their lawyers needed to persuade Moynihan that a hypothetical observer, sitting in the inquiry room, would have reasonably concluded that Morris had already formed prejudicial views. There had to be an 'apprehension' of bias.

Fighting for Morris, the Solicitor-General, Walter Sofronoff, QC, stressed the proceedings were, by their very nature, inquisitorial, and Morris could ask tough questions as he saw fit. Royal commission-style inquiries bear little resemblance to the usual judicial process. Inquiry commissioners are not bound by usual rules; their witnesses may not refuse to give evidence. 'It is one of the weapons in the arsenal of a truth finder to be at liberty to call somebody on short notice or no notice, and certainly in circumstances where that person is not expecting to be called in order to establish facts before false propositions can be cobbled together,' Sofronoff said. Accordingly, Sofronoff argued, a commissioner like Morris was at perfect liberty to call somebody without notice, however upsetting it might have been to the witnesses.

If he could have had a bet on the result, the *Courier-Mail*'s long-time court reporter, inveterate punter Mark Oberhardt, would have put money on disqualification. Others were not so sure.

'We didn't start this course of action to have it aborted halfway through. This inquiry will finish its work,' Peter Beattie said.

Morris remained the preferred commissioner. But, Beattie vowed, a new inquiry would pick up where Morris had left off if he were ousted. The pressure on all the parties was relentless.

As the Supreme Court challenge droned on, Morris conducted hearings in earshot of the din of money being won and lost in the poker machines and on the card tables at the Townsville Breakwater Casino. He had brought the inquiry to North Queensland for three days of hearings. At the breaks when he chain-smoked quickly and deeply, he was anxious for news. He was gambling on a major legal triumph. 'What's the gossip?' he repeatedly asked. Morris was keen for any indication of how things were panning out in Brisbane. At one stage he quipped that Sofronoff had told him: 'Don't be making plans to give up your day job just yet.'

Morris seemed emboldened. And the sensational evidence in Townsville was set to breathe new life into an inquiry that looked like it might totter.

66

Secrets and lies

August 2005

IN the wards and the staffroom at Townsville Hospital, Dr Vladimir Smirnov had sometimes spoken of his colourful past in the former USSR and his lofty status as a bishop in the Russian Orthodox Church. He had appeared concerned, almost paranoid, about the tentacles of the Russian KGB and its covert successors. They had dogged him, he explained, with relentless surveillance and interrogation operations. But for about 250 patients with psychiatric issues, Smirnov, the hospital's eccentric psychiatric registrar, was the person to whom they turned for help.

The man formerly known as Tchekaline Victor Vladimirovich held a lawful authority to prescribe mood-altering medication. He had assessed the mental condition of the patients after listening to their fears and frustrations. He had told them how they should and could be feeling. He had dealt on a daily basis with fragile people whose anxieties could cause them to self-mutilate with knives or attempt suicide by walking in front of speeding cars.

Smirnov had his own unusual ideas and practices. When he visited patients at their homes he appeared more interested in the children, particularly young boys. Medication had calmed the violent tendencies of one of the patients, who had committed murder. Smirnov took him off the pills. Smirnov told other patients, who were clearly mentally ill, that they were perfectly fine. He overruled senior psychiatrists by significantly changing treatment plans. As far as the patients knew, however, Smirnov was a Queensland Health employee, registered by the Medical Board to deal with a range of serious psychiatric illnesses.

Psychiatric patients who complain that their psychiatrist is weird are not, as a rule, taken seriously.

When Jarrod Cowley-Grimmond, one of the lawyers seconded to the Morris inquiry to run behind-the-scenes investigations and interviews, first went to Townsville to follow several leads, he was told about the Smirnov file. It had been concealed by Queensland Health and the Medical Board since early 2003. As the comprehensive file showed, Smirnov was not even qualified to replace bandages. He had crudely forged paperwork to purport that he had done extensive training at Voronezh University in the former USSR. He was a total fake. In all probability his mental problems were more serious than those of his patients.

Smirnov's true former vocation – as a schoolteacher in the USSR – ended years earlier. Despite having no experience or training in medicine or psychiatry, he had been given a green light by the Medical Board and a job with Queensland Health to treat the community's most vulnerable people.

The evidence in Townsville was devastating. It showed that the Board had been warned by the Australian Medical Council and the Royal Australian and New Zealand College of Psychiatrists that Smirnov's documents were 'crude forgeries'. The Board did next to nothing after receiving these written warnings. It did not advise Townsville Hospital. Nor did it start a prosecution. Instead, the Board's deputy, Michael Demy-Geroe, issued a qualified Certificate of Good Standing to Smirnov, who used it to seek jobs elsewhere.

He pitched his bogus CV to a hospital in India. He almost landed a job in the Northern Territory and New Zealand. On the information available to Queensland Health and the Board, Smirnov had committed a string of criminal offences, from fraud to assault, yet he was permitted to slip quietly away.

'He was a plausible rogue?' Morris asked Townsville Hospital's Medical Services Director, Dr Andrew Johnson.

'Yes, you know, basically a conman,' Johnson replied.

When Johnson first discovered by accident the embarrassing truth about Smirnov, the Russian refugee had already left the hospital due to his lamentable lack of knowledge about psychiatry. Smirnov had lasted a year. Johnson crafted a comprehensive strategy to alert Smirnov's patients and come clean with the public. He proposed an audit of the patients and hotlines for anyone seeking urgent counselling. Advisers in Townsville drafted media releases.

Draft parliamentary speeches were also written for then Health Minister Wendy Edmond, who was sent a briefing paper saying: 'Many clinical staff maintain that there exists an ethical obligation on Queensland Health to inform patients that they have been receiving care from a person whose qualifications to provide that care have been found to be invalid. There are a number of patients and their families in the audit who have quite sensitive psychiatric, medical and social situations. Although informing them of these issues may make them more anxious, there are many such patients who would feel that not informing them was a breach of their rights and our responsibilities.'

On 24 January 2003, shortly before the plan was to have been achieved, Steve Buckland sent a strictly confidential email to Terry Mehan, the senior manager in Townsville for Queensland Health: 'Our issue is about the quality of [Smirnov's] performance. In discussions with the Board they refuse to acknowledge that he was not registerable. Game set and match. Therefore there is no official misconduct and no need to report.'

Johnson believed that if he spoke up again, his job might be at risk. 'Certainly at that time bringing bad news was never a good thing. I felt that there was a push to ensure that Queensland Health was "kept off the front page",' Johnson subsequently told Morris.

The conduct of the Board and Queensland Health was, I believed, unforgivable. They had concealed the Smirnov matter in 2003 and they had concealed it from the inquiry in 2005. It would have remained a secret if not for the efforts of Cowley-Grimmond.

> Morris: Over three months of evidence now, we see again and again cases of Queensland Health getting reports about problems here and problems there. And I just wonder if you can see any logical justification for the culture, that seems to be pervasive at least to Charlotte Street, if it is bad news you hide it away in the basement and never tell anyone about it?

Johnson: Commissioner, I think there is a very simple answer and that's the fact that politics has really taken over the delivery of health care to an unreasonable extent.

You know, the reason that we're being prevented from saying things is essentially, I would suggest, for political purposes. No politician likes to have bad news on their watch...the only reason that I can think of for suppressing information is for short term political advantage...

Buckland and Edmond later cited an opinion taken at the time from a senior Queensland Health psychiatrist, who advised it could have been harmful to the patients to learn the truth about Smirnov. It was a compelling defence, but my experiences with Buckland and Edmond influenced my view that their overriding concern was less altruistic. Put simply, it would have been harmful to Edmond and the Beattie Government for the public to learn the truth about Smirnov. The *Courier-Mail* editorial summed it up:

Just as it seems Queenslanders may be inured to yet more tales of cover-up and obfuscation emanating from the upper echelons of the health bureaucracy, along comes a fresh scandal involving people suffering at the hands of a bogus doctor. For many following the course of the commission of inquiry, it would be tempting – indeed it is preferable for some in the Beattie Government – to focus on the wrongdoing of these rogue practitioners and not bother too much with questions about the system that set them loose on the hospital floor.

But this would save from proper scrutiny the culture of arrogance and secrecy that continues to thrive within the senior ranks of the health bureaucracy and which has done so much to damage the public reputation of the state's health system. Queensland hospital workers, the doctors, nurses and clinicians who deal with the public every day are, by and large, performing well under extremely trying circumstances. Their actions did not produce the likes of Jayant Patel or Mr Smirnov.

Rather, these outrages were the fault of the senior health

bureaucracy and successive health ministries, both of which have for some years valued political machinations and economic wrong-headedness over patient care.

Russell Grenning was incredulous when we spoke during the Townsville hearings. A former top political and media adviser, he followed the fortunes of governments with keen interest. His sage advice had helped Joh Bjelke-Petersen's corrupt government remain in power in Queensland until it was thrown out in the wake of the Fitzgerald inquiry. Grenning, now safely ensconced at the Law Society of Queensland where he rubbed shoulders with judges and lawyers, could see the Beattie Government going the same way. 'Honestly, there are some stories so bizarre, so incredible, that you couldn't make them up, but every day they're coming out of the inquiry and we're hearing them and seeing them on the 6 pm news. It is politically devastating,' he said.

It angered me that in early 2003, several months before the arrival of Jayant Patel, the Medical Board and Queensland Health were aware they had been duped by Smirnov, yet they failed to improve the abysmal systems to screen applicants from overseas seeking jobs as medical practitioners in Australia.

I asked Philippa Harris, co-ordinator of the Townsville-based North Queensland Mental Illness Fellowship, her opinion. She said Queensland Health, which partly funds her organisation, had been 'absolutely neglectful and irresponsible': 'We are gobsmacked by what has come out and distressed that Queensland Health chose not to act in the public interest, particularly when the local managers wanted it out in the open.'

There was something else about it that bore striking similarities to the Patel case: Smirnov's personnel file was adorned with glowing references. 'He clearly has considerable experience in psychiatry...I believe he has much to teach us about psychiatry as performed in Europe and it would be a considerable loss if people such as him are not recognised as specialist psychiatrists in Australia with his very considerable experience,' wrote Dr Brian Boettcher, a Queensland Health mental health director.

Another senior psychiatrist from the organisation, Dr Leon Petchkovsky, wrote: 'It should be said that he is a man of the highest possible standards of integrity, tried in the fires of life. He is an experienced and trusted colleague and I have no hesitation in recommending him for any consultant level posting he might apply for.'

67

The long wait

August 2005

STARTING with the Vladimir Smirnov scandal, August saw a flood of damning revelations which caused massive political damage and led to pleas from medical staff and the public for a complete overhaul of the health system. Having cracked the Smirnov cover-up, the Health inquiry's lawyer-cum-investigator, Jarrod Cowley-Grimmond, began to unravel Queensland's public hospital waiting lists.

Premier Peter Beattie had for years pointed to these lists as proof that Queenslanders enjoyed one of the world's finest health systems. People spent less time on these lists awaiting surgery in Queensland, he boasted, than in any other state. For years, doctors had been telling me and other journalists the reverse. They insisted the political boasts were untruthful. Before patients who needed surgery, such as a cataract operation or a hip replacement, could make it onto the official published waiting lists, they had to graduate from another waiting list. This was an undisclosed list.

As Dr David Molloy, the head of the AMA in Queensland, had told Tony Morris in the second week of the inquiry, patients could remain on the concealed lists for as long as eight years. But the public only ever saw or heard about the much shorter waiting lists of those people who were booked in for surgery, having finally seen a specialist.

Premier Beattie, his former health minister Wendy Edmond and her successor Gordon Nuttall had always been aware of the other lists. But they ensured that members of the public were only given figures from the shorter lists. Beattie confidently asserted a few weeks after Molloy's evidence: 'Not only are our waiting times the shortest, but we are admitting more patients into our hospitals for treatment than anyone else.'

The campaign of deceit was undone when the secret lists were unearthed by Cowley-Grimmond. Confidential Queensland Health documents showed that more than 108 000 people across 29 regions statewide were waiting for an appointment to see a specialist at a public hospital; they were on the concealed lists the Beattie Government had not previously acknowledged in public displays of breast-beating. Queensland had a public health system unable to meet demand and stretched well beyond its capacity, yet for years the politicians had hidden the evidence.

Morris drew an analogy between Queensland Health's waiting lists and fashion swimwear: 'There's no interest in speed or comfort or protection or safety. It is simply a matter of revealing as much as possible that people want to see and covering up anything that's going to cause public disquiet.'

Shortly before my deadline for the completion of a lengthy Saturday article on the disclosure of the lists, I spoke to Beryl Crosby. She had just returned from a Bundaberg meeting with fellow members of the Patients' Support Group. Despite the best efforts of various ministers and their advisers to win Crosby over, she had refused to succumb. Crosby told me:

> It's a disgusting, covered-up mess. From the time the Jayant Patel issue broke and everything we have heard and learnt since, we thought nothing more could shock us but now these waiting lists have come out. If they had been open and transparent in the beginning, the public would have seen the problems and understood them better.
>
> It is depressing but this inquiry has also been a worthwhile exercise because the system would only have got worse. It was like a boil. When it burst with Patel, all this gunk started coming out. Until it has all oozed out, it will never begin to heal. But how do you heal it?

The doctors offered a variety of answers. Fundamentally, they wanted the administration and political leaders to stop treating hospitals like units of commerce. They pleaded for the system to be properly funded to give patients good outcomes and slow the flow of doctors and specialists to the private sector. When Dr Jason Jenkins, a vascular surgeon at Royal Brisbane Hospital, gave evidence he despaired at the lack of top-level initiative and leadership. He pointed to an expensive abundance of increasingly powerful bureaucrats with little insight into health care but finely tuned antennae for the political and executive line on damage control. Jenkins said:

> It becomes an intolerable place to work when you are being told to stop admitting because there are no beds.
>
> The patients are piling up behind us and we can't keep up with it. They're losing legs, they're losing their lives, rupturing aneurisms because they haven't been seen in outpatients and that's a factor of funding.
>
> Every day we get a message on our pagers 'Discharge patients. Beds critical. No admissions without approval'. That's what you get every day at the Royal Brisbane Hospital on my pager. It's become an intolerable place to work because you can't actually work.
>
> You're told to stop spending money because there's no money, stop putting in the best graft for the patient because we've used up our prosthetics budget. Put in a business case if you want to get something else done.
>
> We were told the other day that all the business cases just get thrown in a box at Charlotte Street because there's no money to actually deal with them. We want to work, but we're not allowed to work a lot of the time because there's not the money to actually fund this system.
>
> And at the moment, the general consensus in the public hospital system is our leader doesn't go into battle for us. When we ask for help, we get none. The only help we get is when there is a crisis because we don't want to end up on the front page

of the *Courier-Mail*. And I mean, we're playing politics with health.

Health is people and the problem at the moment is where we're messing with it with politics. They need to speak to clinicians and ask them what needs to be done, not have administrators telling us what clinicians should be doing.

You know, I sometimes think we're playing for a different team. We're playing for the health team and they are playing for the budget team. So I guess we're being made toothless tigers in a system which is being run by administrators. I mean, one of the problems is they don't come to us to ask us how to fix the problems. Half the time they tell us how to fix the problems. A lot of the time that involves actually more administration and less patient care.

Earlier Morris had asked Chief Health Officer Dr Gerry FitzGerald: 'Is there some difficulty with the proposition that the taxpayers who pay for the health system in this state, and the members of the public who utilise public hospitals, are actually entitled to know that there is a problem in the hospitals rather than having it gather dust in a filing cabinet in Charlotte Street? When do we stop this system of shooting the messenger and hiding the evidence rather than putting it out in public so that things can be done about these problems?'

On 20 August, angry voters punished Beattie. His two Labor candidates were crushed by huge margins in by-elections. The health crisis had become a major political crisis. Malcolm Cole, the *Courier-Mail*'s state political correspondent, reported: 'The Beattie Government faces its first serious electoral test at the next state election, after voters handed it two shattering defeats in weekend by-elections. The leaders of all three major political parties said the massive swings against Labor in its formerly safe seats of Chatsworth and Redcliffe proved the next election was an open contest.'

Lawyer and political commentator Stephen Coates described the future for Beattie as potentially terminal because 'unless he can slay dragons and put on a sparkling electoral performance, he faces a fall from power – in disgrace'.

68

The doctors

August 2005

DOCTOR Geoff de Lacy peered at the woman's abdomen and tried to disguise his immediate bewilderment. He looked again and shook his head. There was no mistaking what had happened. The question was why.

The woman had been operated on by Jayant Patel for a hernia. He repaired it. She returned to him with a bowel obstruction, not an unusual complication from a recurrent hernia. But Patel's technique of hernia repair was unique, not something de Lacy, a well-qualified surgeon in private practice in Bundaberg, had ever seen before.

One of the problems common to hernia repairs is inadvertent damage to other anatomical structures. When the woman went back to Patel, the small bowel was vulnerable. It would have been unfortunate, but not unacceptable, for a single stitch used in the hernia repair to pass through her small bowel. But something bizarre had happened. If de Lacy had not seen the needle patchwork with his own eyes, he would not have believed it possible. He observed that stitches had passed through 20 loops of the small bowel. He wondered if it was incompetence on a remarkable scale. Or something else. Something deliberate.

'What it represents in my experience is the most ham-fisted attempt at repairing a hernia I'd ever seen,' de Lacy said. 'It's certainly possible to catch up a loop of bowel during closure of an abdomen. I've found it impossible to envisage how you could go through the bowel with every stitch and not notice unless you were looking out the window, you know, rather than at the patient, and there have been a lot of other examples of the sort of errors of that magnitude.'

The evidence of de Lacy at the inquiry was riveting in a macabre way. It made me wonder about Patel's motive. If he were to mount an insanity defence, arguing that he had lost his mind, some of his botch-ups and clinical decisions as described by de Lacy would be easier to understand.

Toni Hoffman suspected that Patel might have caused the complications to some of the patients so that, when they returned to his care, he would know how to fix the very problem he had caused. 'It's a sickness. He craves attention and adulation. He wants the other doctors to think he's brilliant. He was prepared to ruin healthy organs to make himself look good as the surgeon doing the repair,' she told me.

More than 150 patients and their medical files were examined by de Lacy in the weeks and months after the Patel story broke. The more de Lacy, who had performed dozens of corrective procedures, looked at their injuries and the documentation, the more he realised how dangerous and dishonest Patel had been for the two years he was at the hospital:

> One of the points that I'd like to make if I could was that I'm not certain that the magnitude of his errors, the number of problems that he's had, the number of deaths that he's had has ever been sort of appropriately compared to what we might have expected him to have, and these things aren't just things that happened to an average, general surgeon, at all.
> They're not 10 times what you might expect. They're more like 100 times what you might expect.

De Lacy had decided there was no rational explanation for the number of patients Patel insisted on taking to theatre or the complexity of the operations he performed. Many of these patients should have been sent home; they were too frail or sick to undergo major surgery. 'He saw operations as an end to themselves, not as a way of treating patients, not as a way of improving their health in my opinion,' de Lacy said.

Tony Morris asked whether, in de Lacy's observations of Patel's handiwork, the surgeon was at the low end of an acceptable degree of competence. De Lacy replied:

Far worse. Far worse. I've looked after complications in the last four months that I've never seen before.

I've had an opportunity to sort of assess his decision making both pre-operatively, intra-operatively and post-operatively and it was terrible. Terrible care doesn't necessarily result in terrible outcomes. It just results in an increased likelihood of those outcomes being terrible. And, for example, with patients who had cancer removed, whether they will or will not have their cancer back in five years and you can generate a statistical risk of that happening. They certainly don't have symptoms of cancer at the moment but because of what Dr Patel has done or not done, they have got an increased risk of their cancer coming back in five years.

He explained how, when a segment of a hollow tube is removed – a typical example being part of a large bowel that contains a bowel cancer – two ends have to be joined together again to re-establish the continuity of the gastrointestinal tract. In technical terms the join is called anastomosis, a key part of the operation. After an operation, the recovery of the patient often hinges on whether the join leaks or heals. He continued:

If it leaks, the contents of that tube, in this case the bowel, spills out into the rest of the abdomen, with peritonitis and death if they don't have another operation…and certainly there were many examples in Dr Patel's surgery. Anastomoses do leak in the best hands. They don't all leak. And certainly the number of leaks that I have seen would be, you know, grossly excessive.

I didn't see any evidence that he judged his outcomes at all. If there was a problem…then it was inadequate suture material, or the practising in a third world hospital, which is how he described Bundaberg Base Hospital, or something else, some other issue, some reason, the patient had done something wrong, or whatever.

And I suspect, you know, from talking to a lot of these patients and assessing his work, that he never had judged the outcomes he had, having these problems certainly in the States, it seems for 10 or 20 years, and he spent his whole career not fixing up these fairly basic problems because they weren't his problems, they were somebody else's problems.

Before he became involved in looking after Patel's patients, many of whom no longer trusted the public health system, de Lacy doubted the stories I had written about Patel's incompetence. He suspected the allegations being made by the nurses and the patients were exaggerations. Having met Patel a few times in the hospital, de Lacy regarded him as arrogant and controlling, but the opportunity to witness his surgical techniques had not arisen. But his view changed:

> ...I have got a different opinion now. My opinion now is that the real story of what was going on there was worse, that the number of patients was, you know, 10 to 100 times more than I thought there would be, and that the type of complications that were allowed to happen there were gross by comparison to what I was expecting.
> We certainly didn't know that he was the subject of numerous inquiries overseas, but he did. And a lot of these issues – the [subverted] mortality and morbidity meetings, the failure to transfer patients, his relationships or lack of relationships with other staff, were explainable in my opinion by just a desire not to have his work checked for fear of this, I guess.

Of the 150-plus former Patel patients seen by de Lacy, fewer than 20 were well managed by the former Director of Surgery. The overwhelming majority were victims of a standard of care below that of a reasonably competent surgeon. De Lacy cited the example of a middle-aged woman:

> Numerous investigations were done and Dr Patel came to the conclusion that the patient had a diagnosis called ischaemic colitis, which is poor blood supply to the bowel. She had an operation which would have been appropriate for someone

with ischaemic colitis, but was not appropriate for someone with Crohn's disease, which is what she actually had. She had a very difficult post-operative course but survived.

She has been left with most of her bowel having been removed...her day-to-day lifestyle is that she passes between 12 and 20 loose bowel motions per day. She was 85 kilograms, she's now 56 kilograms. All of these people have those magnitude of problems. It is a long litany of medical problems.

Before he operated on the patients to attempt to correct the problems Patel had created or worsened, de Lacy regarded Patel's notes as slipshod. After a number of operations, de Lacy no longer had faith in Patel's notes. They were fundamentally dishonest, like the man himself. The notes repeatedly and falsely purported that various risks and complications were explained to the patients or that there were no problems after theatre. De Lacy said:

A lot of it is rubbish. There must have been somebody dying on the surgical ward all of the time and there must have been horrendous complications physically being managed on the surgical ward all of the time. Those closest to him were most threatened by him. And he spent most of his energy intimidating or otherwise isolating his practice from them.

There are systems in place, albeit faulty ones, to try and prevent this happening, and my personal opinion is that this tragedy wouldn't have occurred unless there was both active subversion by the individual and complacency at best by the supervising body that was supposed to identify these problems.

In my opinion there was a predisposition in the system to allow a rogue surgeon to be placed in this position of power and allowed free reign.

Whereas de Lacy witnessed serious surgical complications, Dr Peter Woodruff, the primary expert witness, was struck by an unusual omission after his examination of patients' notes, charts and x-rays. In 47 000 pages of material related to 221 patients – a small sample of the

1500 men, women and children as young as six treated by Patel in his two years at Bundaberg – Woodruff could not find a single letter or document written by Patel to seek the opinion or advice of another specialist or doctor. Worse than that, there was not one letter from him about his management of his patients or their outcomes. As Ralph Devlin, the lawyer for the Medical Board, put it, Patel had operated in 'splendid isolation'. 'I have no hesitation in saying that his performance was incompetent and that this performance is far worse than average or what one might expect by chance,' said Woodruff, a vascular surgeon.

Although he regarded Patel's complication rate as frightening, Woodruff·was determined to remain objective, dispassionate and impervious to the horror stories. Woodruff was also limited by the terms of reference of his Queensland Health-sponsored review. He examined no bodies, only documents, many of them the work of a surgeon with a record of dishonesty. In the absence of the patients, Woodruff gave Patel the benefit of the doubt in a number of cases.

As a leading figure in the Royal Australasian College of Surgeons, Woodruff had seen first-hand the reluctance and fear of politicians to introduce major healthcare reforms. The politicians were always worried about a voter backlash. Woodruff told me how he had once made an irrefutable case for systemic change to a former federal health minister, Dr Michael Wooldridge. 'Yes, you're right. We're going' to get onto it straight after I have removed the old age pension,' Wooldridge replied.

Woodruff had been around operating theatres long enough to know surgical mistakes were inevitable and, in many cases, acceptable. The practice of surgery was not a benign undertaking. Provided you were honest and corrected your technique or reconsidered whether the approach was even justified, occasional errors of judgement would not normally lead to disqualification. In surgery, Woodruff knew of colleagues who were defensive to the point of concealing mistakes or pretending they didn't occur. Pride and the aggression of personal injury lawyers were contributing factors. But Patel was a puzzle. Woodruff at first struggled to understand the motives of the surgeon, whom he regarded as intelligent and industrious.

Late one evening, the answer came as Woodruff used his laptop computer to scroll through the list of patients who had died or suffered serious injury. It suddenly occurred to him that the worst cases involved those procedures which Patel had been banned from performing in the United States.

'And I wonder whether this is not the missing piece of the mosaic that I was ignorant of...I wonder if his motivation for doing these quite outlandish operations is not to try and reassert in his own mind that what he's been precluded from doing in Oregon he is in fact capable of doing, and that he is, in effect, re-credentialling himself if only in his own mind,' Woodruff said.

After so much speculation, the pinpointing by Woodruff, de Lacy and another senior surgeon, Dr Barry O'Loughlin, of many examples of atrocious care for the patients of Bundaberg was distressing. Tony Morris was reminded of something attributed to Sir Arthur Conan Doyle, Scottish practitioner and creator of the character of Sherlock Holmes: 'When a doctor goes wrong he is the first of criminals. He has nerve and he has knowledge.'

My concerns revolved around the knowledge of the other doctors with whom Patel had worked closely. I had difficulty understanding how nurse Toni Hoffman, who had no surgical training and had never seen Patel operate, knew instinctively that he was dangerous – and did something about it – yet several doctors in Bundaberg who worked beside the Director of Surgery did not. Did the other doctors believe that Patel had virtues? Was the silence part of the culture spoken of by Woodruff?

It was the view of the Chief Health Officer, Dr Gerry FitzGerald, that the anaesthetists were in the best position to judge the competence of a surgeon. But Dr Martin Carter, the anaesthetist in charge of the Intensive Care Unit at Bundaberg for the two years Patel was Director of Surgery, was at pains in his evidence to absolve himself of any responsibility. Carter said:

> I knew [Hoffman] had concerns about Dr Patel's competence. Unfortunately for an understanding between us, the idea of what we're in a position to do about these sorts of things is different between nurses and doctors.
>
> It takes a long time for one to work out whether you can actually prove almost effectively in a court of law that the person

you are talking about is incompetent to do what they are saying they can do and stop them doing it.

I mean, if you as a barrister or solicitor were continually losing cases, nobody would go to you, but at least you wouldn't be, sort of, losing anything other than your livelihood here.

In terms of a surgeon or a physician or a psychiatrist or whatever, you know, how do you know when they're missing things that they shouldn't miss or whether what's happening is, basically, beyond anybody's sort of care?

Tony Morris: You told us very candidly that you didn't like the man, you found him brash and abrasive and so on. Was it your sense that there was almost a degree of megalomania in it, that he thought he had come from America to show this little country town how surgery is done and he just saw no limits to what he could or should do?

Carter: I think that probably would be a reasonable way of expressing it, certainly more polite than mine.

Carter saw himself as responsible for keeping the patients alive, pain-free and unresponsive during surgery, monitoring the vital signs and ensuring the flow of appropriate medication. 'It is very difficult to also monitor the surgery at the same time,' he said. 'In my opinion, Dr Patel was not the worst surgeon that we had at the hospital. He was not the best surgeon but in my experience there have been worse at the hospital.'

Unfortunately, nobody at the inquiry asked Carter to identify those surgeons whom he rated as more incompetent than Patel. Nor was Carter asked whether he had taken steps to bring those unnamed surgeons to the notice of authorities.

69

The collapse

1–2 September 2005

AFTER 50 days of public hearings, more than 5000 pages of transcript evidence and the unearthing of maladministration as well as negligence in surgery at Bundaberg Hospital and elsewhere, Tony Morris, QC, was close to the end. The inquiry chief was considering major reforms that might save countless lives.

The legal action by Peter Leck and Dr Darren Keating threatened to sabotage the reform agenda. Near the end of the month-long wait for Supreme Court Justice Martin Moynihan's decision, Morris had become desperate to stave off an inglorious end to his delicately poised inquiry. He assured Leck and Keating that he was not proposing to make findings against them. He extended a similar undertaking to the former health ministers, Wendy Edmond and Gordon Nuttall and the sacked director-general, Dr Steve Buckland, and his deputy, Dr John Scott. They all basked in immunity. As Morris placated key witnesses and aimed to blame the system for the obvious shortcomings, I wondered if there was anyone left to be held responsible for this health disaster.

A legal contact had confidently told me Moynihan would oust Morris and kill the inquiry. The assertion was based on a cryptic comment he was said to have made: 'A picture tells a thousand words.' The cliché was a reference to the hours of footage subpoenaed from the television stations that showed Morris responding emotively, sarcastically and caustically while questioning Leck and Keating. The footage lent devastating force to the Leck–Keating bid, but ironically it was only available due to the unusual decision of Morris to allow cameras into the inquiry in the first place.

Before the fiftieth day of public hearings, Richard Douglas, SC, a dogged but unfailingly courteous lawyer, had joined the fray to help the flagging inquiry team. Douglas was fresh and methodical. He pushed hard for political explanations for the subterfuge that had been practised with the waiting lists for surgery. He understood how political paranoia about the lists was part of the explanation for the Bundaberg Hospital disaster and the culture of concealment in the health system.

'Do you agree that to wax lyrical in press releases about short waiting times for elective surgery without referring in the same breath to the particulars of the unofficial list is, to put it at its lowest, misleading?' he asked Edmond. Essentially, Edmond argued that it was much more complicated and that she had originally intended to release all the lists when sworn in as health minister. But she had soon realised they were political dynamite.

The inquiry had been a lawyers' picnic at a cost to taxpayers of more than $100 000 a day. But at that stage the patients and their families had not experienced emotional or financial compensation. They feared the prospect of the inquiry being shut down by Moynihan. Karen Orreal, the mother of Shannon Mobbs, the boy whose leg was amputated, said:

> Our lives have been catastrophically changed by what has occurred. My son has been forced to endure a further eight operations. He will have to learn to walk again with the aid of a prosthetic limb. We have to live with the constant thought that my son's leg could have been saved if he had received appropriate medical treatment. It is almost unbearable for me to have to hear the evidence as I am tortured with thoughts of 'if only my son had not been exposed to Dr Patel and had been transferred to a Brisbane hospital...'

'Just one hour until either the guillotine comes down or the gates open,' said Angus Scott, one of the inquiry's legal sleuths, on the afternoon of Thursday 1 September. My friend and colleague Amanda Watt perched over the reporters' desk in Court 15 waiting for the decision. The gloomy room was crowded; there was tension and muffled murmuring until Moynihan entered. He was so impassive he might have been pronouncing on a neighbourhood dispute. Matter-of-factly, as if he made similar rulings every other day, he found in favour of Leck and Keating. Moynihan ruled Morris had, indeed, shown 'ostensible bias'. Amanda and I reeled.

The finding surprised Premier Peter Beattie, but it outraged Queenslanders. Evening polls by the TV stations drew record responses from viewers who overwhelmingly condemned the judgement. Beryl Crosby said it best. 'I feel like I've been hit with a brick,' was her comment.

Des Bramich's widow, Tess, who went to almost every day of the public hearings, was distraught. 'I feel they are trying to bury this, that it is about politics again and not the patients, but I will never rest,' she said.

Toni Hoffman sent me a message she wanted forwarded to Morris: 'When the ruling came down today, there was personal outrage from the staff at the hospital. I am extremely angered that Premier Beattie has allowed this inquiry to be sabotaged. It was an honour to be a part of at least what we attempted to do, to make Queensland Health a safe place to work and, more importantly, a safe place to be a patient.'

Despite his earlier pledge to appoint another inquiry chief in the event of Morris being ousted, Beattie seized on the chance to end the political pain. Since Jayant Patel became a household name just 18 weeks earlier, Beattie had lost his personal standing, a mountain of political capital, two by-elections, a health minister and a handful of top administrators. The health department was in meltdown. And now the public blamed him for a judicial finding. He decided that there would not be a second inquiry, breaking his earlier promise.

Morris was sipping coffee with his parents, Graeme and Jan, in a George Street cafe when his friend, lawyer Tony Barlow, tipped me to their whereabouts.

'All is not lost,' Morris said. 'If there is any personal disappointment, it's because I feel that I have let down all of these people.'

Jan Morris: 'I think you got too emotionally involved.'

Morris: 'No, as one of the patients said in the journal of record [the *Courier-Mail*] this morning, how could you not be biased when you see and hear what's going on and Peter Leck and Darren Keating are not making any explanation for it? They were not losing their spouse or their limbs or their bowels. The supreme irony of all this is the [legal action] by Leck and Keating was to protect their reputations, and I just wonder what good it's done to their reputations.'

Graeme Morris commended a cartoon in the *Gold Coast Bulletin*. It depicted Leck and Keating saying to maimed patients of Patel: 'Oh yeah! You think you suffered. When the Commissioner asked us questions, he didn't say "pretty please with sugar on top", the big meanie!'

But Beattie ruled out an appeal. Despite compelling legal submissions by Gerry Mullins, the lawyer for the patients, who urged the appointment of a new inquiry head to direct the near-complete show to its conclusion, Beattie had given instructions to end it. The spurious justification cited was that all the evidence had been contaminated. There would be no substitute inquiry chief. No findings. Just costly failure. To soften the blow, Beattie put the final touches to a generous compensation deal for the patients. If the money was right, maybe they would keep relatively quiet.

Keating, almost expressionless in the public hearings, was seen laughing by one of my colleagues on George Street after the verdict. Leck's solicitor Patricia Feeney, who felt strongly that her client was harshly treated by the inquiry, looked delighted with the outcome as she strolled from the courts complex.

In the absence of another inquiry, I was depressed. Although it was hard to admit openly, in my heart I knew Morris went too far and had at times played favourites. He had become the major performer of a drama so strange, no one could have dreamt it. Like many a brilliant man before him, his successes were spectacular and his failures disastrous.

A number of key witnesses were adamant that the extravagant behaviour of Morris had persuaded them to give evidence. 'It is precisely Mr Morris's particular style that gave me the confidence to come forward and speak the truth without fear,' Dr Charles Nankivell told me. 'I support him without reservation. I agree fully with Dr Peter Cook's comments about it being a once in a lifetime opportunity.

Indeed, when I retire and look back on my medical career, I will regard that having contributed to this inquiry and thus to have helped all Queenslanders to an improved health system will be a major highlight.'

Many of the lawyers and judges around town believed Morris had made a fool of himself and got everything he deserved. Key inquiry staff, particularly the hardworking and talented lawyer Damien Atkinson, who knew the evidence down to the finest details, were crestfallen. 'What a waste,' lamented Wayne King, one of the investigators. But Morris was only briefly daunted. Having ensured his place in history, he began writing a detailed report about the inquiry, the hospital and the personality of Patel. Perhaps Morris felt guilty for failing to finish. 'He needed more than vindication: he needed respect; he needed admiration; he needed to be valued,' Morris wrote in the report he presented to a Federal Parliament committee. It was a paragraph that might also have described the ousted inquiry commissioner. He continued:

> Those whose opinions did not matter to him, especially amongst the nursing staff, were lucky just to be ignored.
>
> Some of the junior medical staff praised his care, enthusiasm and generosity as a teacher – quite conceivably, the image of a respected pedagogue was one which suited Patel's ego – but any who had the temerity to question his judgement or ability were swatted away like insects.
>
> Thus he surrounded himself with sycophants and flatterers, when he could find them; and was otherwise content to work with people who had the good sense to keep their opinions to themselves.

Geoff Davies

8 September 2005

BERYL Crosby sounded upset and frustrated when we spoke over the weekend. The patients for whom she advocated were in retreat as a result of Peter Beattie's lightning trip to Bundaberg to outline the generous compensation package and cajole key public figures like Toni Hoffman. 'He's talking them around,' a glum Crosby told me. She had been excelling in a crash course in politics and leverage since being thrust into a role as leader of the support group, but wanted nothing less than a new inquiry, and she threatened to organise protest marches until she got her way.

Although Beattie sounded determined to avoid any further scrutiny of the health system, he had underestimated the public anger at the turn of events. His hasty adoption of the Supreme Court's ruling was a mistake; it fuelled the suspicions of many Queenslanders who, unfairly, blamed Beattie for the inquiry's shutdown. His backbenchers, already petrified by polling showing they faced defeat unless public sentiment could be swung around, were deluged with complaints from voters. Even critics of Tony Morris believed the inquiry's total shutdown was overkill.

Geoff Davies, QC, a newly retired Court of Appeal judge with impeccable credentials to head any new inquiry, was also in that camp. Having watched the first inquiry unravel, the unsentimental Davies was unsurprised by Justice Martin Moynihan's ruling. But Davies was troubled by some of the misinformation being spouted, such as the claims that all the evidence from the Morris inquiry was 'contaminated' and therefore of no use.

Steve Austin, the 612 ABC Radio presenter, used his morning show to interview another retired and highly respected judge, James Thomas, who methodically destroyed the claims about all the evidence being contaminated. There was no legal reason why a new commissioner could not resume hearings. With one of the excuses for not restarting the inquiry now discredited, Beattie, unhappily, bowed to the public demands. The most logical choice was Geoff Davies. 'We've listened to the people and I don't see that as a crime or a sin. Too often, politicians don't have the guts to listen to the people. Well, I have,' Beattie said unsmilingly.

Senior judges and lawyers could not understand why Davies had not been asked in the beginning, back in April 2005. But after the Morris collapse, friends told Davies he would be mad to take it on. He weighed the decision for a couple of days before saying yes. 'I could see the unsatisfactory state of affairs. And I don't criticise the judge's decision to terminate the commission of inquiry – on the contrary, I think it was the correct decision – but I could see the terrible position Queenslanders would be in unless something was done,' Davies told me.

Before his retirement early in 2005, I had interviewed Davies about aspects of the law he believed needed urgent reform. 'I want to let go of the day-to-day work I've been doing. I don't like, for example, doing criminal appeals which involve mostly sex cases. I find them distasteful. It's a very important job to do and I've tried to do my best, but I do want to be involved in what I believe are necessary reforms to the legal system. Systemic reforms. It's one of the reasons I've retired early,' he said. His openness and thoughtful proposals were refreshing. Although he expressed himself carefully to avoid a mini-rebellion on the bench, Davies was concerned that political patronage rather than intellect and acumen too often determined the appointment of judicial lightweights. He could see the courts being stacked with mediocrity. The perils for litigants were obvious because poor judges meant miscarriages of justice became inevitable. Davies called for an independent and transparent commission to help select judges.

It was one of the stories I filed before investigating the Jayant Patel scandal, and Davies had suggested I seek comment on his proposals from the former federal attorney-general, Michael Lavarch. I suspected

Lavarch was still peeved at my stories on alleged vote rorting in his former electorate. It was a good guess. When I telephoned him, the new dean of law at Queensland University of Technology, he told me my journalism stank and had never done a scrap of good for anyone. His hostility and his comments were cutting. The episode proved my theory that journalists were hopelessly thin-skinned even as they made inferences or reported facts that could ruin or damage the lives of other people.

But Davies understood that if the media took up an issue, politicians usually followed and then change might be possible. He spoke candidly of his concern about the right to silence. He believed that a jury should be permitted to draw adverse inferences in relation to an accused who exercised a right to silence. He was also agitating to change the law to permit the use of evidence illegally obtained. Although criminal defence lawyers vehemently disagreed with Davies and regarded some of his ideas as heresy, nobody doubted his intellectual force.

On the first day of the Commission of Inquiry, Mark II, in Court 34, everyone bowed respectfully and stood to attention when Davies entered. The shenanigans were over. It was as though a strict but fair headmaster with no tolerance for the naughty pupils had come to restore order to class.

'I'll start with appearances,' said Davies, as he surveyed the lawyers seeking permission to do battle before him. 'This is, of course, a public inquiry, and unless I make any order to the contrary, all proceedings will be made public.'

Peter Leck and Darren Keating felt sick. Their lawyers had won the battle, but now the two hapless hospital administrators were about to lose the war. After the shutdown of the first inquiry, Leck's spirits soared from depression to elation. It appeared that both men had trounced the system and would not even lose their jobs despite their incompetence.

Neither Leck nor Keating had anticipated the public backlash and political backflip that led to the inquiry arising anew from its own ashes. Their folly in not accepting the last-ditch offers of immunity from Morris, and thus saving his inquiry and themselves, became the talk of the legal community. Now, all bets were off. Davies was not bound by any previous undertakings or offers and he was in no mood for deals. He and the legal team of David Andrews, SC, Richard Douglas, SC, Damien Atkinson and Errol Morzone devised a strategy. They needed to hear evidence from the most important witnesses, culminating with Keating and Leck, tie up dozens of loose ends and produce a major report with far-reaching findings and recommendations.

Leck's lawyers and psychiatrists were determined to keep him out of Court 34, citing the mental health condition that had worsened after the grilling by Morris. 'Individuals suffering from such a Major Depressive Episode and Generalised Anxiety Disorder would be expected to have difficulties with concentration and memory. Cognitive processes would be expected to be slowed and the organisation of his thoughts would be expected to be impaired,' said Leck's psychiatrist, Dr Martin Nothling.

Although sympathetic to Leck's situation, Davies ruled that he must give evidence. The patients quietly applauded.

Davies at no stage relished his role as commissioner, but his professionalism, measured low-key handling and vast experience put the inquiry back on track. He was inscrutable and poker-faced; the antithesis of Tony Morris.

When the story of Patel first broke, Davies had followed it from his New Farm apartment with avid interest. The incompetence of the surgeon and the system fascinated Davies in his retirement. On a trip to the United States while the Morris inquiry was ongoing, Davies had spoken to American friends about the revelations. They were scarcely interested, he found, until the following day when the *New York Times* carried a lengthy story about it on its front page. He brought it home as a memento. Now, after a life's work in law, Davies was poised to make a major impact on the health system.

His persistence and the dogged work of Richard Douglas in extracting secret Cabinet papers, confidential emails and covered-up hospital reports showed clearly that the culture of concealment was fostered at the highest levels by Beattie himself, although the Premier denied it.

One of the most damning documents was a 12 November 2002 memo written by Cabinet liaison officer Brad Smith about a secret decision to suppress a series of reports which had been intended for public release to show how all the hospitals and their staff were performing. Smith wrote to the then heads of Queensland Health, Rob Stable and his deputy Steve Buckland:

> Neither the proposed public report which was attached to the Cabinet Submission nor any of the 60 individual Hospital Reports are to be distributed to *anyone*. Senior management can be briefed on the outcomes of the quality measurements and the contents of the documents but they are *not* to be given copies of any of this material.
>
> The Department of the Premier and Cabinet advised that the Premier has emphasised that Cabinet does not want this material released or circulated in any way.

For years, the Beattie Government and its predecessors, including the former Coalition Government, had used Cabinet to hide thousands of sensitive documents. The method was simple. Under the provisions of the Freedom of Information Act anything taken to Cabinet was exempt from disclosure. The extent of the abuse of Freedom of Information was revealed when Michael Clare, a former Cabinet senior staffer, testified he had to find a refrigerator trolley to wheel cartons of documents in and out of Cabinet, ensuring they would be withheld from the public for 30 years. The procedures were subsequently streamlined with legislation permitting documents to be deemed to have been taken to Cabinet without the bother of actually wheeling them in.

When Davies wrote to Beattie and Opposition leader Lawrence Springborg inviting them to either put up evidence to rebut probable conclusions about their egregious conduct or accept the potential adverse findings, Beattie replied: 'I am prepared to act to continue my Government's record of openness and accountability.'

Davies dismissed the glib line as nonsense. He began exposing the politicians' deviousness and hypocrisy, even as the Premier and his followers protested their innocence.

Forensic scrutiny

WHEN Dr Steve Buckland's partner asked what he would like for Christmas 2005 the sacked former director-general knew immediately. 'I want 2006,' he groaned.

Like many of the casualties of the Jayant Patel scandal – patients, nurses, doctors and bureaucrats – Buckland arrived to give his evidence at Court 34 looking meek and beaten. He had spent weeks compiling an exhaustive statement with dozens of attachments, and now he just wanted to put it all behind him. Buckland believed that the ills in the health system were the product of a lack of money. Combined with political interference, the worsening health of patients, a workforce shortage and doctors reluctant to admit mistakes, it was little wonder Patel had gained a toehold at a regional hospital. 'I did not create the public health system in Queensland and the "bureaucracy" that goes with it. No individual did,' he said. 'No individual is especially responsible for its failures. No individual can take credit for its successes. Until we get beyond the culture of blame of blaming individuals and groups for the shortcomings of a system, we will not get very far.'

I recalled his willingness to blame one of the most junior doctors, Andrew Doneman, over the death of ten-year-old Elise Neville, when serious system problems highlighted by that tragedy were unresolved. Beryl Crosby, still toiling tirelessly as leader of the Patients' Support Group, recalled Buckland being happy to permit Patel to continue in Bundaberg, even though he would not have let the surgeon operate on him.

Buckland wanted to resume his career as a medical practitioner 'and avoid the politics of the health system from now on', but inquiry lawyer Richard Douglas needed some answers.

Douglas: I want to make this suggestion to you – and I ask you to carefully consider it before you give your answer – I suggest to you that your decision on 24 March 2005 to, in effect, refrain from taking any step forthwith to suspend Dr Patel from undertaking clinical duties at Bundaberg Hospital involved a dereliction of your duty as Director-General?

Buckland: Sir, I reject that absolutely.

Douglas: I'm seeking to elicit from you, in respect of a decision to which you are party, in the conduct of Queensland Health during your time as Director-General, how bad a surgeon has to be…in order to move the Director-General to cross the Rubicon and suspend that person?

Buckland: I would have to be concerned to the point where I thought that the individual was dangerous, that patients were dying unnecessarily, or that there was some other major event in terms of the surgeon's either mental or surgical capacity.

In the days before Buckland gave evidence, his sacked deputy Dr John Scott, his career in tatters, was melancholy while recounting political meddling in the health system. When asked if he had identified any deficits in his own performance as a senior bureaucrat, Scott, the man who had two months earlier elevated a trivial dinner party of journalists at Bundaberg's Indian Curry Bazaar restaurant into a matter of urgent review by the Premier and the Crime and Misconduct Commission, took time to answer. 'I think probably that if I look back in retrospect, I would say that I probably was more of an activist for the Government and the Minister than perhaps I should have been,' he said softly. We shook hands on his way out.

We heard from Dr Con Aroney, a leading cardiologist who had quit the public health system because of his disgust with management's approach to patient care. Aroney regarded some of his former bosses as 'sociopaths' for their inability to grasp the nettle. We heard, too, from Dr Rob Stable, who served as director-general for eight years and left just before everything hit the fan. He absolved himself of responsibility for the mess.

Dr Gerry FitzGerald, the disarming and mild-mannered Chief Health Officer, attracted sympathy from patients, and key figures including Toni Hoffman. Although he had misled me and others about Jayant Patel, it was difficult to dislike FitzGerald, a man who came across as caring and sincere. His failure to respond properly to the Patel crisis was something Commissioner Geoff Davies would not gloss over.

> Davies: You knew he had 25 times the complication rate, or prima facie it appeared that he had 25 times the complication rate for a very normal piece of surgery. What more do you want to protect the potential patients of Bundaberg Hospital?
>
> FitzGerald: A more detailed investigation of those cases.
>
> Davies: And in the meantime you let him continue to practise and perform surgical procedures?
>
> FitzGerald: I would always seek to try and protect the patient wherever possible.
>
> Richard Douglas: What you did was you protected Dr Patel rather than the patients?
>
> FitzGerald: Well, that was not the intent.
>
> Davies: See, one possible view that I could form, doctor – and I am not saying for the moment that I have formed or that I am – is that you were deliberately concealing this unfavourable data in the hope that because Dr Patel was likely to leave reasonably soon, it would all go away?
>
> FitzGerald: Well, that was not my consideration at the time.

Away from operating theatres and wards, in this adversarial court-room where a misstatement might be seen as deliberately misleading, the doctors were no match for the lawyers. The clinical dissection continued day after day, disposing of the foolhardy, the true believers, the yes-men. It was a warm-up for what should have been the climax, the appearance of Bundaberg Hospital's managers Peter Leck and Dr Darren Keating, but by the time they arrived, so much blood had been spilled that it was possible to feel sorry for them.

Keating must have felt betrayed and foolish for defending Patel, who deceived him along with almost everyone else. Keating had become a laughing stock; worse, he faced prosecution. His best strategy at the inquiry was to stick to the one he had adopted all along, and maintain that Patel was not too bad. The surgeon, safely back in the United States, had tried to call Keating at one stage but hung up before making contact. Douglas urged Keating to consider more than one proposition 'carefully'. 'I suggest to you…' Douglas began, and we knew the question would require the outflanked witness to agree or disagree that his conduct amounted to a 'gross dereliction of duty'. The questions were like scythes. Another severed head plopped into the basket.

Gerry Mullins, the lawyer for the patients, and John Allen, the lawyer for the nurses, mopped up. 'When you look back now, do you agree there was a raging fire of Dr Patel's incompetence?' Keating responded: 'I don't believe so. I could not see a major trend, taking into account the number of complications and concerns in each of these different areas.'

Allen had stayed on a true and steady course for the truth throughout the public hearings. He put to Keating that he was lying for saying he would have permitted Patel to operate on him at any time at the hospital. 'It is honest,' Keating insisted. 'It's not the truth,' Allen barked

What would it take for someone in a position of responsibility to own up and admit fault? 'Look, I'm sorry, I am partly responsible for all of this and I deserve censure.' But there was little contrition in Court 34. Nobody did anything wrong.

Having destroyed the first inquiry, a move that backfired, and then failing with a legal argument that his fragile psychiatric condition should preclude him from giving any evidence at the second inquiry, Peter Leck and his lawyers had a small win – orders to shield him from the media throng. But Davies needed Leck's sworn testimony. At this late stage with just a few days until the curtain fell, Blind Freddy could piece together most of what had gone wrong in Bundaberg. Davies, however, could not make findings against individuals until they had been given an opportunity to state their cases and respond to questions. Leck was afforded every courtesy by his inquisitors, none of whom wanted to cause him further mental distress.

When Davies asked if it occurred to Leck 'at any stage to consider suspending Dr Patel from surgery', the humiliated hospital boss said he relied on Keating's opinion.

At the lunch break, Beryl Crosby and her friends in the Patients' Support Group, Tess Bramich, Lisa Hooper and Doris Hillier, rushed to the other end of George Street to Parliament House, to hear the vanquished inquiry chief, Tony Morris, deliver a speech: 'The Black Death in Queensland Health'.

Morris, in robust form despite his judicial trouncing, credited Justice Martin Moynihan for turning 'a lawyer, a member of the most distrusted and reviled profession in our community, into a popular and even heroic figure'. Earlier, he borrowed a quote from his wife when he quipped to me: 'As Alice likes to say, we're bitter but not twisted.'

EIGHTY kilometres away at Southport on the Gold Coast, other pressing health issues were all too personal. My sister Rebecca methodically distilled the latest information about our mother Diana's condition.

Frustratingly, the results from a biopsy of a tumour 7–8 centimetres long were inconclusive. The endocrinologist suspected it was malignant, but the oncologist differed. 'However, it is my understanding that Dr Feather has some doubts as to whether there may be cancer in the lung which may explain some of her respiratory problems,' Rebecca wrote to Mum's GP, Dr Jim Abrahams. 'Whilst in hospital, she lost about 10 kilos, however, she has started to eat again and now has the strength to walk to the bathroom. Last week we were advised to get

Mum's affairs in order due to the status of her health, however this week we have a different story altogether and we honestly don't know what is going on as the various medical teams/doctors don't communicate with each other or us.'

72

An ill wind

25–26 October 2005

COVERING the once-in-a-lifetime scandal of Jayant Patel and the wider story of how political interference and bureaucratic incompetence conspired against a health system was demanding, but never boring.

We were witnessing a near-revolution in health care with two Commissions of Inquiry (the first one spectacularly shut down) and a massive boost in funding for the hospitals and their staff. There would be a new and improved complaints commission, unprecedented transparency and a commitment to proper audits of deaths and injuries to prevent another Jayant Patel.

The outcomes were remarkable but a fluke. At so many different stages before the Patel story broke, coincidental events and chances became the links in a chain that was not apparent as it formed. If just one of those links had failed, there would have been no result. The links were independent of each other, yet essential to the final result. What if Toni Hoffman had given up? Or not heard about Elise Neville, the little girl who fell out of her bunk bed? What if Hoffman's local Member of Parliament, Rob Messenger, had put her concerns in the too-hard basket? Or if Des Bramich had not died in Bundaberg Hospital? What if I had never held suspicions about both the competence of the Medical Board and Overseas Trained Doctors? Or if nurse Karen Jenner had not made a casual remark at Hoffman's house about Patel not becoming a bad surgeon overnight – that he must have left a trail of human wreckage elsewhere.

There was no doubt the *Courier-Mail*'s revelations back on 13 April 2005 were the catalyst for public outrage about Patel and the trigger for the inquiries. If Queensland Health had not chosen to cover up its knowledge of Patel's bans in the United States, the Beattie Government would not have been on the back foot. If the heads of Queensland Health had simply confessed everything immediately, beating me to a ridiculously straightforward Internet check, they might have escaped much of the public anger and the investigative blowtorch. After years of official secrecy, the cover-up had hopelessly failed and now everything was exposed. Once again, a rough adage of my profession, namely 'the screw-up is always in the cover-up', had been confirmed. It was irony.

The doctors, nurses and readers of the newspaper who had stayed in contact with me believed the lives of many patients would be saved or improved by the promised reforms.

On 25 October 2005 I returned to my desk at the *Courier-Mail's* offices in Campbell Street, Bowen Hills with its view of the Royal Brisbane Hospital, feeling melancholy. The assignment I had taken on with my hard-working and good-humoured colleague Amanda Watt was almost over. She decided this was a cause for celebration. She had been calm, professional and supportive right to the end. As I responded to emails I tried to come to terms with the end of the inquiries and the start of a new challenge – whatever that might be. No matter how many rocks I might turn over in future, nothing would match the power, scope and impact of the Patel scandal.

For Premier Peter Beattie, it was a momentous day. He heralded one of the major spin-offs, which he hoped would prevent his government from being thrown out.

My colleague Malcolm Cole wrote:

A raid on future budget surpluses and public service pay rises will fund the $6.36 billion Beattie Government plan to fix Queensland's ailing health system and revive its own political fortunes.

Months of political turmoil that began with the Bundaberg Hospital scandal earlier this year culminated with the delivery of Queensland's first state mini-Budget.

Premier Peter Beattie said while the massive funding and reform package had been forced by the extraordinary failures in

Bundaberg, the changes would flow through to every facet of the state's health system. Queenslanders will pay for the changes through higher taxes and lower budget surpluses over the next four years.

'Well mate, you've cost this state $6.4 billion. How do you feel?' my colleague Craig Johnstone joked on returning from the mini-budget announcement. 'When all our power bills go up Hedley, we can send you the bill,' said Tess Livingstone, another colleague.

My mother, Diana, was in the Gold Coast Hospital and watching the TV news about the health crisis. Her condition was poor; the specialists were divided on how she would fare with the tumour in her adrenal gland. We feared the tumour was malignant and possibly inoperable. She was losing weight and had little energy. Her high cheekbones were now prominent because of the weight loss. She had lost her hair and replaced it with an expensive wig. My mother was a beautiful woman and had always strived to look her best. Her appearance worried her more than the probability that she had a terminal condition.

My mother was a wonderful storyteller. She could tell classics – family squabbles, workplace triumphs, meetings with the rich and famous – although the facts were usually in dispute. She was also a natural stirrer. Perhaps that's why she took credit for her son choosing journalism. Was the craft not a combination of stirring and story-telling?

I drove back to Brisbane after each visit feeling guilty that I was not doing more to understand her condition or find the best specialists to help her. The nurses told me she watched the TV news on the night of 25 October. All the bulletins led with the massive boost in funding for the health system.

I left my desk earlier than usual: I had been asked to talk about the Jayant Patel story to the Sunnybank Private Hospital's Annual Medical Council dinner. My talk at the Tattersall's Club in the city started with Elise Neville. She was more than a link in the chain. The death of this little girl, the campaign by her parents, Gerard and Lorraine, and the hideous failure of the health and regulatory system to repair itself, even while prosecuting an inexperienced and exhausted doctor who had erred in treating a head injury, had a profound impact on me, Hoffman and many others. In the end, Elise's death was not pointless. Like the deaths of the children at Bundaberg Hospital in 1928, it led to positive change.

That night I dreamt that my mother had died. When I woke in the early morning, I felt uneasy and decided I would spend the day at her bedside.

'Where's Mummy! Where's Mummy?' my daughter Sarah yelled as she clambered across the sheets. My wife, Ruth, was not in our bed. She had gone down to Alexander, our son, when he cried out during the night.

It was a little after 6 am on 26 October 2005 when my sister Peta called. She was distraught. 'Hed, Mum has just died. The staff from the ward called me. They're so sorry. They don't know what happened.'

73

The findings

Brisbane, 30 November 2005

'HE didn't miss anyone,' volunteered one of the inquiry's lawyers, Jarrod Cowley-Grimmond, outside the Brisbane Magistrates Court. Other lawyers, who had fought since May to put the best possible light on the poor conduct of their clients, were walking away, grim-faced, with a 538-page maroon-coloured document titled *Queensland Public Hospitals Commission of Inquiry Report.*

Cowley-Grimmond was right. Inquiry Commissioner Geoff Davies, who at that moment was presenting the poisoned chalice to Premier Peter Beattie as the TV cameras filmed their forced smiles, had not played favourites. He was as tough on the political leader who asked him to conduct the inquiry as he was on the minions whose incompetence cost lives. Apart from the tragedy at Bundaberg, he reported on crises in hospitals in Hervey Bay, Townsville, Rockhampton, Charters Towers and Brisbane. Davies did more than pinpoint the guilty parties. He urged national leadership, an overhaul of funding strategies and major reforms to the health bureaucracies and regulatory bodies.

The Beattie Government and the former Coalition

Davies found a 'culture of secrecy' fostered by successive governments had been a major cause of the Jayant Patel scandal and unsafe care in the health system. 'It involved a blatant exercise of secreting information from public gaze for no reason other than that the disclosure of the information might be embarrassing to Government,' Davies ruled.

Campaigns of concealment at the highest levels of the government were contrary to the public interest, misleading and deadly. The culture, encouraged by politicians, 'filtered down to Queensland Health staff and, through them, to administrators in public hospitals', resulting in a failure to act decisively on safety. He ruled:

This culture started at the top with successive governments misusing the Freedom of Information Act to enable potentially embarrassing information to be concealed from the public. All this reflects poorly on the politicians involved in the stewardship of Queensland Health.

Unsurprisingly, Queensland Health adopted a similar approach, and because inadequate budgets meant that there would be inadequate health care, there was quite a lot to conceal.

Again unsurprisingly, the same approach was adopted by administrators in public hospitals, and this, in turn, led to threats of retribution to those who saw it as their duty to complain about inadequate health care.

Davies criticised the former Coalition Government, the Beattie Government and former Labor health ministers Gordon Nuttall and Wendy Edmond.

Queensland Health

The lives and care of patients in the public health system had been compromised for years because of chronic under-funding, Davies ruled. He advocated national leadership on health funding to prevent the collapse of the public system which, he found, was unsustainable unless more patients paid for their care.

'And it is also wrong, in my opinion, to assume that the other States are providing an adequate and safe system,' he said. 'Even more concerning is that the lower cost in Queensland in delivering health care services has come at the cost of lowering the standard of health-care to one which is grossly inadequate and dangerous.'

By relying on unqualified doctors to perform complex surgery beyond their competence and by 'dumping inadequately trained doctors' into hospitals, patients were put at risk. 'In my view it is an irresistible conclusion that there is a history of a culture of concealment within and pertaining to Queensland Health,' Davies ruled.

The Medical Board of Queensland
Davies ruled that the Board's incompetence had led to 'large numbers of overseas trained doctors practising in this State without meeting the standards required of Australian-trained doctors'. This was particularly disturbing as the Board and its major stakeholders had been aware for several years that the registration system for Overseas Trained Doctors 'was in crisis'.

'Any reasonable enquiry would have revealed that Dr Patel had lied in the application about his disciplinary history. If that had been revealed, the dishonesty alone should have persuaded the Board that Dr Patel was not a suitable person for registration. The Board, effectively, made no independent inquiry,' Davies ruled.

Dr Steve Buckland
Davies blamed the sacked director-general for fostering a culture of concealment and suppression, and compromising the safety of patients by attempting to deny or ignore serious clinical issues linked to dangerous doctors. He found Buckland 'failed to take any appropriate action to suspend [Dr Patel] from duty, or providing surgical services, or further restrict his scope of practice...or cause any further investigation of Dr Patel's conduct until April 9, 2005, after Dr Patel had left the country. Each failure, in the circumstances, was deliberate or careless and incompetent and unreasonable.'

He ruled Buckland was inclined 'to criticise the critics and to conceal the criticism rather than to deal with the problem'.

Dr Gerry FitzGerald
His approach to the audit he led into Dr Patel in early 2005 and his interpretation of its alarming findings of a significantly higher complication rate were 'quite inexplicable', Davies ruled, adding Dr FitzGerald acted 'deliberately or carelessly and incompetently'.

'Permitting Dr Patel to continue to practise and then leaving it to the Medical Board of Queensland to take whatever steps they thought necessary, was a course designed to minimise publicity and in effect conceal the truth. The interests of the patients were ignored,' Davies said. 'Dr FitzGerald failed to take any step to restrict Dr Patel's surgical practices through suspension, limitation of practice, or restriction of duties at the hospital, whether temporarily or otherwise, when such advice was reasonably appropriate and warranted. In my view Dr FitzGerald had it in his mind from the outset that it was likely that Dr Patel would not remain in practice in Australia beyond 31 March 2005. This was likely to put an end to the issue. He did this against the background of knowing that from 22 March 2005 the issue had become a political one, it being raised in Parliament by Mr Messenger MP...'

Dr Darren Keating

Davies recommended a police probe into evidence that Bundaberg Hospital's Director of Medical Services deliberately misled state and federal agencies in relation to Patel's status and abilities. Keating 'persistently ignored or downplayed the seriousness of complaints' and had 'performed his duties carelessly or incompetently'.

'When the matters are considered together, they lead to the view that there was a strong element of orchestrated incompetence, or wilful blindness, in Dr Keating's response to complaints about his Director of Surgery,' Davies ruled. 'I find that Dr Keating deliberately diminished or downplayed complaints about Dr Patel. He declined to initiate inquiries into Dr Patel where, at the very least, serious concerns had been raised, and he promoted or acquiesced in a perception amongst staff that Dr Patel was protected by management because he was valuable.'

Peter Leck

For performing his duties 'carelessly or incompetently' the hospital's District Manager should face disciplinary action, Davies ruled. Leck permitted Dr Patel's promotion to Director of Surgery before anyone had checked his skills.

Leck had not set up a system to vet the credentials of doctors at the hospital and, accordingly, 'the formal qualifications, training, experience and clinical competence of Dr Patel, amongst others, was not assessed and the opportunity was lost for such a committee to discover Dr Patel's disciplinary history and take appropriate action'.

'Upon learning of complaints and concerns about Dr Patel's competence, Mr Leck failed to ensure that they were investigated properly,' Davies ruled. 'Like Dr Keating, Mr Leck's conduct in my view evinces, if not a policy of calculated concealment, an attitude that discouraged any frank discussion of clinical issues within the [hospital].'

Toni Hoffman

In paying tribute to people 'whose care, passion or courage was instrumental in bringing to light the matters covered here', Davies singled out the nurse manager of the Intensive Care Unit at the hospital. 'She might easily have doubted herself, or succumbed to certain pressures to work within a system that was not responsive. She might have chosen to quarantine herself from Dr Patel's influence by leaving the [hospital] or at least the Intensive Care Unit,' Davies said.

'Instead, and under the threat of significant detriment to herself, Ms Hoffman persistently and carefully documented the transgressions of Dr Patel. It was her courage and persistence which, in the face of inaction and even resistance, brought the scandalous conduct of Dr Patel to light.'

Jayant Patel

The missing surgeon was found to have been a pathological liar who performed operations beyond his competence and beyond the capacity of the hospital and its staff. 'As a result of negligence on the part of Dr Patel, 13 patients at the [hospital] died and many others suffered adverse outcomes,' Davies ruled.

'Dr Patel unreasonably failed to transfer patients to a tertiary referral hospital within an appropriate timeframe, causing adverse outcomes for many of those patients. On many occasions, Dr Patel failed to adequately record in patient files the true details concerning material facts including the surgical procedures undertaken, complications arising from surgery, wound dehiscence, infections, the course of post-operative care and reasons for post-operative return to surgery. Dr Patel failed to refer 13 reportable deaths to the Coroner.'

Davies recommended police consider charges of manslaughter, negligent acts causing harm, grievous bodily harm, assault occasioning bodily harm and fraud. He found that Patel had virtues. He was 'not without skill, intelligence, and an aptitude for learning, and might well have thrived in a larger hospital where he was closely supervised. Staff attested to the fact that Dr Patel worked tirelessly'.

74

Dear Dr Patel

Portland, Oregon, July 2006

FOR most of the long flight to the United States my imagination ran riot. In my mind's eye I was driving a hire car to an address I had memorised, and knocking confidently on the heavy front door of Jayant Patel's impressive mansion. Like Paul Barry from *60 Minutes* the previous year, I would stride across the manicured lawn and declare: 'Dr Patel, we know you're there.' As a photographer steadied for the 'gotcha shot', an unsmiling Patel would unbolt the door and invite us in for an exhaustive interview.

It was a long shot but stranger things had happened since this bizarre scandal first erupted. Stefanie Balogh, the *Courier-Mail*'s Chief of Staff, and Toni Hoffman were positive. 'Just remember this – his ego is so huge that he would love to talk about what happened and blame everyone else,' Hoffman told me. 'I think he wants to talk. It's only his lawyers who have stopped him.' The patients and their families, the doctors and nurses, the politicians and the bureaucrats – they would be morbidly engrossed in even the most self-serving explanation from Patel. So far, his story remained untold. It was the final chapter. He might as well lay it out with the reporter who had made a study of his career.

Having decided days earlier to resign from the newspaper after seven years there, I had another motive. An exclusive Patel interview would be an appropriate way to finish. He had been in legal limbo since a Queensland Police brief comprising more than 35 000 pages of evidence went to the Director of Public Prosecutions, Leanne Clare, in February 2006. His Brisbane solicitor Damian Scattini said the entire saga had been horrendous for his client. 'How do you imagine he feels about it all? He takes it all very seriously and it's been a nightmare for him,' Scattini said.

Terry O'Gorman, the civil liberties lawyer, said: 'He's been dubbed Dr Death for a period of 12 months or more. He's been the centre focus of a royal commission in which a whole lot of evidence, not admissible in a court of law, has been led. It is my view that he cannot get a fair trial.'

Hoffman and the patients, however, remained confident he would be extradited for a trial in the Supreme Court in Brisbane. The detectives from the Homicide Squad were adamant that she would be a key witness for the prosecution, while Police Commissioner Bob Atkinson had visited Bundaberg to reassure grieving families that the case was a high priority.

The 13 deaths attributed to Patel from evidence in the inquiry run by Geoff Davies had risen to 17 in the ensuing months. Prosecuting Patel over so many deaths would increase the workload for the police and the lawyers, so Atkinson opted to whittle the number to a handful of manslaughter and grievous bodily harm cases where the evidence was strongest.

As Patel pondered his future waiting for a knock on the door from a US Marshal with extradition papers, or an opportunistic reporter with a digital recorder, Hoffman suffered a breakdown. The stress had finally caught up with her. Ordered to take a long break from work, she watched a TV news clip on 6 June – Premier Peter Beattie had upped the injection of funds into the health system to almost $10 billion after polls tipped electoral disaster. 'This means more elective surgery, more responsive and better resourced emergency departments, expanded public and community health activities and, ultimately, a healthier Queensland,' Beattie said.

'TELL me, what is happening? When are they going to bring him to Australia?' Jim Kronenberg, the Oregon Medical Association's effusive manager, asked for an update within moments of meeting at Portland's Hotel Deluxe. In a long career working with physicians he had never encountered anything as strange as the Patel scandal.

'What happened to the unfortunate folks in Australia was a real shock to us here. This guy would have worked in every Kaiser Permanente clinic in Portland. He has worked with scrub nurses and (anaesthetists). He has assisted surgeons and supervised surgeons,' Kronenberg said.

Doesn't that make it worse? That he worked for a long time with many qualified people, and yet it took years for him to be stopped?

'Well, I have a theory. I'm left to conclude that with all the surgeons with whom he worked, none of them saw enough. They saw a mistake here and there,' Kronenberg answered. 'And they often say things like, "well, I wouldn't have done it that way". But that's the thing – there is not always a precise and scientific way, every time. The human anatomy is different. I used to think we were all set up the same way, but no. Take a woman's uterus. There are big ones, small ones, long ones, wide ones. So after saying, "I wouldn't have done it that way", a reviewing surgeon will next say, "but I can understand why it was done that way".'

THE Oregon Board of Medical Examiners in downtown Portland has an impressive sign above its reception desk: 'Mission: To protect the health, safety and well-being of Oregonians by regulating the practice of medicine in a manner that promotes quality health care.'

One of the Board's investigators, Don Short, had been asked to greet me and decline requests for information about their most infamous registrant. The chairman, David Grube, would that day invoke an order signed by Patel to prevent reinstatement as a surgeon until he 'proves to the satisfaction of the Board that the criminal and administrative process against him in Australia is complete and that all penalties or conditions imposed by that jurisdiction have been satisfied'.

Short was tight-lipped. He had been told to say nothing about recent contact with either Patel or his criminal lawyer, Stephen Houze, who had flagged a long battle with Australian authorities if extradition proceedings were started.

'DO you think he will be extradited back to Australia?' asked John Dulley, sitting in his favourite room, filled with sports memorabilia –

Red Sox baseball gear, football helmets, celebrated covers of *Time* and *Life* magazine – in the family home in a heavily wooded suburb south of Portland. He pointed to an x-ray in a frame on the wall. 'There's the clamp that Patel left inside me.'

'Can you imagine that being left inside someone?' asked his wife, Tracey. The stainless steel clamp measured 20 centimetres from tip to handle. 'They did such a good job hiding all this. There's a gag order on his law suit. And they tried to sell it as a mistake, a terrible accident that happened in a learning situation.'

In 1992, Dulley, then a 27-year-old restaurant cook, suffered from ulcerative colitis. He underwent a procedure to have his colon removed after being reassured by the confidence and apparent ability of his surgeon, Patel. When Dulley left the Bess Kaiser Medical Kaiser Center to go home ten days after the surgery, he was doubled up with pain.

'They told me in the hospital that they had "nicked my urethra" and had to repair it,' Dulley told me. 'I went home and I was having trouble urinating. I was urinating through my rectum. I told one of the interns what was going on. And then they discovered the clamp. The intern told me "this is a surgeon's worst nightmare". He said I should get an attorney.'

Patel had left the sexually active man permanently impotent. He required five major operations by other surgeons to repair some of the damage from the first procedure by Patel. The settlement of Dulley's legal case in 1994 should have been reported to the Oregon Board of Medical Examiners by the Kaiser group, but it withheld the information. He has wondered how many patients might have been better off if the Board had begun investigations at the time. He hoped Patel would be severely disciplined. 'What I think would really hurt him most is him having to explain what he did to people he thinks are beneath him. He would hate that. I just know it,' Dulley said.

SUSAN Goldsmith swung her Chevrolet Tracker onto the freeway and headed north, peeling off for the last five minutes of the journey to Patel's house in the Bronson Creek estate where the houses are larger and more expensive.

'I know he's around. I don't know if he's around this second, but I'm told he hangs out at the Starbucks in Washington Square,' the heavily pregnant investigative journalist for the *Oregonian* newspaper told me. 'You know, I had so much trouble finding doctors willing to talk to me – even those doctors who worked with him and knew about his problems. I don't know what it's like in Australia, but here there's like this culture of secrecy with the doctors. I went to one of the local doctors' association meetings and they broke into a jog to get away from me. It was unbelievable. I was like "what is wrong with these people?" If you are a sicko in this profession, you will be protected. Patel found the right profession, and then he found the right specialty where there are a lot of complications.'

'What is our strategy?' I asked. 'Do you want to pull over and talk about it?'

'Let's just bowl up and knock on the door,' she replied. So we did. She knocked. I called out.

There were many questions. Why did he keep operating in Bundaberg when it must have been obvious that his patients were suffering? How did he cope knowing of the suffering – the deaths, maiming and psychological trauma? What would he like to say to those affected?

I went back to the house five times and telephoned repeatedly. But nobody answered.

Epilogue

BERYL Crosby looked shattered. Wired with devices to monitor her heart, Crosby was still rushing around helping others when she should have been resting in the weeks before Premier Peter Beattie called a circuit-breaking state election for 9 September 2006. The doctors at Bundaberg Hospital were worried about her high blood pressure as well as her conflict with Rob Messenger.

The unflagging advocate for the patients and the fearless politician were no longer allies. Messenger believed that many of the several hundred patients, and perhaps Crosby herself, were being unjustly treated in Australia's largest compensation program for medical negligence. It included free legal and medical advice and relatively generous payouts for the physical injuries and psychiatric stress arising from Jayant Patel's surgery.

'I'm devastated,' Messenger told me when I visited Bundaberg for a late-July meeting of the Patients' Support Group. 'Beryl's line is that I'm just being political. She believes I'm using this to advance my political career – and that's a big kick in the guts for me. Beryl and I no longer have a relationship. She believes the compensation system is operating fine.'

Crosby, who had been sped to hospital by ambulance the previous week after collapsing from stress, could no longer cope with Messenger's interference. 'Patients are walking out of our meetings. We have had five now who say they won't come back because of him,' she explained. 'People are angry with him. He's grandstanding. I think he's doing it because he believes he's winning votes, but little does he know that he's losing them. I don't care if he burns up all the goodwill he had, but I care that he's upsetting the patients. It's sad. It's bedlam. We were great friends.'

I had a hunch that the evening meeting of the Patients' Support Group would herald news about the efforts to extradite Jayant Patel from Oregon to Australia. The patients hoped the appearance of the Attorney-General, Linda Lavarch, meant a breakthrough.

Others were sceptical. 'I don't believe that Patel will ever be bought back to Australia because I think he would implicate too many other people,' said Karen Orreal, the mother of teenager Shannon Mobbs who lost his leg and almost lost his life.

When I spoke to Gerry Kemps' widow, Judy, at her retirement villa at seaside Bargara, she was determined to see the surgeon stand trial. 'I think Gerry was meant to go the way he did, to put a stop to all the carnage. But even now, I'm having anxiety attacks. They're scary. I'm taking antidepressants,' she said. 'The police reckon they are going to have news soon. I'm glad they've made Gerry one of the manslaughter cases. I feel as if he's contributing. I get so angry when people say "oh, they won't ever get Patel back here". I feel like slapping them. Of course they'll get him back. When the trial starts, I want to be in the front row. I will go every day.'

A little after 7 pm in a conference room at the Brothers Club, Lavarch and a small entourage took their seats. Her media adviser, Paul Childs, quipped about new quality controls. 'We don't appoint anyone now without first Googling them,' he said. Lavarch pledged that her door would remain open for anyone with complaints about the compensation. She was adamant the ongoing efforts of the Director of Public Prosecutions, Leanne Clare, and the police to bring Patel back for a criminal trial were completely independent from her office.

'I can't go down and say "hurry up". They need to be independent', Lavarch stressed. 'They need to be given all the time they require to investigate all the matters. You can categorically trust the office of the DPP to ensure that every matter is progressing well. You have all been courageous. And the fact that you care about each other sends a very loud message to all of Queensland about what a great community this is.'

The patients stayed for tea and biscuits. Nelson Cox looked as fit as a fiddle. Shannon Mobbs, the youngest victim, beamed as he walked on his new prosthetic leg. Marilyn Daisy, down the back in her wheelchair, was unwell, although she did not let on.

AFTER an election campaign that went disastrously for the Opposition, Premier Peter Beattie romped to victory at the polls on 9 September. A few months earlier, he was worried: 'In the end, health could be the death of me. We've got a fight on our hands. But it's a fight we can win.' But Beattie had faced up to a disaster that, I suspected, he knew was partly of his own making. He started an unprecedented process of reform. He was braver than any other Australian politician confronted with a health crisis.

The political pundits who had predicted serious pain for his Labor government attributed Beattie's fourth-term triumph to the voting public's disgust at the strife-torn Opposition, which failed dismally in its attempts to capitalise on the Jayant Patel scandal. One of Labor's few losses was in the retiring Nita Cunningham's once-safe seat of Bundaberg.

As I settled into my new role at *The Australian* newspaper, reliable sources hinted at something that seemed incredible. Through his lawyers, Patel had secretly offered to return voluntarily to Brisbane before the state election. Weeks of highly confidential talks between his legal defence team and the DPP had culminated in Leanne Clare recommending to Linda Lavarch that the Patel deal be approved. It was an extraordinary opportunity. It would have saved years of costly and uncertain extradition proceedings. As part of the package, Patel's lawyers Damian Scattini and Stephen Houze had sought undertakings from Clare and Lavarch that bail would not be opposed at an initial court appearance in Brisbane. If a magistrate agreed to grant bail, Patel would fly back to Oregon and remain at his home until the start of his criminal trial in Brisbane's Supreme Court. He had offered to give up his passport and report to Portland police.

Queensland's best legal minds told me on and off the record that Lavarch should have snatched the deal, particularly as Clare and her top

prosecutors, David Meredith and Ross Martin SC, had urged acceptance after exploring the fine details.

'How is the public going to be served by getting Dr Patel back in
two or three years? People die, people forget who operated on whom.
Time defeats proper outcomes and once people's recollections are
taxed, people who should be convicted are not convicted,' Richard
Douglas SC told me. I thought of the elderly Judy Kemps.

The evening after Marilyn Daisy's death at Bundaberg Hospital in
October, I called Lavarch's mobile phone. I already knew the deal had
failed. I knew that Lavarch stubbornly refused to support it despite the
DPP's lobbying. Her surprise decision after consulting Beattie behind
closed doors was final. The Office of the DPP was unimpressed. Patel
was dumbfounded when Scattini told him of the Queensland
Government's veto. For more than a year, politicians had been
demanding his scalp. Some proposed hiring bounty hunters. Now he
was being told 'stay away'.

I was in no doubt that the decision had been influenced by political rather than legal reasons. The return of Patel could have been disastrous for Beattie, so close to the state election. Labor had directed its
small-target campaign away from health. The politicians had concealed
the deal's existence even as they spoke in public about the need for a
trial and closure for patients. But the subterfuge was almost over. When
Lavarch answered her mobile phone and nervously defended her decision, the front page of the *Australian* was already being drawn under the
headline: 'Beattie scuttled Dr Death deal'.

The news stunned and appalled the patients, particularly Beryl
Crosby, who recalled Lavarch's visit in late July when she insisted her
office had nothing to do with the 'independent' DPP. When she
addressed the patients that evening at the Brothers Club, Lavarch had
already rejected the Patel proposal four weeks earlier. The story in the
Australian developed momentum and provoked widespread anger.
Beattie and Lavarch were accused of misleading State Parliament;
Scattini broke his silence and forced Beattie to retract false claims;
Crosby demanded the release of all relevant documents. In the same
week, Marilyn Daisy was laid to rest. After apologising for covering up

information and misleading the public, Lavarch quit as Attorney-General on 18 October, citing depression.

A warrant seeking Jayant Patel's arrest was taken by Queensland police to a Brisbane magistrate on the afternoon of 22 November 2006. The warrant, a formal trigger to start an extradition process, listed numerous proposed charges including manslaughter, grievous bodily harm and fraud.

The news of the development overwhelmed many of the patients and their relatives. Beryl Crosby was kept busy briefing her members and doing interviews with journalists. Judy Kemps broke down. Her husband was named in the warrant as one of the three manslaughter cases.

Mostly, my sources believed Patel would not be coming back – or, at least, not for a long time. The Director of Public Prosecutions, Leanne Clare, publicly warned that the extradition proceedings would be complicated and time-consuming. But, as Crosby told the patients, it was a start.

JAYANT Patel's favourite restaurant in Bundaberg, the Indian Curry Bazaar, has been busier than ever. Tourists ask Pam Samra to sell the placemats. She has retailed dozens as souvenirs.

Having rescued the inquiry, Geoff Davies has become a key adviser on health to the Beattie Government and the Royal Australasian College of Surgeons. Queensland Health now boasts an independent Health Quality and Complaints Commission with 'more powers, more resources and more responsibilities'; hundreds of extra places for doctors; transparency on surgery performance and waiting times; and one thousand extra nurses.

Toni Hoffman has another award: Whistleblower of the Year. The citation says she put herself on the line to save lives. She has been to lunch with the Governor-General, to dinner with the Queen and had cocktails with the Prime Minister.

Dr Gerard Neville and his wife Lorraine have been looking ahead. When told of their daughter Elise's special role in the Jayant Patel scandal, they wept.

Endnotes

Abbreviations used in the endnotes are as follows:
BBHCI: Bundaberg Base Hospital Commission of Inquiry
QPHCI: Queensland Public Hospitals Commission of Inquiry

Prologue   General information and quotes have been obtained from the Report of the 1928 Royal Commission of Inquiry into the Fatalities at Bundaberg, headed by Dr Charles Kellaway. Other information is attributed in the text.

Chapters 1–3   General information and quotes have been obtained from the author's interviews with Gerard and Lorraine Neville and their affidavit material filed in the Health Practitioners Tribunal of Queensland. Additional material came from Freedom of Information searches of Queensland Health. The author also relied upon statements of Caloundra Hospital staff and investigation reports by independent medical experts.

Chapter 4   General information and quotes have been obtained from the author's interviews with Toni Hoffman and members of her family and friends.

Chapter 5   General information and quotes have been obtained from the author's interviews with Dr Sam Baker and Dr Chris Jelliffe. Other material came from testimony and statements at the BBHCI and the subsequent QPHCI.

Chapter 6   General information and quotes have been obtained from the reports and investigative files of the Oregon Board of Medical Examiners.

Chapter 7   General information and quotes have been obtained from statements, attachments and testimony to the QPHCI. Other information comes from research and interviews by the author.

Chapter 8   General information and quotes have been obtained from the author's interviews with Dr Sally Ehlers and reporter Susan Goldsmith in Oregon. Direct quotes are attributed within the text.

Chapter 9   General information and quotes have been obtained from testimony and statements to the BBHCI and the QPHCI, as well as the author's interviews. References to the *Bundaberg NewsMail* are attributed in the text.

Chapter 10   General information and quotes have been obtained from testimony and statements to the BBHCI and the QPHCI, as well as the author's interviews with hospital staff.

Chapter 11   General information and quotes have been obtained from the author's interviews with Dr William Craver in the United States. Other material came from statements and testimony to the New York State Department of Health, the New York Office of Professional Discipline and the New York State Board for Professional Medical Conduct. Correspondence from Dr Raymond Hinshaw came from the Oregon Board of Medical Examiners.

Chapter 12–14   General information and quotes have been obtained from testimony and statements to the BBHCI and the QPHCI, as well as the author's interviews with hospital staff.

Chapter 15   General information and quotes have been obtained from the author's interviews as attributed in the text. Other material comes from a report into Overseas Trained Doctors by Dr Denis Lennox and email correspondence as attributed.

Chapter 16   General information and quotes have been obtained from the author's interview with Dr Ross Cartmill. Other information came from articles in the *Courier-Mail* and the *Cairns Post* as attributed. The reference to Dr Steve Buckland's letter came from an attachment to his statement to the QPHCI.

Chapter 17   General information has been obtained from the Bundaberg and Districts Historical Museum. Other material and quotes came from the author's interviews with Pam Samra, Toni Hoffman and Carol Elliott, and evidence to the BBHCI.

Chapter 18   General information and quotes have been obtained from testimony and statements to the BBHCI and the QPHCI, as well as the author's interviews with hospital staff.

Chapter 19   General information and quotes have been obtained from the Hansard record of State Parliament, testimony and statements to the BBHCI and the QPHCI, as well as the author's interviews with Rob Messenger and hospital staff.

Chapter 20   General information and quotes have been obtained from testimony and statements to the BBHCI and the QPHCI, as well as the author's interviews with Tess Bramich, Mark Bramich and hospital staff.

Chapter 21   General information and quotes have been obtained from testimony and statements to the BBHCI and the QPHCI, as well as the author's interviews with hospital staff.

Chapter 22   General information and quotes have been obtained from the author's interviews with Gerard and Lorraine Neville and their affidavit material filed in the Health Practitioners Tribunal of Queensland. Additional material came from Freedom of Information searches of Queensland Health. The author also relied upon statements of Caloundra Hospital staff; and investigation reports by independent medical experts.

Chapter 23   General information and quotes have been obtained from testimony and statements to the BBHCI and the QPHCI, as well as the author's interviews with hospital staff. The author also relied on correspondence with Toni Hoffman.

Chapter 24   General information and quotes have been obtained from testimony and statements to the BBHCI and the QPHCI, as well as the author's interviews with hospital staff. Other information relating to Elise Neville came from the ruling of the Health Practitioners Tribunal.

Chapter 25   General information and quotes have been obtained from testimony and statements to the BBHCI and the QPHCI, as well as the author's interviews with hospital staff. Other material came from the author's interviews with Judy Kemps.

Chapter 26   General information and quotes have been obtained from testimony and statements to the BBHCI and the QPHCI, as well as the author's interviews with hospital staff and Karen Orreal.

Chapter 27   General information and quotes have been obtained from testimony and statements to the BBHCI and the QPHCI, as well as the author's interviews with hospital staff.

Chapter 28   General information and quotes have been obtained from testimony and statements to the BBHCI and the QPHCI, as well as the author's interviews with hospital staff. Other information comes from the author's interviews with Dr Gerry FitzGerald and the widow of Mr Harry Petrohilos.

Chapter 29   General information and quotes have been obtained from testimony and statements to the BBHCI and the QPHCI, as well as the author's interviews with Toni Hoffman and Rob Messenger.

Chapter 30   General information and quotes have been obtained from testimony and statements to the BBHCI and the QPHCI, as well as the author's interviews with Rob Messenger, Toni Hoffman and Malcolm Cole. Other material comes from Hansard, the record of State Parliament.

Chapter 31   General information and quotes have been obtained from testimony and statements to the BBHCI and the QPHCI, as well as the author's interviews with hospital staff and his contact with newspaper colleagues including Graham Lloyd. Other material comes from the *Bundaberg NewsMail* and the *Courier-Mail* as attributed.

Chapter 32   General information and quotes have been obtained from testimony and statements to the BBHCI and the QPHCI, as well as the author's interviews with hospital staff and Beryl Crosby. Other information comes from various media outlets as attributed and Hansard, the record of State Parliament.

Chapter 33   General information and quotes are the author's recollections of contact with his wife's family in Mackay. Other material comes from correspondence with Toni Hoffman.

Chapter 34   General information and quotes are the author's recollections of contact with his wife's family in Mackay and a friend, journalist David Murray.

Chapter 35   General information and quotes have been obtained from testimony and statements to the BBHCI and the QPHCI, as well as the author's interviews with Rob Messenger. Other information comes from *Doctor Q*, the magazine of the Australian Medical Association Queensland, as attributed.

Chapter 36   Quotes are attributed in the text to correspondence between the author and Toni Hoffman.

Chapter 37   General information and quotes have been obtained from testimony and statements to the BBHCI and the QPHCI, as well as the author's interviews with hospital staff and Rob Messenger.

Chapter 38   General information and quotes have been obtained from testimony and statements to the BBHCI and the QPHCI, as well as the author's interviews with hospital staff. Other quotes are attributed in the text.

Chapter 39   General information and quotes have been obtained from the author's interview with Toni Hoffman and her friend, Karen Fox, as well as testimony and statements to the BBHCI and the QPHCI.

Chapter 40   General information and quotes have been obtained from the author's notes from contact with the media advisers to the Health Minister Gordon Nuttall. Other information and quotes came from testimony and statements to the BBHCI and the QPHCI.

Chapter 41   General information and quotes have been obtained from the author's interviews wth Dr David Molloy, Rob Messenger, Tess Bramich, Chris Blenkin and Dr Peter Woodruff. Other information and quotes came from testimony and statements to the BBHCI.

Chapter 42   General information and quotes have been obtained from testimony and statements to the BBHCI and the QPHCI, as well as the author's interviews with hospital staff.

Chapter 43   General information and quotes have been obtained from the author's contact with Brendan McKennariey and an interview with the Health Minister Gordon Nuttall.

Chapter 44   General information and quotes have been obtained from the author's contact with Maria Woodruff, wife of Dr Peter Woodruff. Other information came from the author's interview with Toni Hoffman and contact with Gordon Nuttall's media adviser, David Potter.

Chapter 45 General information and quotes have been obtained from the author's interview with the Chief Health Officer, Dr Gerry FitzGerald.

Chapter 46 General information and quotes come from the author's recollections of reporting in Childers in June 2000 and in Bundaberg in April 2005. Other quotes come from the author's interviews with patients and relatives as attributed in the text. Information and quotes related to the decisions of Dr Gerry FitzGerald and Peter Leck come from testimony and statements to the BBHCI and the QPHCI.

Chapter 47 General information and quotes have been obtained from the author's interviews with Pam Samra and, subsequently, Toni Hoffman, Karen Jenner and Karen Fox. Two other nurses have requested anonymity.

Chapter 48 General information and quotes have been obtained from the author's interviews with patients Nelson Cox, Ian Fleming and Beryl Crosby.

Chapter 49 General information and quotes have been obtained from correspondence to the author as well as from newsroom recollections. Other information came from interviews with Toni Hoffman, Dr Gerry FitzGerald and Jim O'Dempsey, as well as testimony and statements to the BBHCI and the QPHCI.

Chapter 50 General information and quotes are attributed in the text.

Chapter 51 Quotes were obtained from transcripts of interviews with Dr Jayant Patel as attributed in the text. Other information and quotes came from the author's interviews with Gordon Nuttall, Rob Messenger and Toni Hoffman, and psychiatrists Dr Warwick Middleton and Dr Ian Curtis. The author also relied on testimony and statements to the QPHCI, the BBHCI and State Parliament. The accounts from colleagues who attended a public meeting were adopted.

Chapter 52 General information and quotes have been obtained from the author's interviews with Toni Hoffman and her mother, Marie. Other sources are attributed in the text.

Chapter 53 General information and quotes have been obtained from the author's interviews and correspondence with Tony Morris. Other sources are attributed in the text.

Chapter 54 General information and quotes have been obtained from Hansard, the record of State Parliament, as well as the author's interviews with people including Tony Morris and Premier Peter Beattie.

Chapter 55 General information and quotes have been obtained from the author's interviews with Beryl Crosby, Dr Sally Ehlers, Toni Hoffman and hospital staff. Other sources are attributed in the text.

Chapter 56   General information and quotes have been obtained from the New Jersey State Board of Medical Examiners and the State of New York Department of Health. Other material was obtained from the BBHCI, the Health Rights Commissioner David Kerslake and the author's interviews with medical sources in Cairns and political sources in Brisbane.

Chapter 57–58   General information and quotes have been obtained from the testimony and statements to the BBHCI.

Chapter 59   General information and quotes are attributed in the text.

Chapter 60   General information and quotes have been obtained from the author's interviews in India with Rahul Bedi and former colleagues of Dr Patel as attributed in the text. Other information relating to the journalists' visit to Portland came from the author's interviews with Tuck Thompson as well as published accounts of certain events, attributed in the text.

Chapter 61   General information and quotes are attributed in the text.

Chapter 62   General information and quotes have been obtained from testimony and statements to the BBHCI. Other material came from the author's observations and interviews as attributed in the text. Material relating to the Supreme Court challenge against the BBHCI came from affidavits filed as part of the case.

Chapter 63   General information and quotes have been obtained from the author's interviews with staff of the BBHCI, the patients and their lawyers, as well as testimony and statements to the BBHCI and the subsequent Supreme Court challenge.

Chapter 64   General information and quotes have been obtained from the testimony and statements to the BBHCI. Other information relating to the dinner party at the Indian Curry Bazaar is attributed in the text.

Chapter 65   General information and quotes have been obtained from the transcript of the Supreme Court challenge before Justice Moynihan, as well as evidence and statements to the BBHCI.

Chapter 66–68   General information and quotes have been obtained from evidence and statements to the BBHCI as well as the author's interviews with people attributed in the text.

Chapter 69   General information and quotes have been obtained from the author's interviews with people including Graeme, Jan and Tony Morris; and Toni Hoffman. Other quotes are attributed in the text.

Chapter 70   General information and quotes have been obtained from the author's interviews with Beryl Crosby, Geoff Davies and Michael Lavach. Other material came from testimony and statements to the BBHCI and the subsequent QPHCI.

Chapter 71   General information and quotes have been obtained from testimony and statements to the QPHCI. Other material came from contact between the author, his sisters, and medical practitioners.

Chapter 72   General information and quotes are attributed in the text.

Chapter 73   General information and quotes have been obtained from the QPHCI report. Other quotes are attributed in the text.

Chapter 74   information and quotes are attributed in the text and have been obtained from the author's interviews and research while visiting Portland, Oregon.

Epilogue   General information and quotes have been obtained from the author's interviews with people including the Attorney-General Linda Lavarch, Premier Peter Beattie and lawyer Damian Scattini. Other information came from Hansard, the record of State Parliament, and various statements at media conferences.

Acknowledgements

I owe special thanks to my father, Hedley Robert Thomas, my wife, Ruth Mathewson, my best friend from childhood, Martin Leonard, and the best nurse in the country, Toni Hoffman, for their unstinting support and advice.

Many sources – doctors, nurses, public servants, lawyers and friends – have my everlasting gratitude. I will not make your work any more difficult by publishing your names. You know who you are. Your information and expertise were invaluable.

I hope, however, the following will not mind being mentioned: Dr Gerard Neville and his wife, Lorraine, Dr Ingrid Tall, Dr Marsh Godsall, Dr Peter Woodruff, Dr Iain and Mary Mathewson, Dr David Molloy, Dr Sally Ehlers, Rob Messenger, Geoff Davies QC, Tony Morris QC, Richard Douglas SC, David Andrews SC, Damien Atkinson, Errol Morzone, David Groth, Gerry Mullins, Ian Brown, Damian Scattini, Brendan McKennariey, Jarrod Cowley-Grimmond, Tim Lunn, Beryl Crosby, Tess Bramich and Judy Kemps. Thank you.

I am indebted to Matt Condon for motivating me to write the story and helping when I was in despair. We go back a long way, mate.

Reporter Amanda Watt and photographer John Wilson were marvellous. I thank, too, the *Courier-Mail*, News Limited and CEO John Hartigan and my print and TV colleagues – Jane Hodgkinson, Rahul Bedi, Susan Goldsmith, Graham Lloyd, Tuck Thompson, Phil Norrish, Danielle Isdale, John O'Brien and Claire Forster.

To the National Press Club and its fantastic staff, particularly Maurice Reilly and Marietta Rudolf-Troeth, as well as Medicines Australia: cheers.

Finally, I would like to express heartfelt thanks to Sue Hines and Andrea McNamara from Allen & Unwin and editor Jo Jarrah for making the manuscript a reality.